D0449007

PENGUIN BOOKS

## GOOD INTENTIONS

An award-winning writer, Bruce Nussbaum served in
the Peace Corps from 1967 to 1969. Currently senior
writer at *Business Week*, he is also the author of *The
World After Oil: The Shifting Axis of Power and Wealth*.
Mr. Nussbaum is married and lives in New York City.

# GOOD INTENTIONS

How Big Business and the Medical
Establishment Are Corrupting the
Fight Against AIDS

# Bruce Nussbaum

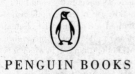

PENGUIN BOOKS

PENGUIN BOOKS
Published by the Penguin Group
Viking Penguin, a division of Penguin Books USA Inc.,
375 Hudson Street, New York, New York 10014, U.S.A.
Penguin Books Ltd, 27 Wrights Lane, London W8 5TZ, England
Penguin Books Australia Ltd, Ringwood, Victoria, Australia
Penguin Books Canada Ltd, 10 Alcorn Avenue, Suite 300,
Toronto, Ontario, Canada M4V 3B2
Penguin Books (N.Z.) Ltd, 182–190 Wairau Road,
Auckland 10, New Zealand

Penguin Books Ltd, Registered Offices:
Harmondsworth, Middlesex, England

First published in the United States of America
by The Atlantic Monthly Press 1990
Published in Penguin Books 1991

1   3   5   7   9   10   8   6   4   2

Copyright © Bruce Nussbaum, 1990
All rights reserved

Excerpts from a *Village Voice* article reprinted with permission from *Reports from the holocaust: the making of an AIDS activist* by Larry Kramer, St. Martin's Press, 1988.

THE LIBRARY OF CONGRESS HAS CATALOGUED THE HARDCOVER AS FOLLOWS:
Nussbaum, Bruce.
Good intentions: how big business and the medical establishment are corrupting the fight against AIDS/Bruce Nussbaum.—1st ed.
Includes index.
ISBN 0-87113-385-7 (hc.)
ISBN 0 14 01.6000 0 (pbk.)
1. AIDS (Disease)—Research—Political aspects—United States. I. Title.
RC607.A26N88   1990
362.1'9697'9200973—dc20        90–1054

Printed in the United States of America
Designed by Laura Hough

Except in the United States of America,
this book is sold subject to the condition
that it shall not, by way of trade or otherwise,
be lent, re-sold, hired out, or otherwise circulated
without the publisher's prior consent in any form of
binding or cover other than that in which it is
published and without a similar condition
including this condition being imposed
on the subsequent purchaser.

To Leslie
M.P.B.

The Road to Hell Is Paved with Good Intentions

# Contents

# CONTENTS

# Introduction

This is a book about medicine and medical scientists, the men and women who develop drugs to treat disease. I didn't begin the book angry but I did finish it that way.

Despite my twenty years as a journalist, much of it covering business and finance for *Business Week*, I was not prepared for the behind-the-scenes realities of big-time medical research. Even after the wild and woolly eighties, where greed became a Wall Street theology, the corruption was startling.

On Wall Street, the financial crooks, the insider traders, knew for the most part that they were cheating, breaking the law. The games they played were new—the LBOs, the hostile takeovers, the greenmail. But the corruption itself was as old-fashioned as embezzlement.

Nothing of the sort exists in medical science. In that arena, people have good intentions. They believe they are doing good works for the general health of the nation. Indeed, personal corruption is still rare, although faking experimental data appears to be on the rise.

The corruption in medical science goes much deeper. It derives from the very way the Food and Drug Administration, the National Institutes of Health, and the dozen or so elite academic biomedical research centers work with private drug companies.

An old-boy network of powerful medical researchers dominates in every disease field, from AIDS to Alzheimer's. They control the major committees, they run the most important trials, they determine what gets published and who gets promoted. They are accountable to no one. Despite the billions of taxpayer dollars that go to them every year, there is no public oversight. Medical scientists have convinced society that only they can police themselves.

Yet behind the closed doors of "peer review," conflicts of interest abound. These are not perceived as conflicts of interest by the scientists themselves. The researchers are convinced that they have only good intentions. This book will show that medical science is the graveyard of good intentions. It will indicate how medical science, in its own unique way, may turn out to be the Wall Street of the nineties.

*Good Intentions* is about AIDS. It could be about cancer or heart disease or any other major disease. The social, political, and financial structure of the biomedical research behind each one is similar. Acquired Immune Deficiency Syndrome is relatively new. The deals, the arrangements, the conflicts of interest are therefore more open to the observer. They are only just now being constructed.

AIDS is also a killer. It strikes young people in the prime of their lives. The AIDS virus is infectious. Anything that gets in the way of quickly developing safe and effective treatments is monstrous. Against this background, the behavior of medical science is thrown into stark relief. A long history of cancer would illustrate the same issues and problems.

Part One of the book introduces the main players in AIDS research at the NIH, the FDA, and Burroughs Wellcome Company, sponsor of AZT, the only antiviral drug ever to have been approved against AIDS. It discusses how the disease devasted the gay communities in cities around America and how a few brave individuals and local doctors fought back on their own, ignored by the biomedical powers that be.

Part Two is about conflict. It shows how a vast medical underground is being built that does alternative medical research and offers people with AIDS unapproved drugs. ACT UP, founded in New York, and Project Inform, based in San Francisco, have put intense pressure on the FDA, the NIH, and the drug companies to change. At times, they find themselves in a peculiar coalition that includes conservative Republican members of the Bush administration, the editorial board of the *Wall Street Journal,* and several big pharmaceutical companies tired of the ghastly regulatory stranglehold of the FDA. At other times, they find themselves at war with these tactical allies.

Part Three shows the success of this underground, which is, however incomplete, setting the stage for a complete overhaul of the American medical system. A new medical research agenda for fast drug development has been proposed that will, if implemented, affect all diseases, not just AIDS. But opposition from the small band of reactionary medical scientists opposed to any change appears likely to sabotage the initiative.

Seventy-five percent of the material in these pages was obtained through over one hundred interviews conducted between 1988 and 1990 in New York; Washington, D.C.; Bethesda and Rockville, Maryland; Raleigh, North Carolina; and a number of other cities. Nearly all of the major figures in the book were interviewed in person, some more than once, a few many times. Only one medical scientist refused to grant an interview, and that person's point of view was obtained from a colleague in close contact with that person in the late eighties.

A number of sources preferred to remain anonymous. As an outsider to the gay community, I was struck by how many gay men remain in the closet. These men are, for the most part, conservative individuals working in mainstream professions—bankers, lawyers, stock traders, football players, investment advisers, policemen, politicians, entrepreneurs, corporate managers, soldiers, and journalists as well as scientists. A good percentage of them vote Republican. Some of these sources would speak only off the record. There were other sources who requested anonymity because they were in politically vulnerable positions at the NIH, the FDA, and elsewhere.

The offices of Congressmen Henry Waxman (D.-Calif.) and Theodore Weiss (D.-N.Y.) were extremely helpful. So was former Senator Lowell Weicker (R.-Conn.). These men played key roles in defending the nation's health system against the ravages of Reagan administration cutbacks. The general public has no idea how close that system came to being destroyed by nearsighted ideologues. The measles epidemic now sweeping the country is a consequence of their actions. It is man-made, caused by cutbacks made in the early eighties. The rear-guard action led by Waxman, Weiss, and Weicker to save what they could is a moving drama.

There is no reconstructed dialogue in this book. The hundreds of hours of interviews were transcribed personally into a computer. Often the tone of voice, the hesitations, the pauses in conversation are more important than the actual words. This, hopefully, was captured.

In the grand tradition of journalism, quotes have been changed to save the ungrammatical from themselves. Dr. Leslie M. Beebe, a professional linguist, taught me that people don't talk the way they write. They don't speak in grammatical sentences. It only looks that way in books. Leslie has done much more. Her caring, her encouragement, and above all her love saw me through the dark days of reporting and writing this book. She has been a constant source of strength, joy, and beauty since I met her in the graduate library at the University of Michigan, half a lifetime ago.

I would like to thank Stephen Shepard, editor-in-chief of *Business Week*, who was more than generous in providing a leave to do this book. He also reminded me, a few years back, that I appeared to enjoy writing a bit more than editing.

Good writers are rare; good editors are rarer still. I wish to thank Ann Godoff, my editor at Atlantic Monthly Press, for her advice in shaping the narrative story, in highlighting the good stuff and culling the bad. My agent, Esther Newberg, at ICM, was brilliant in teaming the two of us up. She's the best matchmaker in the business.

Thanks too to my parents, Henry and Sylvia Nussbaum, who brought the *New York Times* home every Sunday when I was a kid. They got me started.

Bruce Nussbaum
May 1990

# PART ONE

# BEHIND THE SCENES: DRUG REALPOLITIK

The scientist sat in his office raging on into the cold night. Outside, a rare Maryland snow covered the campus of the National Institutes of Health, the nation's top biomedical research center. His four-door Honda, parked in front of a sign that read, DIRECTOR, NCI, was already covered in two inches of white.

Burroughs Wellcome, a foreign drug company, was stealing his discovery, he said. *His* discovery. He'd risked his life, and the health of his wife and children, by handling the deadly virus, while *they* were mumbling about "lack of safe facilities."

It was nothing less than a theft of credit, he said. It was immoral, he warned. They haven't told their investors the real history of the discovery of the drug. They lie. "It is their policy to denigrate and nullify the contributions of others," he said. "They trivialize us as the gnomes of Bethesda."

Sam Broder, M.D., sat back, drained of his anger for the moment. His dark brown hair curled around his collar. He wore a mustache, a signal in his insular world that Sam Broder was a sophisticated man, more than just a lab bench nerd.

Broder cocked his head to the right, breathed deeply, gathered up steam, and plunged on with the amazing accusation. If he was right, this was going to be one of the greatest scandals ever to hit medical science.

The drug was AZT and the disease was AIDS, but what Broder was suggesting could change the way drugs for cancer, Alzheimer's, heart disease, transplants—everything in medicine—get developed.

Broder knew why Burroughs Wellcome was rewriting history. It was the power of credit. Whoever controlled the official history of AZT apportioned the credit for its development. Broder believed that Burroughs Wellcome needed to grab all the credit for AZT to explain the drug's $10,000-a-year price tag, practically the highest ever on a drug. With 1.5 million people infected with the AIDS virus in the United States alone, Broder knew that AZT could become the most profitable drug in the history of pharmaceuticals. Billions of dollars, not millions, were at stake.

Broder also knew who was behind this move to steal his credit. David Barry, Burroughs Wellcome's vice president of research, was the real culprit. Suave, smooth, a Yale man, Barry epitomized "Eastern Establishment" to Broder, a Detroit street kid.

The fight had been going on for years, stormed Broder. The battle had played itself out in the pages of the *New York Times*. First there were editorials condemning Burroughs Wellcome for profiteering, making obscene profits off the sick and dying. Then there were letters from Wellcome defending itself by using a company version of AZT's history in which Sam Broder was nowhere to be seen.

Tapping his finger against the top of the table, Broder looked down and was quiet. Burroughs Wellcome and David Barry might need the credit for AZT to support their claim to big profits. But Sam Broder needed that scientific credit too, for something just as important. Pride.

As he left, walking into the dark winter night, Sam Broder was still visibly furious. His last words, almost to himself, were: "They shouldn't have made us all into schmucks. . . ."

David Barry, M.D., read the *New York Times* editorial and he boiled. Outside his office at the Burroughs Wellcome headquarters in the gently rolling green hills of Raleigh, North Carolina, the temperature neared eighty.

AZT'S INHUMAN COST, screamed the headline. This was the second blast by the *Times* editorial board in ten days and the third time in a single year the paper of record had accused Burroughs Wellcome of profiteering. Barry couldn't believe it. No other private company in the history of the country had ever come under that kind of attack by the *Times*.

Each and every time the newspaper took Wellcome to task for charging too much for AZT, it wrote a specific version of the history of the drug.

4

This last one, on August 28, 1989, was typical. "In 1984, Samuel Broder of the National Cancer Institute encouraged companies to submit possible anti-AIDS drugs for screening by a special test developed in his laboratory. Burroughs sent in AZT, a compound it happened to have on its shelves after studying it for another purpose."

The first editorial blast, back in the summer of 1988, had gone so far as to basically accuse Burroughs Wellcome of grabbing the drug from the NCI. It said that AZT's "effectiveness against the AIDS virus was shown in 1985 by the National Cancer Institute's Samuel Broder, who developed a special screening system and tested AZT at Burroughs's request." Then the *Times* concluded that "by the time the Government thought of applying for a patent on the drug it had invented and tested, it found Burroughs had done so first." There was a vaguely criminal innuendo in that.

Barry thought he knew who was behind the editorial attacks and he said so: Sam Broder. The *Times* was repeating, virtually word for word, Broder's version of the history of AZT's development. It starred Sam Broder, he said. Very coolly, Barry observed how strange it was that those guys up at the NCI were always trying to hog the credit. "First it was Robert Gallo who insisted he discovered the AIDS virus, even though I and everyone else I know believe the French got to it first." Now it was Broder with AZT. "Maybe it's because government scientists make less money than scientists who work for private industry that they feel the need for so much credit," said Barry. "They always see themselves as being much more important in the scheme of things than they really are."

Just look at who was on the front page of the *Wall Street Journal* and the *Washington Post* when AZT was found to work against AIDS, said Barry. Sam Broder, not anyone from Burroughs Wellcome. But who organized the trial? Who paid for it? Wellcome scientists, not the government's. The NIH didn't put out a dime for that trial, even though I personally asked, said Barry. They were so slow, he added, shaking his head. We couldn't wait for them.

Sure Sam had been a great champion of AZT inside the federal bureaucracy, Barry acknowledged. Broder wasn't called "Mr. AZT" for nothing. But the brutal truth is that Broder had been the *third* scientist Burroughs Wellcome had sent AZT to for testing, not the first. Broder didn't discover AZT. He merely *confirmed* that AZT was active against AIDS in the test tube. "Someone else, at Duke University, saw in vitro activity first," said Barry.

So where did the *New York Times* get its version of events surrounding AZT? It had to be Broder and his cronies. No one knew the *real* history of the drug. No one was willing to listen to *him*. "You can easily get the impression that we were an innocent bystander in the development of AZT," he said. "Sam Broder's stamp is on everything."

If the currency of medical science is credit, then he who writes the history of discovery apportions that credit. Yet credit can go to bolster reputations, advance careers, and win Nobel Prizes, or it can be used just as well to rationalize prodigious profits made off terminally ill people.

That is what is at stake in the bitter battle between Sam Broder and David Barry. Their fight reveals an ugly truth about America's medical system. It is a polite fiction that scientists at the NIH and the drug companies work for the public health. They really work for credit and cash.

# ..1..
# The Choice Is AZT

It was butt-kicking time for Sam Broder. You could mess around in the laboratory for just so long. Then you had to get the drug into humans. It was the only way to see if the damn thing really worked. But which drug should he put into humans first?

Those idiots didn't understand. Scientists all over the country were whining that there weren't any anti-AIDS drugs. How can you treat the AIDS retrovirus anyway? It was impossible, they said.

They think they're so smart, thought Broder. All his life Broder had seen people trying to show how smart they were by saying "That's impossible." All his life Broder had been proving them wrong.

Broder knew better this time as well. He knew that there was a gigantic menu of drugs that might work against AIDS. Contrary to common belief, there were probably two dozen compounds that looked good in the test tube. What those idiots didn't understand was that this was the whole problem. Which one do you pick?

It was late winter 1985, and time was running out. The epidemic was into its fifth year. The government had done nothing. People with AIDS were screaming. Congress was mad. And Broder's lab was in revolt.

It wasn't safe, what Broder was doing. He was putting his people at risk and he knew it. They felt threatened. They were handling live AIDS virus without the proper containment facilities, and no one knew how contagious the virus was. Most of his staff wanted out. All of them had families. Every time they came down with a fever or one of their kids got sick, they thought it was AIDS. They were terrified.

Broder's "boys," his two brilliant lab assistants, stuck by him. The three would start work at the crack of dawn, stop when the rest came in, and pick up late at night just to prevent the other staffers from being exposed to the live virus.

Now they were exhausted, stressed out. They had tested hundreds of drugs. Maybe twenty looked good in vitro—in the test tube. It was time to go with one.

Mitch Mitsuya, Broder's Japanese postdoc with the best hands in any lab anywhere, liked Compound S. That baby really popped when they tested it out. It wasn't the first drug to work in Mitsuya's assay. It hadn't been the last one. But it was the most impressive.

Compound S had everything going for it. That's another thing those idiot scientists didn't understand, thought Broder. Drug development was a *practical* matter. He couldn't develop a drug in his lousy eight hundred square feet of lab space. It cost big money, millions, to test a drug on hundreds of humans. It took clout to get a drug through that damn bureaucracy they call the FDA. It took *drug realpolitik.*

So on March 1, Broder flew down to Raleigh, North Carolina, to talk to the guys at Burroughs Wellcome Company who had sent Compound S to his lab. He walked into their weird headquarters that looked like some intergalactic space station and confronted David Barry, the head science honcho. "Look, are you serious about this drug or what?" Broder demanded. "Because if you're not gonna be serious, if you're not gonna go all out with this drug, I'm gonna tell you something. *We're gonna stop testing your stuff!*"

Broder told Barry that he didn't have the time to get jerked around. He couldn't just test a compound and not go anywhere with it. People were dying, fella, he said. "Is you is or is you ain't my baby?" asked Broder.

Broder thought he held the trump card. He knew Mitsuya had invented the only quick test for anti-AIDS drugs. If Barry and Wellcome didn't come across, they would be frozen out for good. Decision time, guys.

As he was fighting the good fight with Wellcome in Raleigh, Broder's boys tried to keep themselves busy in the lab back in Bethesda, Maryland. They had seen this kind of fight before: Broder, charged up with enormous enthusiasm, championing a drug he believed in, a drug tested in his lab, driving headlong against the forces of inertia. But this was different. In the past, Broder's fights had been against government bureaucracy. Now he was

8

up against perhaps a more powerful opponent, a private company. Things were bound to get loud and dirty down there. But when it came to scientific crusades, Sam Broder had shown a knack for winning. He prided himself on being a realist. He knew exactly where to point the lance. And how to push hard.

In science, there are career-making diseases. AIDS is one of them. For Sam Broder and his generation of scientists who came of age professionally in the late seventies and early eighties, AIDS has been the seminal factor determining their success or failure in life.

There's no secret about why. Money. In the fifties, it was polio that received the big government research bucks. In the late sixties and seventies, cancer got the billions. Young, ambitious scientists tend to follow the money trail.

Sam Broder followed that trail first into cancer, then into AIDS. Others took different career routes before steering into AIDS. All agreed on one thing, however. If there were Nobel Prizes to be won for research done in their lifetime, they would go to men and women who had made their reputations in AIDS.

Broder was to become the consummate eighties AIDS scientist. The disease was tailor-made for him. He wrapped the moral urgency of an epidemic around his own ambition and rode it to the top of the hill. While his colleagues were still fighting the old diseases, stroke and cancer, he saw early on that AIDS was the new frontier for science, or at least scientific research. It was all open spaces, big money, and institutional no-man's-lands. Nobody was in control, no one person held the reins on funding, no one had a lock on career advancement. It was all there just for the grabbing.

Broder was one of the first to grab his share. With his overwhelming enthusiasm and his killer instinct for the appropriate phrase that would destroy his adversaries in meetings, Broder cut his way to the scientific heights.

Of all the scientists who were to become well known in the eighties fighting AIDS, it was Sam Broder whose face would appear in more newspaper stories, more magazine profiles, and more TV spots than any other. He would come to be the very symbol of the great progress of science against the monster disease. The good guy. And he would do it by ramming through a second-rate, mediocre drug called AZT, the first and only billion-dollar AIDS drug. He was so identified with this single drug that by the beginning of the nineties, Broder would actually be known as "Mr. AZT."

The man who would come to embody a war against a deadly epidemic was born in 1945, just after another holocaust. Both of Samuel Broder's parents were concentration camp survivors. He was raised in Detroit in the booming postwar fifties when fins were in and big-car sales sizzled like steak on a backyard grill.

Broder's parents ran a diner, and while they were putting in fourteen-hour days, their son was getting A's in public schools at a time when the schools still provided upward mobility for immigrants and the working class. He looked like the proverbial "boy genius," a pudgy little kid with glasses, not much into sports.

But that didn't mean he wasn't aggressive and it didn't mean he wasn't tough and it didn't mean he wasn't streetwise. Broder had learned to be all those things growing up in Detroit. And more. The knowledge served him well in the brutal world of science politics.

Broder didn't go to an Ivy League college. He went to a state school, the University of Michigan, just an hour and a half away from his parents in Detroit. As a state resident, he didn't have to pay very much to attend Michigan, and Broder was actually able to make a few bucks since he was constantly winning scholarships with his grades.

"Big Blue" wasn't Harvard, Yale, or Princeton, but it was as close as a second-generation immigrants' son without riches or connections could expect to get. Besides, the U of M liked to bill itself as the Harvard of the Midwest.

Broder was in that part of the sixties generation that somehow managed to miss getting touched by the sixties. It wasn't an easy thing to do. Broder was on the Ann Arbor campus when it was a hotbed of radicalism and counterculture. President Kennedy had launched the Peace Corps from the steps of the Student Center. SDS was hot. Lyndon Johnson's War on Poverty was in the news. Vietnam was simmering. The air around the Quad, where all the undergraduates hung out, was full of the sweet smell of marijuana and the electric sounds of the Rolling Stones and the Beatles. But Sam Broder was in the library studying, living his parents' dream of their son becoming a doctor, a respected man, a professional. He graduated

Phi Beta Kappa in '66, immediately enrolled in the U of M's medical school, and started taking classes on the North Campus, a few miles down the road from the Quad.

The '68 Chicago Democratic convention street riots came and went, Bobby Kennedy was shot, Johnson sent a few hundred thousand troops to Vietnam, and the Doors were still singing "Light My Fire" while Broder cracked the med books and checked the plumbing of cadavers. His sixties were very different from the *Big Chill*'s.

From the start, Broder was a talker. He wasn't merely verbal; he was a master at argument, a genius at debate. Broder used his mouth as a nonviolent weapon. His gift of gab gave him enormous power to rout his enemies, in and out of the classroom. His intellect made Broder smart. His verbiage made him powerful.

Power was important. Broder didn't try to be "nice." That wasn't his style. In fact, he wasn't afraid to be outright bellicose. He discovered early on that if you were difficult, people were more inclined to respect you. Being difficult was a way of amassing personal power. It fit right in with his argumentative abilities. Broder could shut people up by the force of his logic, by the strength of his energy, and by the condescension in his voice.

Broder's voice actually revealed a good deal about his real ambitions. When he left Detroit, he left behind a lower-middle-class street accent for a more standard "American" midwestern speech. His voice went a bit high-pitched sometimes, especially when he got excited about something in science, which was about every ten minutes. But it was nonethnic and nonstigmatized. This voice, Broder's powers of argumentation, and a good sense of humor broadcast a message: "I'm really smart, I'm really good, and I'm really going places." It was a very attractive message and Broder had no trouble getting followers over the years.

Broder got his M.D. in 1970. He spent the next two years, the height of the Vietnam War, doing his internship and residency in medicine at Stanford University in Palo Alto, California.

A year after President Richard Nixon signed the National Cancer Act into law in December 1971, Sam Broder took his first job at the National Cancer Institute in Bethesda, Maryland, just outside Washington, D.C. It was the largest of all institutes at the National Institutes of Health. With $20 billion pouring in to cure cancer by the end of the decade, this was where science was really happening. Broder never left.

Broder joined the Commissioned Corps of the Public Health Service.

11

Lots of young doctors did at the time. Not everyone at the NIH wanted to wear the white, navylike uniforms of the PHS, but joining up did have advantages. In the early seventies, the most important was that it allowed you to serve your country—it *paid* you to serve your country—without being forced to shoulder a gun in Vietnam. All that Broder had to do was look a little silly every Wednesday when members of the corps had to wear their whites. It was actually a kick in a way.

Sam Broder was very good at the care and feeding of powerful men. He was particularly good with people reputed to be "impossible." With their help, he spent the seventies on his own personal march up the ranks of the NCI. He joined as a clinical associate, became an investigator in 1975, and was a senior investigator a year later.

The seventies were the heyday of funding for the NCI, thanks to Nixon and the Congress. They were the scientific equivalent of the Roaring Eighties on Wall Street. Money just rained down, and whoever was smart enough to catch a downfall did very well. Sam Broder did perhaps the best. When it ended for cancer and AIDS became the next research nirvana, Broder simply jumped ship.

The Bulldog liked Broder. Vincent "Bulldog" DeVita was the director of the NCI, and there was a lot behind the moniker. People who worked for him spread the word that this guy was mean, a miserable man who asked the impossible of people. He never forgot who crossed him, or so went his image. DeVita's nickname also derived from his being incredibly tenacious. He never let go, no matter how heavy the pressure or criticism.

DeVita built his scientific rep by pioneering in chemotherapy. He believed in "full-dose" chemo, really aggressive treatment against cancer. These highly toxic chemicals designed to kill cancer cells often debilitated patients—a kind of full-dose poison. DeVita got into a big fight with doctors around the country who refused to pour on the chemo in an effort to blast the cancer to hell. They said their patients couldn't take it. They thought DeVita was heartless and cared more for statistics than for people. They felt he was more interested in flipping through charts of cancer survivors to show Congress and the president how he was conquering cancer than he was in the individuals stricken with the disease. Their suffering, both from the treatment with highly toxic drugs and from the cancer, was of little interest to DeVita. Or so the doctors said.

DeVita's high-dose chemo became standard operating procedure at the NCI under his reign. It would also have a major impact on the treatment of AIDS. The first infections associated with AIDS were treated with full-dose drugs. Unfortunately, it often turned out that lower doses were much more effective against this particular disease. But that wasn't discovered until several years into the epidemic, after a number of people had died because of their treatment.

DeVita saw himself in Sam Broder and liked what he saw. Broder fought like hell for what he wanted, and he wasn't afraid to go up against his colleagues. Broder was tenacious—just like DeVita. He could be deliberately abrasive—just like DeVita. He was cocksure—like DeVita. He was shrewd—like DeVita.

DeVita liked Broder's brio and quickly became his "rabbi," his mentor within the NCI. In 1981, the year AIDS was first identified, DeVita appointed Broder associate director of the Clinical Oncology Program of the National Cancer Institute. He would soon be director of oncology and deputy clinical director right under DeVita. His laboratory was in charge of supervising the protocols for new drug trials, for diagnosing whether new drugs or combinations of drugs were safe and effective, and for general treatment against disease.

This placed Broder in the most strategic of positions. He was, in essence, able to direct and speed up the development of any drug he chose to champion. He was gatekeeper of AIDS treatments, the arbiter of scientific fashion and code. With the seventies' flood of money for cancer beginning to taper off, a second medical gold rush was about to begin. Broder, in the new white captain's uniform that came with his promotion, was to be at the very center of the fight against AIDS.

But it was a battle that few in the NIH wanted to embrace. It took two more years for the pooh-bahs of American science to decide to take AIDS seriously, and by the time they did, the French were in the lead.

In April 1983, the Centers for Disease Control in Atlanta reported that approximately three thousand people had contracted AIDS and one thousand had died from it. At that point, the NIH decided it had to get serious. Despite the growing epidemic, the NIH acted only after Dr. Luc Montagnier at the Pasteur Institute in Paris began telling American scientists that he had isolated the AIDS virus. He called it LAV, for Lymphadenopathy-Associated Virus.

The cover of *Newsweek* that Monday, April 11, was the first of what would be nearly a dozen covers throughout the eighties on AIDS. The pressure to do something was mounting fast. Congress was getting more

13

demanding, gay lobbying groups were more active. Since January, the country at large had been reacting strongly to reports of the first AIDS cases in blood transfusion recipients. It looked as though AIDS might break out into the wider heterosexual community. This really got middle-class America frightened. Finally, something just had to be done.

Peter Fishinger, deputy director of the NCI, called a meeting of the new NCI Task Force on AIDS. Standing next to him was Dr. Robert Gallo, the discoverer of the first human retrovirus and the most famous scientist at the NCI. Broder was there. So were Dr. William Blattner, Dr. James Goedert, and Dr. Robert Biggar from the family section of the NCI's cancer epidemiology unit. Richard Krause, the director of the National Institute of Allergy and Infectious Diseases (NIAID), didn't attend. He sent a representative.

Gallo spoke after Fishinger. He said that the French were claiming they had found a virus that caused AIDS. He believed that the real virus, whether it was the French one or another, was a human retrovirus, the kind he had discovered back in 1978. Gallo announced that he was now going to put all his lab's resources into proving this hypothesis. And he was going to do it within one year.

They didn't have to be asked. Everyone there knew why they had been invited. Gallo needed them. They considered it an honor and immediately pledged their support. Gallo was going to lead them into a glorious scientific battle against the French. The NCI even had a head start on all the other American research centers. It had already done some research on AIDS because of the rare cancer, Kaposi's sarcoma. KS was one of the first symptomatic opportunistic infections of AIDS detected back in 1980. There had even been a conference at the NCI on KS in 1981. To them, the NCI was the natural place for AIDS research, especially if Gallo was right and the disease was caused by a retrovirus. Gallo had done his pioneering work on retroviruses at the NCI.

Sam Broder made sure that of all the scientists in that room, he would be the most important to Gallo. As head of oncology, he had close contact with Building 10, the big hospital on the NIH campus formally called the Clinical Center. A growing number of its beds were filling up with AIDS patients. Broder was in a position to control priorities. While cancer theoretically had top priority, Broder told Gallo that he and his AIDS research would come first. The commitment was an extremely important exercise in power that made Gallo's research much more efficient.

Broder curried Gallo's favor even further by hiring for his own lab a Japanese postdoc who had specialized in the type of human retrovirus discovered by Gallo. HTLV—Human T-cell Leukemia Virus—was widespread in southern Japan, causing a rare leukemia. The shrewd appointment was a nod to Gallo's importance and served to tie Broder to him.

Gallo was a man not much burdened by other people's feelings. His arrogant, dismissive personality antagonized a huge number of scientists at the NCI, including many doctors who worked at the hospital. Some doctors stopped cooperating with him. They distanced themselves to the point where most refused to allow their lab technicians to take tissue samples over to Gallo's lab.

Sam Broder literally became the bridge between Building 10, the hospital, and Gallo's lab. He hand-carried tissue samples from AIDS patients directly to Gallo. The press would later cite this as one more example of how Broder cut through the red tape at the NIH. It was, but it was something else as well—an exercise in the care and feeding of powerful, difficult men.

Broder tied himself to Gallo for the next year. The NIH grapevine marveled at how he was able to get along with Gallo. Gallo embodied the worst aspects of the "scientific personality." He had a suffer-no-fools temperament and a temper he found no reason to control.

But Broder was ambitious and, although quite young at the time, smart enough to know that this was his best shot. He was going to make AIDS "his" disease. The only question was whether AIDS would be "good" for Broder in the way that some wars are "good" wars for some men. Would it propel Broder to a higher station in life?

At the end of his year working closely with, but always in the shadow of, Gallo, Broder found his reward. The government announced that Gallo had isolated the AIDS virus. It was part of the family of human retroviruses that Gallo had discovered back in the seventies, the HTLV group. Gallo would now turn to finding a vaccine for the terrible disease. Broder would turn to treating AIDS.

Six years later, in the spring of 1990, the NIH would launch an unprecedented investigation into Robert Gallo's discovery. Allegations, published in the press and heard in Congress, charged that Gallo's AIDS virus was actually the French virus discovered a year before his own announcement. It was possible that either the French virus had contaminated Gallo's laboratory by mistake, or that Gallo actually had taken the

15

virus and claimed it as his own. The NIH turned to the National Academy of Sciences and the Institute of Medicine to review the evidence.

By that time, Sam Broder had moved out from Gallo's shadow and far away from his power. He wouldn't be touched by the growing tempest at the NIH.

Right after the announcement that Gallo had found the AIDS virus, Broder had switched priorities totally. AIDS was opportunity knocking for Broder. AIDS would become Broder's focus, if not obsession, for the rest of his career.

It was the spring of 1984, and Broder called a meeting. Robert Yarchoan was there. He was a talented scientist who had just joined Broder's lab. Yarchoan had a remarkable resemblance to Broder, down to the mustache. Dani Bolognesi, a respected virologist and old friend of Broder's from Duke University, was there. So were Deputy Director Peter Fishinger and a number of other scientists. This was to be the big brainstorming session.

It was now clear that a retrovirus was the cause of AIDS, Broder began. He wanted everyone to start thinking about antiretroviral drugs to fight this disease. They needed to start a program of screening compounds right away so they could get drugs into patients as soon as possible.

Broder went on to say that there were plenty of candidates around, no matter what anyone said. Retroviruses used an enzyme called reverse transcriptase to reproduce. The literature suggested that compounds already existed that might work against this enzyme. Let's start there, he said. Right now the most important thing to do was to prove that AIDS was a treatable disease.

This was critical because "there was a belief at that time that retroviruses were inherently untreatable," Broder said later, recalling that period. It was true of all viruses. Scientists almost universally believed that nothing could be done. Bacteria were independent organisms that infected people and could be cured with antibiotics that pinpointed the invading microorganisms and killed them without hurting the rest of the human body's cells.

Viruses, including retroviruses, were weird. Completely different. They were simple, primitive life-forms composed of DNA—genetic material enclosed in a shell. They invaded the host cell and took it over by integrating its DNA with the DNA of its victim. The virus and cell became one living organism. How, scientists asked, could you kill the virus without killing the cell? So viruses can't be cured. It became a self-fulfilling prophecy.

Drug companies also accepted the prophecy, and fewer and fewer government research centers, academic labs, or pharmaceutical companies did any research on viruses. It was useless. It didn't pay. It certainly wasn't in fashion. Even Gallo was going to focus on a vaccine, not a treatment. "There was enormous pessimism at that time," Broder remembers. "Our goal was to confound the prophecy that retroviruses could not be treated." Confound the prophecy.

Broder needed a breakthrough. Testing drugs for activity against a virus is time-consuming skut work. The longer the test takes, the fewer the number of compounds that can be tested in a given amount of time. Impatient as always, Broder needed a faster drug-testing assembly line: "We needed to develop a whole new technology."

Broder did it the "American" way. He turned to a Japanese. It wasn't an unusual tack. Starting in the mid-eighties, thousands of Japanese flooded the NIH, hoping to find the magic American scientific elixir they felt their country somehow lacked—creativity. They came generally as "postdocs," after they had received advanced degrees in their own countries. Their goal was to study with the "greats," learn how to do leading-edge research, and rub off some of that magic creativity onto themselves.

The foreign scientists fit into the NIH social structure. The lab is the building block of all professional and personal life in Bethesda. Behind the redbrick walls of the buildings on the campus, the NIH is nothing but a series of laboratories. Each is run by one powerful lab chief who is the creative spirit. Working under him—and it is a "him" 90 percent of the time—are five to ten people. Nearly all have either a Ph.D. or an M.D. Some lab chiefs have dozens of people working for them. One or two have up to a hundred.

The mentor-protégé relationship dominates the lab. It is very personal, intense, and often emotional. People work late into the night and over the weekends. As experiments are run, day and night blend into each other. Each lab, therefore, has its own personality. A lot of folklore has grown up around "lab life" at the NIH. Some of it has a sexual component, but more often it revolves around ethnicity.

A great number of lab chiefs are Italian and Jewish scientists. Most are like Broder, street kids from working-class families who used the public school system to get out of tough neighborhoods in cities like Detroit, Chicago, New York, and Pittsburgh. They made it on their "smarts." They are big on ego, short on social amenities, and driven to be "the best." Being ethnics themselves, they are also taken to making ethnic generalizations. It is not uncommon to hear "guinea" and "Jewboys" tossed about in casual conversation at the NIH. Usually it's within the context of friendly scientific competition. Often it's in terms of admiration. But not always.

The Russian, Israeli, and French visiting scientists are considered to be very creative by the lab chiefs. The Japanese are said to have "magic hands" that are excellent at running tests and generating data. They are terrific lab workers, but not particularly good at breaking new intellectual ground.

The gossip at the NIH says that the best labs are the "J-J" labs—labs in which Jewish chiefs direct the research and Japanese run the tests. Of course, the Italian lab chiefs insist that "I-J" labs are the best. Everyone agrees that the strong suit of the Japanese is their precision, cleanliness, hard work, and patience. The Japanese may beg to differ.

Sam Broder had one of the best J-J labs at the NIH. In 1982, he hired Hiroaki Mitsuya fresh out of Kumamoto University. Mitsuya had both an M.D. and a Ph.D., very unusual in America, even rarer in Japan. He told Broder to please call him Mitch, as it was a hell of a lot easier for him to pronounce than Hiroaki, which seemed to catch in the throats of most Americans.

Mitch saved Broder. When Broder needed a faster test to screen drugs against live AIDS virus, Mitsuya did the work. The test, or assay, needed to contain several things. First, it had to have a new "cell line," human cells that would literally be immortal, living outside the human body for as long as they were cultured. The cells would have to react very quickly to the AIDS virus. Speed was critical.

By the summer of 1984, Mitsuya had a working model up and running. But it was still too slow. By early fall he had it—a fast-reacting assay. The end point to this assay was cell death. If a drug worked against the AIDS retrovirus, it blocked the virus from killing the cells. If it failed, the cells would die within five days. That was fast.

Mitch gave his boss leverage. He created new technology. This was something Broder could bargain with. He could offer it to private companies in exchange for their proprietary drugs. *He* had it. *They* didn't. It was Broder's main negotiating tool when he flew to pharmaceutical companies to generate interest in developing AIDS drugs. "We brought them . . . newly developed, rapid technologies for determining whether a drug worked against live AIDS viruses in human cells," says Broder. "At that time there was very little technology available outside this campus."

Broder offered his life as well. He told the drug companies that he was willing to risk his life and the lives of his lab assistants to find a drug that worked against AIDS. Mitsuya and Yarchoan told Broder they had signed on for the duration. They were with him. "Essentially, no pharmaceutical company was set up to deal with live AIDS virus," Broder explains. No one, in fact, but Broder. In this Broder believed he was alone.

Broder's lab was on the thirteenth floor of the Clinical Center, Building #10. It was all of eight hundred square feet. He may have been the chief of oncology, but that was all the space he had to work in.

Inside those eight hundred square feet, the pressure to do something was palpable. Broder gave marching orders. Scour the literature. Read the drug catalogs. Ask around NIH. What are the compounds that might work against human retroviruses?

Even as he was issuing his orders, Broder knew that it was useless. It would take years and years to develop a drug within the confines of his own lab. It could be done. It had been done in other labs, with cancer. But it took a very long time.

The only answer was to go outside the NCI, outside the NIH, into the world of commerce and profit. "It became very clear from the total reality of the situation that we would not be able to do it without the collaboration of the private sector," says Broder. "We could not make the kind of progress we needed to make by ourselves."

Factories. That's what he needed. Manufacturing capacity. "If you're gonna have patients, you're gonna have to have kilogram quantities of drug," he explains. "You have to have bulk. What can a pharmaceutical company do that I cannot do? They can manufacture by bulk."

So Broder hit the road. He became a preacher and spread the gospel of profit to the drug companies of America. He told them that there was money to be made in fighting AIDS.

It was a hard pitch. Company executives told him they couldn't figure out how they could make any profit on a disease population that at the time was only three thousand people.

Others stuck to the prophecy: Viruses can't be treated. Kill the virus, kill the patient.

Broder told them that AIDS was spreading very rapidly. The number of people with the disease was going to rise dramatically. The market would explode. There would be money in it for them.

The businessmen basically told Broder he was a fool. "I went to one prestigious pharmaceutical company, hat in hand. I made a special trip, flew up and got about one minute and thirty seconds of a high-ranking officer's time," Broder says bitterly. "It was very disappointing for me. It was sort of emblematic of the issue. There was no real interest in it."

On October 5, 1984, Broder flew down to Raleigh, North Carolina, to talk with the people at Burroughs Wellcome. "Wellcome did not have a retroviral program in the technical sense of the word," he explains. "They had had a viral program." But they were at least open to the idea of working with Broder's lab.

But not too open. The Wellcome officials were worried about that tiny market. "Ironically, that was the first thing Wellcome told me about," says Broder. "I discussed some data with them, showed them what we could do, and said, 'Please get interested. Help me. I will help you. Help me.' "

Then it got a little rough. Seeing that the Wellcome audience didn't exactly jump up out of their seats singing hallelujah, Broder got mad. "They made it clear that on the basis of three thousand patients, there was no way they could practically get involved." That really ticked him off. People were dying and these characters were making profit-and-loss calculations in their heads. "I was consciously abrasive," he says. "As I left I said, 'You know, really, we're gonna have more than three thousand cases. It is gonna be commercially viable for you,' " he remembers, his voice dripping with contempt.

The drug underground angered Broder almost as much as drug company recalcitrance. On a basic gut level, the underground challenged his beloved science, his belief system really.

With nothing coming out of the nation's biomedical research centers, people with AIDS, often with the help of their community doctors, began taking their health into their own hands. They started trying untested drug treatments wherever they could find them.

Tales of the "Dex Kid" began to circulate around the late-night bars and dinner tables of Los Angeles, San Francisco, and New York. James Corti, a registered nurse in Los Angeles, a smuggler of dextran sulfate, ribavirin, and other possible anti-AIDS compounds from Mexico, was an underground hero. Corti's fame grew to legendary proportions, especially on the West Coast.

To Broder, the Dex Kid and the nascent medical underground were a direct threat. Science was not just being challenged, it was being undermined. Broder was determined to stop the underground. "A number of people, for their own need to do something, took a number of approaches that basically were ad hoc self-experimentation," says Broder. "They were simply saying, 'I either don't trust or don't believe in or can't wait for the scientific method to work.' They were saying, 'I will find an herb that I will cook up, I will find a folk medicine. I will find a drug by myself and I will solve this problem. But I don't have to go through the scientific method.' "

Broder believed that science had to show society at large that it was able to respond to the AIDS crisis. If society lost its trust in science because of the epidemic, it would be a disaster, not only for scientists but for the country as a whole. Broder became driven to show that *he* could find a treatment for AIDS. Broder identified himself with science. In his mind, he *was* science. AIDS was *his* challenge. *His* disease.

Broder thought he knew all the shortcuts to drug development. He had seen a lot in cancer as chief of oncology: good drugs that failed because they were improperly developed, mediocre drugs that passed because they were pushed in just the right way.

One thing he knew for sure was that the fastest way to get an anti-AIDS drug into people for testing was to find one that had already been successfully used against another disease. That kind of drug would already have passed all the tests for toxicology, pharmacology, and pharmacokinetics. It would already have been proven safe for human beings and effective at least against one disease. Broder thought he could save six months to a year with this strategy.

Bob Yarchoan, the Broder look-alike, came up with the solution. He was busy chatting up all his buddies at the different NIH institutes. One of them said, "Why not try Suramin?" It appeared to be a reverse transcriptase inhibitor, which could stop viral reproduction, and best of all the drug had been around for sixty years. The big German pharmaceutical company Bayer had developed it when Germany still had colonies in Africa. Suramin was already prescribed to millions of Africans to prevent river blindness. Suramin was full of surprises. One of the first experiments with the drug in Africa had been deemed a failure because the scientists who gave it to people to cure blindness "never saw them again."

When the experiment's subjects failed to come back, the scientists assumed they had either died or remained blind. But a year later, when the scientists returned to try again, they learned that the patients hadn't come back not because they had died or stayed blind, but because they were cured—they could see and went home. But there was one slight problem. Not all of them had been cured. A few had dropped dead from adrenal failure.

Broder asked Mitsuya to see whether Suramin worked against AIDS in the test tube. Mitsuya hadn't yet perfected his assay, but he did have the prototype. It just took longer. When Suramin was put into the test tube with live AIDS retrovirus, the human cells did not die. Suramin blocked the retrovirus.

It worked! This was the one! Broder was so convinced that Suramin could treat AIDS that he immediately ran out and filed for a government patent on the drug. He feverishly worked up a protocol for a Phase I trial—the test of whether a drug is safe to take—even while Mitsuya was still testing Suramin. With the drug now showing activity against AIDS, Broder rushed it over to the FDA. His enthusiasm was enormous. This might just be the first drug able to at least stop the growth of AIDS in people. Patients wouldn't get worse; they might stabilize and live. So far, everyone appeared to be dying. Everyone.

Broder made his case at the FDA. He was very persuasive. "We've got to get it into humans," he kept repeating. There was something vaguely disconcerting about the way he said it—like a mantra. Lots of compounds showed activity in a test tube, but the real test was in humans. Except that Broder used the term "humans" in a most inhuman way—as objects.

The FDA was impressed, and it moved its bureaucratic wheels incredibly fast to accommodate him. The FDA officials hadn't seen such a sense of urgency or such powerful belief in a drug in a long time. By this time, Broder was being called "Mr. Suramin" around the NIH campus.

After the FDA gave Broder the go-ahead he immediately began injecting a handful of AIDS patients in the Clinical Center. The results weren't great. The Phase I safety trial showed that Suramin was toxic, but that it could still be given to people. It was safe enough. There were some positive signs in terms of efficacy. "We thought maybe there was a decrease in the virus load . . . but we weren't sure that that meant anything," says Yarchoan. "It sort of dropped." That was okay. The bad news was that the immune system didn't show any significant sign of improvement. But the cloudy results didn't stop Broder.

Broder's enthusiasm for Suramin was infectious. The gay community,

Congress, scientists—everyone wanted to believe that Suramin just might work. It might be a treatment for AIDS. It could be the one.

The Phase II clinical trial—the test of Suramin's efficacy against AIDS—was held at the AIDS Clinical Research Center of the University of California at Los Angeles. Word quickly got around the L.A. gay community that a drug was being tested that just might save lives. People in the entertainment industry began using their social and political connections to get Suramin. Gay leaders in New York and San Francisco started demanding early release of the drug, even before the Phase II trials had begun.

But Suramin failed. A few months into the trial, it became clear that the drug was not just a little toxic, it was *really* toxic in AIDS patients. Several people in the trial had adrenal failure, the same thing that had killed people in Africa. Talk got into the press that the deaths of some AIDS patients may have been accelerated by Suramin. Dr. Jay Levy of the University of California at San Francisco and Dr. Constance Wofsy, codirector of the AIDS Clinic at San Francisco General Hospital, both said publicly that Suramin was suspected of causing premature death in some AIDS patients because of its toxicity.

Broder's first attempt at finding an AIDS drug had ended in dismal failure. It was a depressing time in Broder's lab; Bob Yarchoan in particular was down. He and Broder had been the ones to inject Suramin into the AIDS patients in the NIH hospital during the Phase I study. He was caught by Broder's enthusiasm for the drug. Now with this failure he crashed.

But not Broder. He felt good. Broder bounced back without missing a beat. At least he had tried something while everyone else was scratching his head. He had *tried.*

The hallmark of Broder's operation was fixed in the sad Suramin affair. Its elements were simple: Find a drug that had been tested for a previous disease. Make sure it had a big corporate sugar daddy behind it. Push the bureaucracy like hell to move it along. And talk it up. Talk it up.

Finally, Burroughs Wellcome came through. They called Broder several months after his trip down to North Carolina and said they were thinking about sending a few compounds over to his lab. Broder, recovering from his Suramin fiasco, went out of his way to promise the company that "we will give you full access to our technology, which you do not have."

That meant Mitsuya's AIDS assay. Plus his staff's courage. "Wellcome at that point could not deal with live AIDS virus," Broder explains. "The concept of live AIDS virus on their campus was just out of the question." Their scientists were so scared they wouldn't touch the stuff until a safe P-3 lab was built. Broder and his "boys," Yarchoan and Mitsuya, were willing to take the risk.

Wellcome sent a few compounds in late '84. Ten in all. The compounds were under alphabetic code to protect the company's proprietary rights and to keep the testing clean of any bias.

One of the drugs that Wellcome sent to Broder's lab really fouled up Mitsuya's assay. "We received a shipment where everything had some sort of toxin in it so that all of our system died," says Broder. The cell line that Mitsuya had so patiently cultivated and cultured croaked. It took time to get the assay up and running again, much to Broder's annoyance. More time lost. Broder's impatience was barely containable. None of the Wellcome drugs was working.

Then in February, Wellcome called to say they wanted to send just one more to Bethesda. It was labeled Compound S. Broder said sure. Okay. Yeah. Yeah. Fine, he said. Mitsuya ran it.

It was active, *really* active against the AIDS retrovirus. Broder was ecstatic. Finally. This compound looked good, very good.

Broder even thought it might be the same compound he had been working on himself in the lab: ddT. He called up Wellcome and asked, Is this dideoxythymidine? No. It's not dideoxythymidine, said Wellcome. Broder didn't know it at the time, but he had made a pretty good guess. Compound S was azidothymidine, AZT. Both ddT and AZT were members of the same chemical family of nucleosides.

But which one should he put into humans first? The whole family of nucleosides showed activity against live AIDS retrovirus in Mitsuya's assay—ddT, AZT, and other compounds such as ddC and ddI. Which one should he pick?

Broder fell back on his hallmark strategy developed with Suramin. In drug development, go with the corporate sugar daddies. Go with great *big* sugar daddies.

The logic was simple. To test a compound in humans, you needed lots of it. Not milligrams or even grams, but kilograms. Broder didn't have a factory to make compounds. As a practical matter, "the only people that could manufacture things are drug companies," he explains. "We could not synthesize drug in bulk to put into human beings without a private sector collaborator. Impossible. We would have just been sitting there."

This was Broder the pragmatist speaking. If other scientists couldn't see the reality of drug development, that was their problem. He could.

Besides, the Suramin trial had hurt his reputation. Broder needed redemption. He had to show the world that science could work against AIDS, against all viruses. He needed to show his critics, the people who showed how *smart* they were by criticizing without doing, that he could confound the prophecy; that he could succeed, that science could succeed.

In Broder's calculus, Compound S looked good. It had the corporate sponsor. Wellcome had a great track record of bringing drugs to market. The company had one of the few big antiviral programs left in the world. It was also very well known in the academic world as one of the biggest private benefactors to pharmaceutical science. Wellcome really spread the money around. There were Wellcome chairs at Johns Hopkins and a number of other American medical schools. There were Wellcome scholarships and Wellcome awards.

AZT also had a past. Wellcome had tried it as an antibacterial drug. It hadn't worked out for use in humans but the company continued to test it as a veterinary drug for chickens, lambs, and pigs. That meant that a great deal of the required preclinical toxicology tests had already been done on AZT. "That took up to six months right off the bat," says Yarchoan. Like Suramin, AZT could be put into people very quickly.

On March 1, 1985, Broder flew down to company headquarters in the Research Triangle Park near Raleigh, North Carolina. He went down there to test Wellcome's real commitment to developing Compound S. He told them, Look, we've got to get drug out. We've got to show that science can do something against AIDS.

Broder bluffed David Barry, who was handling negotiations for Wellcome. He threatened to stop testing all the company's drugs if Wellcome dragged its feet on Compound S. His lab had the only "sentinel technique for deciding whether a drug worked or not against AIDS," he said. Where would Wellcome go if he refused to test their drugs? If they had any ambitions for getting into the AIDS market, they had to go with him. Get behind me now or be frozen out forever. *"We're gonna stop testing your stuff!"* he threatened.

Of course, Broder didn't tell Barry that he had already decided to go with a drug backed by a big corporate sponsor. He didn't say that Compound S was his best shot. Broder didn't let on that he desperately wanted Wellcome to say yes.

Burroughs Wellcome committed. First David Barry had to sell the idea of Wellcome's backing an AIDS drug with millions of dollars. It wasn't the easiest sell Barry had ever made to senior management. At best they were ambivalent. The Wellcome managers in Great Britain were the most difficult to persuade. How can you make a profit on a drug with three thousand patients, they asked? And what was this new disease in America, anyhow?

Barry was able to win the support of his U.S. bosses, Pedro Cuatrecasas, the head of R&D, and William Sullivan, the chairman and president. With them behind him, Barry was able to get London's grudging approval. Wellcome was in for a penny, in for a dollar. Wellcome was in.

"Mr. Suramin" became "Mr. AZT." The enormous enthusiasm Broder had shown for his first drug was now transferred to his second. He became the champion of AZT in Washington, pushing hard for the drug within the NCI, within the FDA, within any bureaucracy that was needed to get this treatment out. There was no "AIDS bureaucracy" at that time at the NIH. Everything was very fluid.

Only two people, Bob Gallo and Sam Broder, were really doing any serious AIDS research in the government. Broder had the most power. He was the only person screening potential AIDS drugs at the NIH. He was chairman of the government's Public Health Service Committee on AIDS Therapeutics. He was in control of the laboratory that decided which potential AIDS treatments to push and which to ignore.

Broder was at the center. He could wire the system for any drug he chose. He picked AZT and ran with it, charging through hurdles, obliterating obstacles. He started getting the word out about AZT, building momentum for the drug. His articulateness and enthusiasm were as important as Mitch Mitsuya's assay. Broder knew that drug development demanded a lot more than a brilliant assay. A new drug needed a voice. It needed a champion. Broder gave it both in Washington.

Broder blitzed through experiments in the lab. Wellcome had an exceptionally large body of data already in house on AZT from its earlier studies on the drug as an antibacterial. It was less than complete, but the company had good numbers on toxicology, pharmacology, pharmacokinetics, and even synthesis.

But the data was not complete enough to apply for an "IND" from the FDA. An Investigational New Drug designation gives permission to test a compound's safety by putting it into people for the first time. More information on AZT was needed for the IND.

Broder whipped his staff into doing more in vitro studies of AZT. He fine-tuned the measurements of AZT's biological activity against the retrovirus. He did studies of lymphocyte activities. He pushed hard, very hard, in the lab.

Wellcome, for its part, buffed up its older, preclinical animal studies. They also did additional work, filling in the gaps.

By June 1985, the data was there. Now the regulators had to comb through it, make sure they thought it was going to be okay, to test it in humans, and give their stamp of approval. This regulatory process normally took months. Ellen Cooper, the head of the FDA's Division of Antiviral Drug Products, said yes in five working days. Less than a week. It was miraculous. A record. A testimony to Sam Broder's enthusiasm.

It was a critical moment. On July 3, 1985, Sam Broder and Bob Yarchoan injected their first AIDS patient with AZT. He was a furniture salesman from Boston named Joseph Rafuse. Then the two scientists waited. An anaphylactic reaction, a massive biological reaction, at this point was not uncommon. It could kill him.

That night, Rafuse spiked a fever. Broder and Yarchoan returned to the NIH hospital and cooled him down. But there was no anaphylactic shock, and the trial could continue.

After a few days, Broder thought he detected a positive response to AZT. "We couldn't be exactly sure, but his platelets went up and his T-4 count rose too." T-4 cells are the key actors in the body's immune system. The AIDS retrovirus attacks them directly, making the number of T-4 cells in a milliliter of blood a good indicator of how the disease is faring. Most healthy people have a T-4 cell count between 800 and 1,200.

Rafuse started feeling better. He gained a little weight.

Broder and Yarchoan went on to the next stage. They began raising the dosage of AZT. This was standard operating procedure, copied from cancer research, and Broder followed it. The object was to find the highest dosage accepted by patients. In cancer, the goal was to kill the most cancer cells in the fastest time possible. The trick was not to kill the patient in the process. The same game was to be played in AIDS research.

Wellcome caused problems right away, according to Broder. First, he was expecting the company to do the clinical pharmacology for the Phase I safety study. "It's common when you're collaborating with a drug company that they help you by measuring serum levels and checking whether the drug is orally absorbed," he explains. It was also common for the company to run tests to see whether the drug passed into the brain. This was important because increasingly, AIDS patients were coming down with dementia. The retrovirus was getting into the brain. For any drug to be useful, it would have to penetrate the brain.

But Wellcome did not want to have any AIDS-infected serum, or blood samples, in their laboratories. They weren't prepared for it. It wasn't safe. "Right around the time we got ready to go," Broder recalls, "my people got a call that said, 'Sorry, you're on your own for the clinical pharmacology. *Don't send us anything.*' "

Broder was dumbfounded. Wellcome's reaction had come totally out of the blue. Now his NCI staff had to gear up to do the pharmacology. "That required sort of emergency reprogramming. It's sort of like you're all psyched up and ready to go and all of a sudden somebody adds another thing to do. Now you have to run the race with lead weights. It just increased the strain that we had."

For the first few patients, Broder did all the pharmacology in his small lab. Wellcome eventually set up a deal with Duke University to do certain pharmacology tests there. Some of the patients in the Phase I safety study were also at Duke. Eventually, Wellcome did the pharmacology at its own facilities. "But at the very early phase, all the burden landed on us," says Broder. "We had to make a quick determination whether the drug got into the brain, whether it was orally absorbed."

Then problem No. 2 hit. Right in the middle of the trial, Wellcome called. " 'We don't have any more thymidine. The study may have to come to a halt. We don't have enough material.' That's what they said to me," Broder recalls.

No thymidine meant no AZT. "While we're moving the study along . . . it was just another unanticipated thing," says Broder. "They just said, 'We don't have enough material.' These are the facts. I'm just giving the facts," he insists.

Thymidine at that time was made out of herring and salmon sperm. It wasn't exactly rare, but not much was made every year. It was relatively expensive. Not many laboratories had it lying around on their shelves.

But the NIH is a big place, and Broder decided he had no choice but to look for a supply of thymidine. He was lucky. "We found a gigantic supply," he reports. More than 100 kilos, nearly 220 pounds, were discovered. Broder sent it down to Wellcome. Gratis. "We didn't charge them for anything," he remembers. "We did not charge them to do any of the studies. They were done as part of the official business of the government."

Sam Broder knew AZT was the one. The drug was safe. The Phase I study clearly showed that. There was some toxicity, but it was tolerable. Broder's faith in AZT went beyond safety, however; he believed the drug was effective against the AIDS virus. He saw patients feeling a lot better. He saw their T-4 cell counts rising. Most of all, the patients themselves were saying they were improving, they were getting better.

This was the one. He knew it. Suramin may have failed, but AZT was going to succeed. "At the end of the Phase I study, the long and the short of it was that *we felt it worked.*"

As his enthusiasm grew with every passing day, Broder began to generate momentum for the drug. He talked up AZT wherever he went. He made it known throughout the NCI. By the fall, the gossip networks at the NIH were humming with word that Sam Broder thought AZT worked against AIDS. He pushed it harder than Suramin. He pushed it with all the enthusiasm that only Sam Broder could generate.

Even before the Phase I safety study was finished back in August, he was telling Dr. Mathilde Krim, a medical researcher who traveled in social circles that included Wall Street and Hollywood, that AZT was terrific. Krim began to talk it up on TV, and people in the gay community began to hear about it. The demand for AZT began to swell exponentially.

Broder felt his job was finished: "We had taken the drug from soup to nuts, from a tissue culture, into humans, and then to the end of Phase I." Beyond that he would not go. It was counterproductive for one man to do more. "People should not believe what *Broder* says without confirming it for themselves," he has said, referring to himself in the third person. Broder on Broder.

Broder had become a transcendental figure in his own mind.

The press played a key role in this transformation, which began in early '85, picked up steam in '86 and '87, and took off in '88, '89, and '90. The visage of Sam Broder increasingly faced Sam Broder across his breakfast table. He was in the newspapers constantly.

The story was always the same: "Heroic scientist risks life to fight deadly disease by discovering new drug treatment." It was almost mythic, or at least an exercise in mythmaking.

Broder tended the myth by cultivating the press corps unabashedly. Wry, knowledgeable, sympathetic, Broder was always available for the pithy quote, the intelligent backgrounder; the story.

Broder was the first scientist to recognize that AIDS was a disease that could apportion credit and glory by the inch—the column inch. The newspaper story, the magazine cover, the TV spot would, when used collectively, determine fame and fortune.

Broder's early favorite was the *Washington Post.* It had the most clout in his circles. It was read by NIH scientists and bureaucrats, by important congressmen who sat on health and science committees, and by the Reagan administration politicos.

But Broder was also able to see himself peering out from the *Wall Street Journal,* the *New York Times,* the *L.A. Times,* and the *San Francisco Chronicle.* The picture was usually one of a man in a white lab coat, head tilted in a serious pose, the definition of sincerity.

Broder sensed from the very beginning that AIDS would be the most politicized disease in the history of the United States, and that the press would play a key role. All this played to Broder's strengths. His superb articulateness, used as a weapon against competitors in the world of science, was transformed into a sound-byte machine richly valued by reporters. The disease raised him from a simple oncologist to a national figure.

AIDS made Sam Broder into a living mediagenic hero.

# ..2..
# The Puppet Master

David Barry was the puppet master, and his favorite marionette was Sam Broder. While Broder was charging around promoting AZT at the National Institutes of Health, Barry was working quietly behind the scenes orchestrating a whole panoply of actors who would ensure the drug's ultimate commercial success.

At the time, Broder had no idea of the role he was playing in Barry's script. He was too busy priding himself on being so sophisticated about the *real* realities of drug development to see just how he was getting set up.

The true pro, however, was David Barry. Quiet, a poised man who spoke perfect Eastern Establishment newscaster English, Barry deftly "ran" Broder by allowing him to give full rein to his own ego and enthusiasm. He was smart enough to let Broder think *he* was the central character in the AZT scenario.

Meanwhile, Barry was cutting the deals with key people at the FDA, negotiating with university research centers, and rounding up his old gang of principal investigators (PIs) who had worked for Wellcome in the past and who might be interested in running yet one more drug trial in the name of science.

Barry's was a virtuoso performance, a George Smiley–style performance, by a master player in the drug development game. The deeds were done before the trails were spotted.


Burroughs Wellcome is the strange duck of the pharmaceutical industry. There is nothing like it in all the world. The company was set up by

31

two American druggists, Silas M. Burroughs and Henry S. Wellcome, in London in 1880. Burroughs died shortly thereafter, leaving his partner the sole owner. Wellcome shaped the company to reflect his own entrepreneurial style and his interest in medical research. Wellcome believed in money and what it could do. He reminded his scientists that profit was essential to lubricating their beloved lab research.

Henry Wellcome's own contribution to the pharmaceutical industry came not in the lab but in sales. He created the practice of "detailing," the training of company reps to go out and bring detailed information on new drugs to their customers, doctors.

The practice continues to this day. Doctors learn more about new drugs from company representatives knocking on their doors with free samples than from medical journals or conferences. No one could accuse Henry Wellcome of not being an innovator.

Wellcome also brought the world the tablet. Before Henry Wellcome, drugs came in the form of powders that had to be stirred into water for consumption. With the more compact form of the tablet, taking drugs orally became much easier. The tablet was a raging success and transformed the entire drug industry.

Admirals Peary and Byrd took tablets with them to the North and South Poles. Wellcome loved the new age of exploration that was opening in the early twentieth century, and he supplied much of the medical equipment to the key explorers. Sir Henry Stanley carried Wellcome medical kits on his journey in Africa. Charles Lindbergh had one with him on board *The Spirit of St. Louis* as it flew the Atlantic.

Wellcome's genius perhaps expressed itself best in the complex financing structure of his company. In 1906, he set up an American subsidiary. In 1924, he established the Wellcome Foundation and consolidated the Wellcome companies in Britain and the United States. In 1936, he established the Wellcome Trust, a charitable trust, in England. Then he put all of the Wellcome Foundation's stock into the trust.

The trust had one ostensible purpose—medical philanthropy. It has grown so large that it is currently the biggest charity in Britain. There was, however, a second, less eleemosynary, reason for Henry Wellcome's financial engineering. Control. By putting all the stock into a trust, he prevented outside investors from buying into his company and taking over. For Henry Wellcome, charity began at home.

In 1955, the Burroughs Wellcome Fund, mirroring the Wellcome

Trust in London, was set up in the United States. It quickly became one of the most powerful forces on the American biomedical scene by providing grants and funding for hundreds of scientists and researchers every year. There are Wellcome chairs in pharmacological studies on many American medical campuses. The American trust gives Burroughs Wellcome a tremendous presence and a good deal of clout in academic medical circles.

The American subsidiary, Burroughs Wellcome, has sales of $1 billion a year and employs forty-two hundred people. Actifed and Sudafed are its most well known consumer products. Worldwide, Wellcome sells products worth $2.2 billion annually and has twenty thousand employees. That puts Wellcome at the bottom of the top tier of international pharmaceutical companies.

In February 1986, within days of giving the first patient AZT in the Phase II trial, the company decided to sell 25 percent of its stock to the public to raise capital. By that time, the cost of developing a new drug in the United States had risen to between $50 and $100 million. Thus Wellcome became a hybrid—a private company with a philanthropic face as well as a charity with a corporate arm. Wellcome is the only one of the top dozen global pharmaceutical giants to have such a peculiar organizational structure.

Only a small percentage of Wellcome's profits are paid out to shareholders. Most of the profits go to further biomedical research. To the men who run Wellcome, profits finance a worthy cause, the development of drugs that save lives. To them, high prices for drugs don't go to feed the conspicuous consumption of the proverbial greedy stockholder. They go to the good guys, the scientists who bring health to the world. How could anyone object?

David Walter Barry was born in Nashua, New Hampshire, in 1943. He went to Yale and majored in French literature. After spending his junior year abroad at the Sorbonne in Paris, Barry graduated magna cum laude in 1965, a year before Sam Broder received his B.A. from the University of Michigan.

Like Broder, Barry stayed close to his undergraduate college. He graduated the Yale University School of Medicine in 1969 and did his internship and residency at the Yale–New Haven Hospital.

In 1972, David Barry joined Broder in donning dress whites as a commissioned officer of the Public Health Service. But instead of going to the NIH, he opted for the FDA and became a staff associate in the Viral Pathogenesis Branch, Division of Virology, Bureau of Biologics. By the time Barry left the FDA five years later, he was acting deputy director of the Division of Virology.

The FDA, of course, was the perfect place to learn the regulatory ropes of drug development from the inside. That knowledge could then be parlayed into a better-paying job by moving to the private sector, which is precisely what Barry did.

Barry published about twenty academic articles during his stay at the FDA. One of them was an article on the "Isolation of foamy virus from rhesus, African green and cynomolgus monkey leukocytes," with P. D. Parkman, M. D. Feldman, and N. R. Dunnick. Paul Parkman was his boss. A decade later, they would meet again.

The low pay and lousy lab conditions drove Barry out of the FDA. His love was virology, but there were very few drug companies left with any kind of antiviral program. From his first month in medical school, Barry, like Broder, had heard the same refrain repeated over and over again: Viruses can't be treated. They integrate with the host cell. Kill one, you kill them both. Treat a patient for a virus and you risk killing the patient. Such was the prophecy.

But in 1974, a Dr. Howard Schaeffer had synthesized a drug that appeared to actually work against herpes, a virus. Barry paid close attention to Schaeffer's work. It was still new and would take years to develop, but the medical literature strongly suggested that Schaeffer was indeed able to confound the prophecy about viruses and create a compound that was nontoxic to the human body yet able to fight a broad spectrum of herpes infections. The company Schaeffer worked for was Burroughs Wellcome. While the consensus was bleating away, Wellcome begged to differ and developed an antiviral.

Barry knew where to find his next job. He joined Burroughs Wellcome in 1977. At the FDA, Barry had done research on influenza. At Wellcome, he switched. The next batch of papers Barry published was on herpes and the antiviral drug Schaeffer had discovered, acyclovir, eventually sold as Zovirax.

Barry did publish one paper that was not about herpes. It was about a rare form of pneumonia that afflicted only children with leukemia. The disease and the chemotherapy treatments the kids received harmed their immune systems. With their bodies' defenses down, the children were attacked by *Pneumocystis carinii* pneumonia (PCP). Wellcome, confounding the prophecy again, pioneered the use of trimethoprim/sulfamethoxazole, or TMP/SMX, in the early seventies as a treatment for PCP. Working with the giant Swiss pharmaceutical company Hoffmann-LaRoche, Wellcome got the compound approved by the FDA. Wellcome's commercial brand of TMP/SMX was called Septra. LaRoche called its brand Bactrim.

In 1980, Barry was working on different mechanisms of getting Septra into people. His paper, "Poor rectal absorption of trimethoprim/sulfamethoxazole in treating *Pneumocystis carinii* pneumonia," reflected his failure in that direction.

Wellcome did, however, come up with an intravenous form of Septra for children who were bedridden. It had applied for approval to the FDA, and while it was waiting, it was offering the drug in its IV form free to doctors for the asking. Wellcome assumed that it would be hearing only from cancer specialists treating leukemia.

In the winter of 1980, Barry began to notice that doctors specializing in infectious diseases, and even some community physicians, were calling in to request the drug for a totally different category of patient—young male adults. Most of the calls came from San Francisco, Los Angeles, and New York.

Barry and others at Welcome were circumspect. Under the FDA restrictions, they couldn't give out IV Septra for just any reason. It was specifically developed to help children with leukemia. How could the physicians be seeing PCP in adults? Wellcome asked for documentation and received it. Lots of it. Each case involved a young man who had *Pneumocystis.* Each person was lying in a bed in a hospital and desperately needed the Septra.

After much internal debate, Wellcome decided to ship the drug out. But the incident remained with Barry. It bothered him intellectually. Something was happening out there. Barry was then head of the Department of Clinical Investigation for Wellcome. At the time, he told a colleague, "We've never seen anything like this before. This is really strange."

By 1982, herpes was on the cover of *Time* magazine. While the AIDS epidemic was silently crawling across the gay landscape of the nation, the country's medical attention was turned elsewhere. Middle-class heterosexual singles were coming down in droves with a sexually transmitted viral infection that produced ugly, painful blisters on their lips and genitals. It was spreading quickly to millions of people.

That year, Burroughs Wellcome brought out Zovirax, Schaeffer's drug that could stop herpes. It didn't kill all the virus in the body, but it could prevent its reproduction. Most important, it could stop the monthly appearance of herpes symptoms. The market was huge and the profit was great. Zovirax, the trade name for acyclovir, was the first antiviral drug that made big bucks. It was so profitable that Howard Schaeffer was promoted and made head of research for Burroughs Wellcome.

Zovirax was the second drug that set bells ringing with David Barry. An intravenous form of Zovirax began to be prescribed for the same set of young adult men who were getting IV Septra. Raging herpes infections were decimating hundreds of them. These infections were unusual. They were extremely severe. Different kinds of herpes viruses even struck the same individual. People were coming down with shingles, herpes simplex of the mouth and genitals, and cytomegalovirus (CMV) of the eyes. No one at Wellcome could remember ever seeing anything like it.

What Barry and others at Wellcome were picking up was a desperate attempt by a small number of courageous community doctors to save the lives of patients sick with opportunistic infections due to AIDS. Their immune systems were shot to hell and nearly every virus, every parasite, every bacterium normally held in check appeared to be growing within them. The doctors had to experiment with what they had. There was nothing else they could do. They began combining Zovirax with Septra or Bactrim in pharmaceutical cocktails to ward off herpes, CMV, and PCP.

The government was doing virtually nothing. No drugs were being tested by the NIH. Certainly no combinations of drugs were being researched. No searches of the medical literature were being undertaken at the NCI to find treatments for *Pneumocystis* or the other opportunistic infections (OIs) appearing with AIDS. Only local doctors, watching their patients die, were trying to do something. They were, in their own way, testing out treatments for AIDS.

David Barry monitored all this at Wellcome, as the demand for other Wellcome drugs, such as interferon, ganciclovir, and leucovorin, suddenly spurted. He realized back in 1980 that a new deadly virus was in town, long before the scientists at the NIH had caught on.

After AIDS was identified as a new disease in 1981, Barry knew that if a virus was causing it, he was in the very center of the fight against the syndrome. At one point in the early eighties, Wellcome drugs made up practically 90 percent of the treatments for the opportunistic infections associated with AIDS. Meanwhile, science had quit working on antivirals. That included most government research centers, most academic laboratories, and most drug companies. Wellcome was far out ahead of the powers that be.

David Barry loved most things French. He had spent a memorable year studying at the Sorbonne in 1964. He received Highest Honors in French literature at Yale when he graduated in 1965. And unlike most American scientists, as the epidemic progressed, he kept up with what the French were doing in AIDS research. After all, the Pasteur Institute was one of the four or five great research institutions in the world.

Barry kept in touch with the French scientists working under Dr. Luc Montagnier at the Pasteur. He learned, for example, that in June 1983 Dr. Françoise Barre had isolated a human retrovirus from an AIDS-infected cell culture. Her discovery came just about a year after the term *AIDS*— Acquired Immune Deficiency Syndrome—had been coined.

Barre's retrovirus was completely different from the Human T-cell Leukemia Virus—HTLV—that Robert Gallo was proposing as the cause of AIDS. Montagnier named it LAV, for Lymphadenopathy-Associated Virus. He immediately sent samples of the virus to Gallo at the National Cancer Institute.

The French, however, had a very hard time over the next year publicizing their discovery. Time and again, Montagnier found himself relegated to the tag end of a conference organized by American scientists, many of whom were supporters of Robert Gallo. Getting articles on LAV published in American scientific journals was equally difficult for the French, although they managed to publish a number of them. Medical and science journals ran articles on both Montagnier's LAV and Gallo's HTLV, some in the same issue. In the United States, it wasn't clear which virus was the cause of AIDS.

Then on April 22, 1984, the *New York Times* ran a story in which an official of the Centers for Disease Control in Atlanta said the French were the first to isolate the AIDS virus. It was isolated at the Pasteur Institute in Dr. Luc Montagnier's laboratory.

The next day, on April 23, Health and Human Services Secretary Margaret Heckler stood up before a bank of TV cameras and announced: "Today we have another miracle in the long honor roll of American medicine and science. Those who have disparaged this scientific search, those who have said we weren't doing enough, have not understood how sound, solid medical research proceeds. From the first day that AIDS was identified in 1981, HHS scientists and their medical allies have never stopped searching for answers to the AIDS mystery."

Heckler then announced that Dr. Robert Gallo had discovered the cause of AIDS. It was a member of the human retrovirus family Gallo had discovered in the seventies. Gallo named the new retrovirus HTLV-III. Not a word was mentioned about the French discovery the previous year or the *New York Times* piece of the previous day.

It would quickly become clear that LAV and HTLV-III were not different viruses but the same one. Montagnier would diplomatically suggest that Gallo's lab had accidentally been contaminated by the LAV samples he sent over a year ago. Other, less gracious scientists would accuse Gallo of stealing the retrovirus. Barry knew the French had discovered the AIDS retrovirus first.

Several weeks after Heckler's bombshell, on June 1, Françoise Barre arrived at the Burroughs Wellcome headquarters to bring Barry and other Wellcome scientists up to date on her progress with LAV. She was very persuasive. There wasn't any question but that a retrovirus was causing AIDS. As the disease spread, the immune systems of thousands of people were failing. That was producing the bizarre *Pneumocystis* and herpes infections in young men.

Wellcome had been part of the fight against this disease from the very beginning, through Septra and Zovirax. Now Barry wanted to go after the retrovirus itself.

It made perfect sense. Wellcome had one of the oldest and biggest antiviral programs around, dating back to the forties. If the number of people getting AIDS would grow fast enough, and the price of an anti-AIDS drug was high enough, a lot of money could be made with this disease.

AIDS was Barry's opportunity, "his" disease. If Howard Schaeffer could make his reputation and rise to head of research at the company with herpes and Zovirax, then maybe Barry could follow with AIDS and his own drug.

One of the first calls Barry made after the Barre presentation was to Dani Bolognesi, a well-known expert on retroviruses at Duke University. Duke was just down the road from Wellcome headquarters. Eight miles down the road, to be exact. Barry was well aware of Bolognesi's reputation as one of the investigators who worked on Wellcome drugs. He occasionally ran into Bolognesi on the Duke campus, where Barry taught as an adjunct professor. But what Barry didn't know at the time was that Bolognesi was also a good friend of Sam Broder's.

On the phone, Barry asked if Bolognesi could "lend a hand in terms of tissue culture samples, viral samples, and so on." At that time, Wellcome didn't have the kind of lab facilities secure enough to work safely with the AIDS virus. It didn't have a lab with P-3 conditions, the kind of safe laboratory facilities that permit work on deadly viruses. But Duke did. So did the FDA.

There are about a dozen ways to measure whether a drug works against a virus. An antiviral test, or assay, is one in which a scientist varies any one of three or four main elements. All assays answer the same question: Is the compound active against this virus or not? No matter how the assay is constituted, the key difference is the end point.

Sam Broder's assay, which Mitch Mitsuya had developed, blocked the killing effect on the host cells. It was designed to protect the human cells against death by the AIDS retrovirus. If a drug was active, it would block the virus from killing the cells. This was Sam Broder's new technology.

Dani Bolognesi had another assay. His was designed to see if the AIDS virus continued to reproduce after a drug was added. If the compound worked against the retrovirus, the virus would not reproduce. It would die. This was Dani Bolognesi's new technology.

Jerry Quinnan, who was head of virology at the FDA, had a third assay. His was designed to use cells chronically infected with the AIDS virus. It was different from Broder's and Bolognesi's in design and end point but not in focus. It too showed whether a drug worked against AIDS in vitro. Quinnan had new technology also.

During the fall and winter of 1984, David Barry sent dozens of compounds from the shelves of Burroughs Wellcome to Bolognesi and Quinnan to be tested. This, as Barry explains it, was standard operating procedure for Wellcome: "We don't depend on any single assay because none of the assays are standardized. That's what we always do."

But that was the second step. Before FedExing drugs to outside labs, Wellcome did some testing of its own. Lacking the P-3 laboratory necessary for work on the dangerous AIDS virus, Wellcome could only run tests with animal retroviruses as a screen for a drug's antiviral activity.

Wellcome made fifteen hundred new chemical compounds a year.

Barry knew that with randomly selected drugs he could expect a "hit" only once in ten thousand tries. The process could take forever. But Barry needed to find a drug that he could get into humans for testing as soon as possible. That meant looking for drugs that had already gone through all the hoops for toxicology, pharmacology, metabolism, excretion, and so on. It was the same logic that Sam Broder used.

First Barry ran through all the Wellcome drugs that were already on the market. If they could hit with one of those, the company would be way ahead of the game. Barry didn't luck out.

He then went down a step and tested the company's "Project Level" compounds. These were drugs already in clinical testing in people. No luck there either. None worked.

Finally, Barry went through all the compounds that weren't project related but that had a certain body of data already gathered from toxicology and pharmacology studies. Bingo. That's where he found activity. There were several compounds that looked promising.

In the fall of 1984, Barry began coding samples alphabetically and sending them out to Bolognesi at Duke and to Quinnan at the FDA. They both began testing the Wellcome compounds against the AIDS virus.

Bolognesi suggested to Barry at this time that he invite Bob Gallo and his old friend Sam Broder to brief Wellcome scientists on their work. He said that Broder had been working with live AIDS virus longer than he had. He might have something interesting to say.

Gallo and Broder flew down to Raleigh in October and took a car to Wellcome headquarters. Each man gave a lecture. "Bob Gallo gave his usual talk about retroviruses and how he discovered them." Barry smiles as he recalls this. "Broder gave a talk about Suramin." The big clinical trial of Suramin had started on the very day Broder flew to Wellcome. "After Sam's lecture, we had some very nice discussions."

Broder really had Suramin on his mind. With his proclivity for boosting whatever drug he was working on at the time, Broder was "Mr. Suramin" at that moment. "Basically Sam said, 'Would you guys like to make some analogues of Suramin?'" No thanks, said Barry. Broder also added that he was working with live AIDS retroviruses in his lab and if they wanted to send him some compounds, he would gladly test them out for Wellcome. Barry said he would think about this second offer. Here was yet a third potential source for testing Wellcome drugs against the AIDS virus.

But Barry did not immediately take Broder up on his offer. First he sent the compounds that were active against mouse retroviruses to Bolognesi and Quinnan. Then he decided to send some of them on to Broder. Barry sent eighteen compounds, A through R, to the Duke and FDA labs and ten compounds up to the NCI. None looked really good.

On November 28, 1984, Barry sent Compound S to Quinnan at the FDA. Its internal designation was BWA509U. It was AZT. Quinnan called back right away. The news wasn't great. According to Barry, "Dr. Quinnan's lab said it was somewhat active." Actually, Quinnan's assay showed almost no activity against the AIDS virus. AZT was a dud, as far as he was concerned.

Barry was depressed. This inactivity was the latest in a whole string of failures. But Barry recommended Compound S to Dani Bolognesi a few weeks before Christmas of 1984, just to make sure.

It popped for Bolognesi. His lab found Compound S to be active against live AIDS virus in the test tube. Barry tried to hold his emotions in check. It was fantastic, but what did he really have? One assay that said no, another assay that said yes. He needed something more.

Early in the next year, on February 4, 1985, Barry sent Compound S to Sam Broder. "We knew that Dr. Broder's lab had been doing good work—as had Dr. Bolognesi and Dr. Quinnan." Barry can be quite polite. "After they had given us some results, we also sent it down to Dr. Broder's lab." Broder, of course, using his new technology, found Compound S to be active against AIDS.

By the time Broder received his sample of AZT at the NCI, Barry already knew it was active against both animal retroviruses and human retroviruses. In short, he knew it was active against AIDS. If any scientist outside Wellcome deserved to raise his hand and take credit for AZT, it was Dani Bolognesi, not Sam Broder. "Sam really made the *confirmation*," says Barry, "and that, you know, really sewed it up."

While Sam Broder was promoting AZT at the NIH, Barry was busy elsewhere, behind the scenes.

At thirty-four, Dr. Ellen Cooper was the youngest head of the Division of Antiviral Drug Products at the FDA that anyone could remember. By 1985 she was in charge of passing regulatory judgment on all the antiviral drugs sent to the FDA by the pharmaceutical industry, the NIH, and the biomedical research institutes around the country. Tall, thin, with short hair, Cooper often wore the kind of dress-for-success attire that was popular with women on Wall Street in the early eighties—blue pin-striped suit with a white or pink shirt and a black or pink bow tie. She spoke with a loud, powerful voice that carried to the back of any large room. She was an exacting scientist who believed in following the traditional rules. The scientific method, with its strict patterns of testing and conditions of proof, was very dear to Dr. Cooper. She believed in it—as many scientists believed in it—with more than a touch of the kind of fervor that some people bring to religion. Beyond that passion, Cooper was cold as ice. In fact, she would soon be known by many as the "Ice Queen."

Barry had known Cooper since way back in the seventies, when he worked at the FDA in the Division of Virology. But he got to know Cooper well only later, around 1982, when he was working on Zovirax. Barry met with Cooper in getting approval for the drug. She was impressed by his mastery of the realities of drug development. "He was very, very professional," says Cooper.

Science is commonly perceived as an exact discipline, full of mathematical formulas and precise rules for doing things. Not true. When science is applied, as it is in drug development, all kinds of judgments come into play. When a drug is submitted for an IND—an Investigational New Drug classification permitting human testing—there are many levels of "completeness," and they vary considerably. Personal judgment by the regulator on just what is needed to qualify for an IND plays a critical role.

Cooper was the designated hitter who made those decisions. Now she had to make them in an atmosphere of crisis. AIDS was spreading fast, and the demand to do something was building in the streets, in Congress, and in the White House.

It took Barry a month after Sam Broder ran AZT in his lab to put together a program of testing designed to get an IND. In March, he phoned Cooper. "I called her up and said, 'Gee, we've got this new drug that might be useful for AIDS. We're thinking of having the IND standards not so complete as you'd normally require for a drug like this, in order to get it quickly into people.' " Barry ran down briefly what he had in mind and asked, "Is that satisfactory with you? Did *you* have any specific plan?"

Funny, Cooper told Barry, she was just talking with her colleagues about whether AIDS drugs should have different requirements than other compounds, given the epidemic and all. Cooper said she didn't have an answer for Barry right then but she would call him back in a few days, after they had hashed it out at the FDA.

Cooper, always punctual, called Barry back just as she promised. The answer to his question as to whether she had a specific plan for IND standards for AZT was, well, yes and no. She said they liked what he had suggested, but they'd like a few more tests. Just a bit more data.

Cooper's call was made just a few days before the start of the first International Conference on AIDS in Atlanta on April 4, 1985. Both Cooper and Barry had been planning on attending, so they agreed to meet and discuss the standards for the IND there. It was, after all, the perfect place for this kind of talk. Everyone who was involved in AIDS research would be in Atlanta. Besides, it would be great, Cooper thought, to get away from her office.

The conference took place three months before the world learned that Rock Hudson had AIDS. It was that news in the summer of 1985 that would finally focus the attention of President Ronald Reagan and the nation on the growing epidemic.

The scientific presentations at the conference were getting a little boring, so Barry and Cooper found a quiet place, sat down, and haggled. Barry started by outlining the studies Wellcome had already done on AZT and those that would be completed by May. Cooper said that was fine, but could Barry do a few additional tests? Their discussion lasted for several hours, and in the end, Cooper and Barry reached a deal that day in Atlanta that helped seal the fate of AZT. The agreement called for a relatively low level of data to be submitted to the federal regulatory agency for the IND.

Barry had a second agenda. He wanted to get the IND as fast as possible so he could begin the Phase I trial for safety. Cooper had the answer. She asked him to supply her batches of data as each test was completed instead of giving her the whole package at the end. That would give her a continuous stream of data. Do this "informally," she said. Whenever Wellcome finished a significant test, send the results to her immediately. In FDA regulatory jargon, she was asking Barry to send her a "best" copy, so that by the time Cooper had the full copy in June, she would have read most of the document.

The scenario worked perfectly. Barry rushed through a two-week dog study, a four-week rat study, and other experiments during April, May, and June. He sent Cooper a number of best copies. Sam Broder helped by doing more in vitro work. By the end of June, the last batch of preclinical data, including the animal "tox" data, was ready. Barry put together the full copy and sent it to Cooper. Since she was already familiar with most of the information, Cooper took only five working days to give Wellcome an IND for AZT. This was something of a record for the FDA. Cooper was impressed with Barry's team performance: "They did it quickly and they were well organized. They've got a company behind them and they know what they're doing." Having a company behind them helped a lot.

The deal Barry and Cooper worked out behind the scenes bypassed a tremendous amount of the formal bureaucratic busywork that other smaller, less-knowledgeable drug makers had to go through in search of FDA approval. Hardly any of them ever received it. They didn't know what to do, whom to talk to, where to go. The list of drugs left out in the cold over the years, drugs that might have proved even more effective against AIDS than AZT, is a long one. It includes AL 721, HPA-23, and up to three or four dozen drugs useful against the opportunistic infections that kill most people with AIDS. AZT was promoted by pros. The others were not. Their sponsors simply were not as drug savvy.

But Barry was a master. He knew exactly what the FDA was willing to accept in testing. He knew the players in the game. He knew the rules. He negotiated personally with the key FDA regulator. Barry "handled" people and process smoothly, professionally, and quietly out of sight. The shame of it was that his only audience was inside Burroughs Wellcome. The outside world only saw Barry conducting the strings here, the brass there. Never the entire orchestra.

Barry's IND application called for a Phase I safety trial at two clinical sites. One was through Sam Broder at the NIH's hospital, the Clinical Center, and the other was Duke University. Barry liked doing research at Duke because he was already familiar with their scientists. Several had worked for Wellcome on previous drug trials. For AZT, Dr. David Durack was the PI, the principal investigator, and Dani Bolognesi was involved in the virology.

But Broder had a problem: politics almost killed the trial at the NCI. The NCI did not want to do the Phase I study in the NIH's hospital under a Wellcome IND. "Because of, if you will, bureaucratic requirements at the Clinical Center, the National Cancer Institute wanted to do the studies under their own IND," Barry explains as diplomatically as possible.

So Barry wrote a letter to Cooper at the FDA, cross-filing the Wellcome IND with the NCI. This permitted the NCI to use the original IND written at Wellcome headquarters in North Carolina. "We allowed them to cross-file our IND," says Barry. "See, it required the sponsor's permission."

On July 3, the first patient to get AZT received it in the NIH's hospital.

Duke administered its first dose to a patient a week later. The IND called for twenty patients to be tested, and Sam Broder was able to round up more, and do it faster, than Durack at Duke. "Sam was very vocal" about AZT, says Barry.

In addition, Barry explains, "Broder had just completed a Suramin trial, which, unfortunately, was not successful." But it did make him well known. Broder had patients referred to him from as far away as Los Angeles and Miami. People with AIDS heard about him and wanted to get into the study. Duke had only North and South Carolina as an AIDS catchment area. The NCI and Duke raced to line up patients. In the end, Broder got thirteen AIDS patients to Durack's seven. But to hear Broder tell it, the NCI had practically all the AIDS patients and did practically the entire Phase I trial. That was just fine with Barry. He was only too happy to see Sam Broder out there talking up AZT.

To save time, Barry divided up the clinical pharmacology work so that the blood samples from patients at Duke were tested at both Duke and nearby Wellcome, while the sera from Sam Broder's patients were tested right there at the NCI. Dani Bolognesi did the virology work at Duke. In this way, Wellcome avoided having to transfer blood specimens with live AIDS virus over several hundred miles. It saved a lot of time and it was safer as well.

Barry had his own lab revolt over AIDS at this time. Many Wellcome scientists didn't want to deal with live AIDS virus. They complained that the company didn't have the proper P-3 laboratory conditions. "They stated so publicly," Barry remembers, "but I and the other supervisors said, 'Too bad. You're gonna have to work with them.' "

Then Barry saw that he would run out of thymidine. Just weeks into the Phase I safety trial, he knew that Wellcome was going to move on and begin a big Phase II efficacy trial. After just a half dozen patients, Barry thought it was clear that AZT wasn't going to kill anyone. There were no unexpected adverse reactions, according to Barry. Broder and Durack reported that there was some toxicity but that it was manageable. There were even a few tentative signs of clinical improvement.

Wellcome had enough AZT to complete the Phase I study. But to do a Phase II, with hundreds of human subjects, Wellcome was going to need a lot more of the drug. Manufacturing big quantities of AZT required much more thymidine. Fortunately, Wellcome knew exactly how much more because it was the major consumer of thymidine in the United States; the company was the biggest producer of the drug trichlorozymidine, which in part was made up of thymidine.

In 1985, only ten to twenty kilograms of thymidine were being processed from herring and salmon sperm. Wellcome knew each and every thymidine supplier around the world. Barry had the company's development people tell them to start scaling up production. He also told Sam Broder about the thymidine shortage about halfway through the Phase I study. "We searched high and low for all existing supplies and it was awful tight," says Barry. "Sam said, 'Well, you know the NCI bought some thymidine a number of years ago because it might be useful against cancer. But it's not panning out. Would you like that?' "

Barry said hell yes and was very grateful for the hundred kilos Broder sent down to Wellcome, though it represented only 10 to 25 percent of one year's supply of the thymidine needed for the Phase II trial. But the history of this shipment has more than one version. "There have been times when it has been presented like we were dead in the water, with no drug, and we just had our thumbs up our ass," says Barry. He doesn't mention Broder's name, but it hangs in the air. In fact, Broder made it sound as if Wellcome ran out of thymidine in the middle of the Phase I safety trial, but that was simply not true.

That is not to say that Barry didn't encourage Broder to wrap his career around AZT. He did. He encouraged it as much as possible. While Barry was working behind the scenes with Dani Bolognesi, Gerald Quinnan, and Ellen Cooper, Broder was out there making public waves for AZT. Even Cooper took notice. "Sam was out on the stump."

Broder's identification of AZT as "his" drug, and his championing of it throughout the biomedical bureaucracy, certainly moved it along while other drugs languished for lack of a sponsor. "Sam was very enthusiastic," says Barry. "He was doing a bang-up job both in the laboratory and in the Clinical Center and from, if you will, the public relations point of view. He was getting the word out, showing people the work, really pushing hard. He was very enthusiastic about it."

Dani Bolognesi agrees with Barry: "To my mind, Sam did not so much do the basic work on this as he became a major thrust to get it through the system, getting the FDA to approve it, like that. Sam was *committed.* He started pushing it very hard."

It was Broder's commitment to AZT, his enthusiasm for the drug, that the people at Wellcome valued so highly. Broder was a highly regarded public advocate for their proprietary drug. They allowed him to associate himself with AZT, to become "Mr. AZT," to be profiled in the *Washington Post* and the *Wall Street Journal*. It suited them. Sam Broder had such *enthusiasm!*

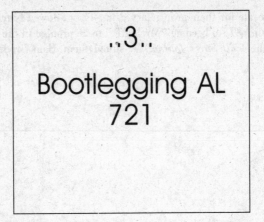

..3..

# Bootlegging AL 721

David Heron was a true believer. You could see it in his eyes. Black, intense, Heron's eyes had a fervor usually associated with religious passion, not cold scientific rationality.

Heron commuted from Tel Aviv, where he lived with his wife, a well-known Israeli painter, to Rehovot, where he worked in the Weizmann Institute of Science. Everybody called it "the Weizmann." It was world class, on a par with the National Institutes of Health in Washington, the Pasteur Institute in Paris, or the Max Planck Institutes outside of Munich and Berlin. Heron was proud to work in one of its best research labs, run by Dr. Meir Shinitzky.

By day, Heron ran experiments, leaving nights free to indulge his real passion, studying Kabbala, Jewish mysticism. On weekends, he would drive up to Safad, the ancient city to the north where Kabbalism was born and where people still practiced it. Most scientists say they search for the truth. Heron joked among his friends that he was looking for the Truth, capital T.

Meir Shinitzky didn't like the people around Heron. The fast Tel Aviv artsy crowd that dabbled in the occult just didn't suit the life of a serious scientist. Shinitzky thought it was crazy for Heron, whom he considered a talented kid, to waste his time with that stuff.

At thirty-nine, Shinitzky was already displaying those personality characteristics that would only intensify during his lifetime. Gifted at making conceptual leaps, he tended to go just a bit further and express them as reality. His brusque manner leant itself to making claims as though they were incontrovertible facts.

48

In the summer of 1979, Shinitzky was doing research on aging. He wanted to restore the memory loss that marks senile dementia, or senility, in old people. As a membrane biochemist, he had a few hard facts to work with. The "drying up" associated with aging wasn't just an old wives' tale. It was literally true. The walls of the body's cells, their membranes, lose their fluidity and become increasingly rigid and hard as people get older.

The chemical culprit behind this hardening of the cell walls was none other than the same compound responsible for hardening of the arteries—cholesterol. Membranes are a mixture of proteins and lipids, or fats. Cholesterol is one of those lipids. The higher the ratio of cholesterol to the rest of the lipids, the more rigid the cell wall.

If he removed some of that cholesterol, Shinitzky could change the properties of the membrane. With a little membrane engineering, he might even be able to increase fluidity and stop the hardening of the nerve cell walls in the brain.

That would stop memory loss, perhaps even reverse it. That could restore memory to the senile elderly. No one had ever been able to do that before. In a way, Shinitzky was attempting to reverse the aging process itself. Anyone who could do *that* would receive a great deal of credit from his colleagues. Enough credit, perhaps, to bring him a Nobel. Just where Shinitzky eventually found his cholesterol-leaching agent would play a major role in the AIDS crisis years later.

The Israeli scientist knew that certain compounds are able to draw cholesterol out of the walls of human cells. He also knew of an unlikely place to find them—in egg yolks. Scientists usually make their compounds out of pure chemicals taken from a bottle in a laboratory. Shinitzky designed his compound out of a natural substance, a food that people could buy at the local grocery store.

But he didn't quite know how to do it. He turned to his lab assistant, Heron, gave him directions and advice, and told him to find a way. It took several months, but Heron did create something that worked. He used a common organic solvent, acetone, and came up with a mixture they named AL 721—Active Lipid with three lipids in a ratio of 7 to 2 to 1. It was crude and difficult to prepare. It also stank. The egg-based compound had a horrendous odor.

The crude concoction was good enough. They began experimenting. When Shinitzky and Heron took brain cells from senescent mice and mixed them in the test tube with AL 721, they could see significant change in the cell walls. The membranes became looser, more fluid. They could measure the cholesterol extracted from the membranes. When they tried it out on live mice, they saw an improvement in membrane fluidity, and there was no evidence of toxicity.

Heron began describing AL 721 as having special, mystical properties. The greater the number of successful experiments with the drug, the more Heron preached about its transcendental nature. Shinitzky grew increasingly irritated with him and this talk of magic. It was all so alien to his way of thinking.

Shinitzky transferred Heron to a lab run by a close colleague, David Samuel, a neuroscientist involved with behavior change, especially drug addiction.

David Samuel was Sir David Samuel, thanks to his service to the British. He was tall and elegant, with a strong British accent when he spoke English. In the extremely informal Israeli atmosphere, where people invariably use their first names, Samuel was known to occasionally correct people—"I am *Sir* David"—without so much as a hint of self-mockery. At the Weizmann his friends sometimes snickered behind his back, but no one made fun of Samuel's abilities. As a scientist, he was first-rate.

Samuel had recently made a breakthrough on the chemistry of drug addiction. He showed that alcohol and heroin addiction physically change the body's nerve cells. An addict's cell walls become rigid, as though the person had become very old. The longer an addict shoots up or the longer an alcoholic drinks, the greater the change in the body's cells, especially the nerve cells. Nerve membranes adapt to the drugs and over time require more and more of them. The greater the dependence, the greater the tolerance and the greater the rigidity of the cell walls. The cause of the rigidity? An excess of cholesterol.

Samuel knew that in drug withdrawal, the pain can be so intense that many addicts can't stand it and revert. After an addict stops taking heroin or alcohol, the body's nerve cell walls take a long time returning to normal. The reason for the delay is that it takes weeks for the excessive amounts of cholesterol to leave the membranes. The tremendous pain of withdrawal is due in large part to these slow chemical and physical changes in the nerve cell walls.

Samuel and Shinitzky hypothesized that if AL 721 could extract cholesterol quickly from nerve cell membranes, the drug might help addicts. Samuel told Heron to set up a series of animal experiments. The results were impressive. The pain of withdrawal appeared to be sharply reduced in the addicted animals. In some, the withdrawal symptoms disappeared immediately.

Heron then killed the animals and analyzed their brain cells. The AL 721 had reduced the cholesterol in the nerve cell walls. Not only did the drug appear to work on processes associated with memory loss in aging, it now seemed to be effective on opiate and alcohol addiction.

Finally, AL 721 was tested on people. A safety trial of six female and three male subjects over age fifty was conducted. Each took fifteen grams of the drug daily for six weeks or more. One took it for six months. The AL 721 was given with a fat-free breakfast or dinner. There were no adverse reactions. None.

Then Samuel took a more fateful step. He conducted a trial with sixteen people who were seventy-five or older to see if AL 721 could reverse the immune suppression that comes with old age. The body's immune system is built on T-4 and other cells that fight disease. They become rigid with age.

Each person was given ten to fifteen grams of the drug every morning for three weeks. All sixteen showed significant improvement in their immune systems. When they were taken off AL 721, their immune systems degenerated back to their original state.

This was too much for Heron. He told his artist friends in Tel Aviv that he had discovered the magic elixir described in Kabbalist literature—a supernatural liquid said to be the chemical equivalent of the laying on of hands. Heron said it cured the sick and prolonged life. This was a heady time for Heron's circle. The crude, smelly, oily compound made out of eggs was transformed in their imagination into an elixir of youth.

Heron's name would appear on many of the initial articles written about AL 721 between 1979 and 1982. But in the end, Heron found himself out of the Weizmann. His talk of magic elixirs was blasphemy at this font of science. Heron disappeared from the scientific scene. He would later turn up in California. Then he was said to have moved into the New Age movement. There were also rumors that he had found a new drug, the *real* fountain of youth drug. Finally there was total silence.

James Jacobson, Jr., was a rich kid. He came from a prominent West Coast family that had moved west from Ohio and built a retailing fortune. A grandfather built a bank. His uncle Lester was a founding member of Fried, Frank, Jacobson, Harris, and Shriver, the well-known Washington

51

law firm that defended Ivan Boesky. His mother was a producer-director in New York and London.

Jacobson was still in his twenties back in the late seventies. He had an MBA degree in international business. From 1974 to 1978, he was a partner in Coach Group International, a Hong Kong–based investment firm. His job was to find United States investments for overseas clients. In 1978 he founded a nonprofit foundation called the FFGB, which sponsored new research in medicine. He was a director of the American Technion Society, which is the Israel Institute of Technology. Jacobson was also a member of the Board of Directors of the Los Angeles Committee for the Weizmann Institute of Science.

Around this time, Jacobson was also dabbling in the film business. His production company was doing a piece on extrasensory phenomena. During the filming, he met Uri Geller. Geller was a frequent late-night TV guest in the United States at this time who had surrounded himself with a group, all Israelis, called The Nine—nine people who were heavily into mysticism. David Heron and his wife were on the periphery of The Nine while Heron was working at the Weizmann. Jacobson first heard about AL 721 through this strange group.

At twenty-eight, Jacobson decided to personally fund the research on AL 721 at the Weizmann in exchange for worldwide licensing rights. The whole thing appealed to him on many levels. He liked the idea of a magic elixir. He wanted to be close to the Israeli mystics. He wanted to do something useful with his inherited wealth. And the idea of being an entrepreneur in the eighties was pretty appealing too. It was a fateful decision. Over the next three years, Jacobson's money was to finance nearly all of the key experiments that showed AL 721 to be a promising drug in treating senility, alcohol and opiate addiction, cystic fibrosis, and immune suppression.

As a result, AL 721 passed into the hands of a tiny one-product start-up company closely held by Jacobson, his uncle Lester, and a few close relatives and friends. The company had few resources, no experience in drug development, and no connections in the highly politicized world of Big Science in Washington, D.C. It lacked everything Burroughs Wellcome had—except for a remarkable drug.

Dr. Bernard Bihari was head of the alcohol addiction center at Downstate Medical Center in New York. He also had a small private practice. Most of his work up to this point had been on addiction, but increasingly his patients were coming down with the AIDS-associated infections that were sweeping the gay community. In early 1982, Bihari got a call from Jacobson asking if he was interested in testing a new drug for treating withdrawal. Bihari checked it out. He found that "there was very good animal literature on AL 721. Mouse and rat studies showed it really relieved withdrawal in laboratory animals."

Bihari met with Jacobson. There was a lot of exciting talk about human trials for the drug. Bihari did some work for Jacobson. Then silence. Jacobson left everything hanging, he had no follow-through. It was the beginning of a series of missed opportunities. "Jake just couldn't get it together," Bihari reports. "I know that when a number of people did work for him, he wouldn't pay them. He still owes me five thousand dollars, and he's a multimillionaire."

Months later, Bihari got a call from a friend, Bill Regelson, a scientist at the University of Virginia who Bihari thought was brilliant. Regelson had also been in contact with Jacobson. According to Bihari, Regelson said, " 'Bernie, do you treat addicts?' I said yes. Regelson said, 'Do you have some with AIDS?' I said sure. Then Regelson said, 'Are you aware that a study's been done showing that AL 721 reverses the immune deficiency of aging in mice?' To that I said no. Regelson said, 'Let me send you a copy. . . . The crucial factor is a change in lymphocyte membrane fluidity. . . . Why don't you read the study and call Jake and get a trial going?' "

This line of inquiry amazed Bihari. Regelson was implying that a treatment for AIDS might be available. Right now! It was the same drug he had been toying with to put into addicts—AL 721.

As his excitement mounted, Bihari called Jacobson again. This might be fantastic stuff, he said. We've got to start testing it. Jacobson listened but again there was no follow-through. He would not commit. Bihari grew frustrated. Increasingly, he was seeing people with AIDS. He could see the epidemic building: "I saw it both in addicts and in a couple of friends who were getting sick with AIDS. I could see a very serious crisis coming. It was obvious to many people by then. But Jake just wasn't interested."

The shiny black Alfa Romeo shot down the Saw Mill Parkway heading south, toward Manhattan. The radio was blaring oldies-but-goodies music, the morning was diamond crisp, and the driver was wearing a huge shit-eating grin. Arnold Lippa was rich.

He was president of Praxis Pharmaceuticals Inc., a little start-up company that had just gone public.* Lippa was now a card-carrying paper millionaire, a true "eighties baby." As he hit the West Side Highway, Lippa was already dreaming of the Jaguar he was going to buy for his wife. It would match the Jag the company was leasing for him next month. Then there was that incredible condo. Lippa couldn't believe he was actually buying a condo from Patrick Ewing, the Knicks basketball star! Ewing had custom-built an "atmosphere room" complete with a sauna. *That* was going to be fun.

Tapping his steering wheel to the tune of "Finger-Poppin' Time", Lippa went over the details of what he was planning to do with this new drug, AL 721. The original idea was to sell it as a food additive in health stores. That would get around the need for FDA approval, which took years.

---

*The corporate parentage of AL 721 is a complex one. Like so many other start-up companies in the eighties, it went through several permutations.

In December 1981, James Jacobson entered into an agreement with the Weizmann Institute in which he personally sponsored preclinical research and toxicology studies on AL 721 in connection with immune dysfunction, age-related memory disorders, and alcohol and drug detoxification. In exchange, Jacobson became the exclusive worldwide licensee of AL 721.

In April 1983, Jacobson formed the Natural Pharmaceutical Corporation (NPC) to further the R&D of the drug and to act as the licensee.

In September 1983, Matrix Research Laboratories Inc. was created. It was a subsidiary of NPC and was put in charge of research and development for a new limited partnership that Jacobson was about to create.

In December 1983, Jacobson put together the Active Lipid Development Partners (ALDP), a California limited partnership that did a private placement and raised an aggregate of $1.775 million to finance AL 721. The limited partners were granted the right to exchange their interest in ALDP for shares of common stock if the licensee of AL 721 should make a public offering. At this point, Jacobson assigned his licensee rights to the Natural Pharmaceutical Corporation, which was the general partner of the limited partnership. Jacobson remained the principal shareholder of NPC.

In September 1984, the Natural Pharmaceutical Corporation became Praxis Pharmaceuticals Inc.

In January 1985, Praxis made an initial public offering, known as an IPO in Wall Street jargon, that raised $3.7 million, and the limited partners of ALDP received common stock in the new public company.

Finally, in June 1987, in order to end potential confusion, the name Praxis was sold to another company with a similar name, Praxis Biologics Inc., for $225,000. The last name of the company that holds all the rights to AL 721 is Ethigen Corp.

At that time, Jacobson was thirty-four years old. He was chairman and chief executive officer of Ethigen. Arnold Lippa was forty years old, and president as well as a director.

As the early Israeli tests had indicated, they could sell it to the elderly as an immune booster for the blood or even as a memory restorative. Lippa knew the damn thing was made out of eggs, so at least it was safe.

He turned off the highway and headed east toward midtown, still thinking about the new drug. Lippa had gotten pleasantly ripped a few days ago with his old buddy Fulton Crews, a lipid biochemist. God, he loved the experience of getting high and talking science. Fulton had yakked on and on about viruses and their shapes. Lippa couldn't remember exactly what he said. Something about how viruses were basically proteins enclosed in membranes. Crews said there were different kinds of membranes. Some were made out of lipids. Fats. These fatty membranes could get stiff. Rigid, as in clogged arteries or the brain cells of senile people. Lippa knew that the Israelis who created AL 721 had shown that the drug could somehow affect this rigidity. So . . . ? Lippa wondered what Crews was getting at. Was he suggesting that AL 721 could be active against viruses?

As Lippa turned into the Parker Meridien Hotel's garage on Fifty-sixth Street, he still couldn't put it all together. It was February 1985, and the Meridien had not yet become a way station for Japanese tourists in New York City. It was a businessman's hotel. It didn't attract the Euro-trash, as the Pierre did. It wasn't as flashy as the Helmsley Palace, but it showed a bit more style than the staid Plaza in the days before Ivana Trump tried her hand at redecorating. What the Meridien had was a fitness center and a great running track on the roof with incredible views of Central Park. The chairman and major stockholder of Lippa's company, James Jacobson, always stayed at the Meridien when in New York.

Lippa walked past the lobby and turned left. It was too late in the morning for the Maurice, with its double-staircased entrance and power breakfasts. Instead, he walked into Le Patio, the informal fourteen-table restaurant. A buffet brunch was being served.

Lippa was the last to arrive. Seated around the table were Jacobson and Dr. Bernard Bihari, a medical researcher with a small private practice in the city. Lippa said, "Hi, Jake," and sat down.

Jacobson began the business meeting, but before he could get into it, Bihari interrupted. He had something very important to say. Bihari blurted out that he had given AL 721 to a patient, a New York city politician. The man had AIDS. "I gave it to him to see what it would do," he said. "It's a safe food substance, isn't it?" It had already been tested out in people in Israel, Bihari added defensively.

Bihari told the enthralled audience that the New York politician was someone they would instantly recognize from the news. The politician had shown a significant improvement in all his AIDS symptoms, Bihari said, including a reduction in night sweats. He gained weight, his energy level rose, and his T-4 cell count stopped falling.

Bihari was deliberately trying to shock Jacobson with the news. He had been trying for months to get Jacobson to finance testing of AL 721. It appeared to have so much potential. But he had gotten nowhere. Now with a scientist on board, Arnold Lippa, maybe he could persuade Jacobson to get trials going. His gambit worked.

Lippa thought this news was incredible. He couldn't believe it. Bihari was saying that AL 721 *did* have antiviral properties. That's what Crews was getting at. It appeared to work against the AIDS virus! Lippa said, "Shit. We've really got something here," according to Bihari. "Don't worry, Bernie, we'll give you credit."

Visions of a Nobel Prize danced in front of Lippa. And dollar signs. Jacobson was quiet. He watched Bihari and Lippa as they talked. They were excited.

Lippa and Jacobson were also in deep trouble. They discussed it at the meeting: The FDA would be furious if it found out that AL 721 was being given to people before going through a safety trial. And think of the liability. What if this guy sued? Praxis was now a public company. It had sold stock. They knew Praxis couldn't go around administering unauthorized drugs.

Lippa swore Bihari to secrecy. He threatened to "sue him up the ass" if he continued to administer the drug to his politician patient. At least, that's the way Lippa remembers it.

Bihari recalls it another way: "Lippa said, 'Will your friend allow us to meet him?' I knew he wouldn't. He was very paranoid. He's somebody that would be recognized. . . . He would not be involved in any way. Lippa said, 'Tell him that if he'll allow us to have a doctor examine him and do lab work, we'll continue his supply of AL 721. Otherwise we won't.' "

Bihari didn't know whether Lippa was bluffing, but he was furious. He never spoke to Lippa again and drifted far away from Praxis, deep into the nascent AIDS medical community movement. In the end he never did get any credit from Lippa on the connection between AIDS and AL 721.

Bihari ran out of AL 721. Within weeks, the politician's night sweats were back. He lost his appetite and he became fatigued.

Then Bihari was able to get another kilo of AL 721. He won't say how or with whose connivance. Bihari's patient's symptoms quickly grew better once he went back on the drug.


Arnold Lippa was the John Belushi of science. He was always hungry—for food, for ideas, for stimulation. He had always been a big eater, a fast talker, a brilliant thinker with a wild imagination. Lippa was a truly prodigal child, with a good dash of sixties antiauthoritarianism thrown in. At thirty-six, he was still the enfant terrible, a grown man who felt he was the boy genius "they" could never quite understand.

Lippa saw himself as the outsider. Unlike Sam Broder and David Barry, Lippa had partaken of the sixties counterculture, and it had had a deep effect on him. But Lippa's contempt for established authority didn't change as he got older. He didn't accommodate. Age didn't bring maturity. Yet like so many who hold convention in disdain, Lippa teetered between rebelling against authority and seeking approval from established figures. He wanted their approval for his eccentricity.

In another time, Arnold Lippa's personality would have made him a political revolutionary or a messianic zealot, but in Ronald Reagan's America he became an entrepreneur. Lippa wasn't much different from Steve Jobs or Ted Turner. He rode the eighties craze for high tech, deregulation, and hot stocks to great personal heights. Arnold Lippa was a man made for the "get-out-of-my-way" capitalism of the times.

He wasn't alone. Scientists and engineers all over the country were bailing out of ivory towers to start up spanking new companies. Genentech, Cetus, Cambridge BioScience were among the dozens of start-ups just in biotechnology. Then there were the computer whizzes and their Apples, Lotuses, Suns, and Microtechs. They formed a new swashbuckling corporate elite the likes of which America hadn't seen since Carnegie, Rockefeller, and Vanderbilt created the country's first industrial base a hundred years ago.

These new entrepreneurs came out of Stanford, Harvard, and MIT, some still clutching their Nobels, in search of the new Holy Grail of science—the Big Buck. Investor demand for new high-tech start-ups was enormous. It was whipped up by an army of stockbrokers and a chorus of press attention. "Buy the next IBM!" they shouted to the public.

Fame fell right behind fortune in the motivation department, and the entrepreneurs were the new superstars. Who wanted to publish in a weighty academic journal when a scientist could be a *Time* cover story? The bookworms of high school were suddenly transformed into the Ferrari-driving visionaries of the decade. Lippa wanted a piece of this. So did dozens of other people who found themselves behind anti-AIDS drugs in the eighties. The drug market was a growth market.

But it was also a closed market. Unlike computers, transportation, finance, and scores of other industries that were deregulated in the eighties, drug development remained locked up by the big guys, the corporate heavies with their links to the NIH, the medical schools, and the FDA. Entrepreneurial brilliance and flash didn't count for much in the big-time pharmaceutical drug business.

Of course, Lippa didn't know this at the time. No one did. AL 721, his drug, was to rise the highest and fall the furthest of all AIDS drugs. By 1986–87, it was being bootlegged by thousands of people with AIDS. Tons of copycat AL 721 were being imported every month from Germany and Japan.

By 1988 it was dead, and without ever really being tested. The list of anti-AIDS drugs that showed potential and died in this way runs to several dozen. All of them, like AL 721, were killed, either by internal incompetence and bitter infighting or by deliberate neglect by the government. AL 721 died from a combination of both. And Lippa's paper millions turned into recyclable cellulose.


Lippa broke with convention early. The son of a rabbi, he married an artist whose parents had emigrated from Italy. The act so provoked his parents that they "sat shiva" for him, the Jewish ceremony for mourning the dead.

Lippa had always been heavy, but at five eleven he could carry his two hundred pounds. His broad face wore a permanent Cheshire-cat grin. Lippa was balding by his early thirties. With his beard, his bulk, and his I-know-something-you-don't-know face, he easily could have passed as an aging Indian guru. Projecting a charismatic aura of "I'll lead you to places you've never been before, and we'll have fun along the way," he never lacked for acolytes.

Lippa received his Ph.D. in psychopharmacology from the University of Pittsburgh. He specialized in biological psychology, the study of how chemicals in the brain affect human behavior—the perfect specialty for a sixties drug-culture academic. But Lippa hated graduate school and couldn't wait to get the hell out. He hadn't shown any greatness in the lab, no "magic hands," but he was incredibly imaginative.

Right out of school, Lippa joined Lederle Laboratories, a division of American Cyanamid. The choice of Lederle marked him as a renegade. Lippa was one of the best in his class; he might have gone to the NIH or some other prestigious research center, but instead he chose to become a commercial scientist. He enjoyed the notion that working for private industry was considered déclassé by many scientists. It appealed to his sense of being outside the Establishment. And then there was the money. His salary at Lederle was more than double what he would have gotten at the NIH.

In the decade Lippa spent at Lederle, 1973 to 1984, he was in constant battle with his corporate superiors. He was completely outside the organizational norm. One year he decided to shave his head completely bald. Just for a change, he said.

But Lippa made money for Lederle. By 1979, he had been promoted to director of molecular neurobiology in its Medical Research Division. Mostly he researched anxiety—how it was produced by chemicals in the brain, and how it could be reduced. Lederle dreamed of finding another Valium, the drug that had made Hoffmann-LaRoche a fortune. Anxiety was the kind of illness that big pharmaceutical companies loved. Millions of people suffered chronically from it. Anxiety was the stuff of mass markets.

Lippa became one of the world's top dozen experts in psychopharmacology. He published widely, spoke at conferences, got paid as a consultant, and was highly respected in the field.

Yet he was itchy. He dreamed of setting up a small "guerrilla" drug firm that would manufacture designer drugs. Lippa felt he could spot market niches faster than the big, bureaucratic companies and beat them at their own game. People working in *his* start-up would be free from the heavy hand of administration. They would have fun at their work. To Lippa, Lederle was stultifying, like grad school, like all institutions.

Lippa's work on the brain led him to research on aging and memory. Alzheimer's disease was capturing the public's attention, and drug companies were rushing to come out with products to treat it. Lippa developed a theory on why specific chemical changes occur when people get old. He predicted that a certain kind of drug would become a therapeutic agent. When Shinitzky and Samuel began publishing their articles on AL 721, Lippa said, "This is the drug I've been looking for."

He went to the money people at Lederle and told them they *had* to buy the licensing rights to AL 721. They weren't interested. The drug hadn't been invented at Lederle and they couldn't figure out how it could be made profitable. That was the final straw for Lippa, the last act of bureaucratic know-nothingism for him.

Moreover, he was ready for a change, ready to transform himself into a capitalist hero for the eighties. In the summer of 1984, he signed on with James Jacobson to become president of little Praxis Pharmaceuticals, whose one product was AL 721. Lippa would receive 110,000 shares in exchange for technology and R&D contracts that he brought with him. Lippa also received options for another 550,000 shares, at a penny a share.

Only one thing bothered Lippa about the deal. Jacobson had promised him total control, but Jacobson didn't designate him as a founder of the company. From the beginning, this would eat away at Lippa. It meant he didn't have full control, and Lippa was a control freak. But for the moment he was happy.

In January 1985, Praxis went public, selling its first common stock on the over-the-counter market. Lippa, along with Jacobson and his partners who had invested in the company early, were able to cash out a good part of their paper holdings for that greener variety of parchment: dollars. A few people were already getting rich off AL 721.

After the brunch at the Meridien, when Bihari said that AL 721 had worked against AIDS in the New York city politician, Lippa immediately championed the drug. Then Jacobson bought in. But Bihari was out.

God. If only Bihari was right, thought Lippa. If AL 721 worked against the AIDS virus, everything would be perfect. Praxis would be a success, everybody with stock would get rich, and Arnold Lippa could win a Nobel Prize.

But Lippa had one small problem. There was no way he could test live AIDS virus in his laboratory. He had rented lab space uptown at City College. No one was going to allow him to mess around with a deadly virus when all these students were walking around. Lippa needed a lab that would test AL 721 against AIDS.

It was 1985 at that time, and Robert Gallo was the most famous scientist associated with AIDS, so Lippa decided to go after Gallo and get him to test the drug. But Lippa knew he couldn't just pick up the phone and talk to the great man. He knew exactly what his presumption would look like to the scientific community. He would be viewed as a psychopharmacologist with no experience in virology working at a tiny new start-up doing research on memory and aging with an egg-based compound no one had ever heard of before. Lippa could almost hear scientists at the NIH laugh and say, "This is crazy. What does all this have to do with AIDS?"

But Lippa had an ace in the hole. David Scheer was on the payroll of Praxis as a consultant, and he was loaded with scientific contacts. In fact, that was basically his business. The son of a Bronx district attorney, Scheer had graduated Harvard. He never finished his Ph.D. and had been a perennial grad student at Yale. Scheer knew science, however—not laboratory science but commercial science. He had a Connecticut-based firm, Scheer & Company. His real occupation was more about venture capital than venturing hypotheses.

Scheer was also a consultant to the rich New York Loeb family. He had been the Loebs' point man when they showed interest in investing in Praxis. Lippa had been impressed with his connections and hired him. Lippa told a colleague that he used Scheer because "he spoke right, he looked right, and he followed orders." Besides, Lippa added, "Everybody needs a preppy front."

Scheer's most important contact was his mentor in the Yale pharmacology department, Dr. Frank Bertino, a man fast on his way to becoming one of the big names in cancer chemotherapy. He knew everybody at the NCI, including Gallo, who was an old friend. Bertino and Gallo socialized quite a bit.

In March, at a party at Bertino's home attended by both Gallo and Scheer, Scheer asked Bertino to act as a go-between, putting Lippa and Gallo together. At first Gallo refused to see Lippa, but Bertino, under heavy pressure from his protégé Scheer, pleaded with him the entire evening. Before the night was out, Gallo gave in to his host, listened to Scheer, and set up a meeting for Lippa at the NCI.

In April, Scheer and Lippa flew down to the NCI at Bethesda, Maryland, for the meeting. Gallo met them in a conference room dominated by a long, rectangular table that could comfortably accommodate twenty people. Gallo seated Lippa and Scheer at one end, then walked the entire length of the table to sit at the far opposite end. Gallo is one of those people who are not burdened by other people's feelings. Gallo's eyes narrowed as he peered down the long table. It was the action of a man sighting his enemy. "Show me what ya got," he said. Lippa began explaining about how lipids affect cell walls and how they might be important to immune function. Gallo interrupted with "That's crazy! Everybody knows that viruses are just proteins." Gallo wasn't particularly angry. He was just being his usual condescending and dismissive self. He gave the idea the back of his hand.

To Gallo and to all virologists at the time, the only important thing about a virus was it is protein. That's what viruses were made of. Membranes had nothing to do with it. It was the insides of a cell, the DNA and the RNA, that counted, not any surrounding membrane.

Lippa and Scheer patiently waited until Gallo was finished with his little tirade. They then gently reminded him that the AIDS virus was a lipid virus and had a lipid membrane surrounding it. Gallo countered by saying that viruses couldn't make lipids, only proteins. Lippa reminded him that retroviruses get their membranes and their lipids when they reproduce and bud from the membrane of the host cell.

"Oh, yeah. That's right," said Gallo. The three then talked about the family of lipid viruses and Gallo warmed up just a little. Then Lippa hit Gallo with AL 721. He told him they had a compound that extracted lipids from membranes. He said he had anecdotal evidence of this compound actually helping a person with AIDS. Lippa then asked Gallo, as smoothly as possible, if he would be willing to help take the first step by testing AL 721 to see if it had any activity against live AIDS virus in the test tube. Would Gallo test it in his own lab?

Gallo waited a beat, then said yes. It wasn't a hard decision to make. He would be doing his friend Bertino a favor. Besides, he knew this AL 721 didn't stand much chance anyway. It wasn't "politically favorable." Gallo himself had set the science paradigm for AIDS drugs by "codiscovering" with the French the retrovirus that was behind the disease. Any scientist seeking a Nobel knew that the game to play was the DNA/RNA game. This stuff affected the membrane, not the DNA/RNA. Who cared?

Lippa quickly sent Gallo a sample of AL 721. A month later, in June, Gallo's lab sent back the results. AL 721 worked to inhibit the AIDS virus in the test tube. It showed no signs of toxicity.

Lippa was ecstatic. He told a friend, "Here is the premier lab in the world telling me *my* compound works." AL 721 was *his* drug now, just as AZT had become Sam Broder's. Lippa felt that with the famous Robert Gallo behind him there was no stopping now.

Lippa then made his second trip down to the NCI to see Gallo. A light-headed euphoria enveloped him as he walked off the shuttle. It had worked! he was thinking. His plan had worked! Now Lippa was going to see Gallo's top lab chief, Prem Sarin, the scientist who'd actually done the tests on AL 721. His gambit with Scheer was paying off. Praxis, and Lippa, had broken into the hallowed world of Big Science.

Gallo welcomed Lippa with a quick handshake and an even quicker introduction to Sarin. He left abruptly. His body language said that Robert Gallo was a very busy man. Sarin immediately went to the data and showed Lippa how well AL 721 had performed in the test tube. A buoyancy pervaded the room. It was full of hope, expectation, and the unstated possibility of fame and fortune.

Sarin started talking about consulting for Praxis. In the words of someone who attended the meeting, Sarin was "wheeling and dealing, seeing what he could make out of all this."

That was okay with Lippa. He was used to it. What he wasn't used to was sloppy work, and he considered what he was looking at to be very sloppy. He thought the notes weren't kept right, the lab itself wasn't neat.

Lippa told Sarin to his face that he wasn't happy with the lab work. Sarin, naturally, defended his work and the two got into a shouting match. It was crazy. A great event had turned poisonous. A golden opportunity was ruined by Lippa's lack of tact. It wasn't an auspicious beginning to a collaborative scientific relationship.


At first Michael May thought it was the normal reaction to losing a job. He felt depressed, didn't have much of an appetite or much energy. The heat and humidity of New York in the summer of 1985 didn't help much either.

But then May began to get strange illnesses: an ear infection that antibiotics couldn't cure; a severe case of athlete's foot for the first time in his life; colds that lasted through the fall and winter. By Thanksgiving he had lost a lot of weight. He felt debilitated, almost feeble.

Over Christmas, May couldn't stop coughing. It wracked his whole body. In January he took the ELISA blood test and tested positive; antibodies to the AIDS virus meant he had been infected.

In February, painful sores broke out on his back. In March, a fungus spread over his arms and legs. Red blotches stained his face. His nights were haunted by sweats and fevers. Nothing stayed down. May knew he was dying.

In April, an Israeli friend sent him a letter saying that the Weizmann

Institute was experimenting with a drug that appeared to help with AIDS. In a wheelchair, with his mother and lover beside him, May took an El Al flight to Tel Aviv. The next day he began taking AL 721. Twice a day, once in the morning and once at night, he spread the oily, smelly stuff on a piece of bread and ate it. His doctor, Yehuda Skornick, told him: "The Americans don't like our treatment. It's too simple for them."

Nothing happened for a week. The euphoria he felt on landing in Israel was replaced by depression. During the second week, May's chronic diarrhea improved. His appetite returned. As the weeks passed, all May's AIDS symptoms gradually disappeared. When he returned to New York at the end of June, May walked off the plane feeling good for the first time in nearly a year. He even looked good. All his blotches and rashes were gone.

But so was the AL 721. By August, the AIDS symptoms began to return. May's T-4 cell count dropped. He took a second flight back to the Weizmann. After a month eating bread "buttered" with AL 721, May's AIDS symptoms disappeared for the second time.

May published his story in the *New York Native* newspaper. The Gay Men's Health Crisis newsletter quoted him. Demand for AL 721 shot up in the gay community.

Sam Broder was the next gatekeeper that Arnold Lippa and AL 721 had to pass in their journey through the government's drug-testing and approval process. Broder had his vaunted new technology to test drugs against live AIDS virus. He was also head of the new drug selection committee that determined which drugs got the green light and which did not.

Gallo assured Lippa he had nothing to worry about. Broder was a great guy, he said. Broder had been so helpful when he was looking for the cause of AIDS. Gallo said he would talk to Broder personally. What Gallo actually said to Broder may never be known. But at that moment, Lippa felt he had Gallo in his corner. He was totally confident as he boarded the Eastern shuttle for his third trip to the National Cancer Institute.

What Lippa was not aware of was that Broder by this time was totally committed to another drug, AZT. AZT had been found to be active in *his* lab. Its giant corporate sponsor, Burroughs Wellcome, had committed itself to spending millions to speed AZT through the system. That was drug development realpolitik. Money, power, and connections were critical. Wellcome had them all. And he, Broder, had the enthusiasm to make it all work.

Broder was in the middle of testing AZT and was revving up for an IND application to the FDA when he got the call from Gallo asking him to take a look at AL 721. That was the last thing Broder wanted to hear. He was incredibly busy. But it was Gallo, so he agreed to see this guy Lippa.

Lippa was not entirely unknown in Broder's lab. Bob Yarchoan had heard of him: "Arnold Lippa was very well known in psychopharmacology," he says. "His name was in a dozen books. He was known in the NIH."

When Lippa arrived and showed Broder Prem Sarin's data, Broder peremptorily dismissed all of it. He criticized each and every piece of Sarin's research. Broder told Lippa it was all worthless. It had to be done in a completely different way.

But Broder said that if Lippa was willing, he would get Mitch Mitsuya to run AL 721 in his assay to see if it really had any activity against live AIDS virus. He told Lippa to send over a sample.

Lippa walked out of the meeting completely shocked. "Broder beat the shit out of us," he recalls. "Here I thought Gallo had set up this entrée for us, and here [I had] a drug coming out of Gallo's lab. I would have thought Broder would have kissed his [Gallo's] ass." That was the last naive assumption that Lippa ever made about the NIH and the way hardball biomedical science is played.

Lippa sent a sample and waited. Three months passed. Still nothing. He called constantly and couldn't get through to Broder. What the hell was happening? After all, the assay took less than a week.

Finally Broder picked up, only to say that no, AL 721 did not show any in vitro activity against AIDS virus. It didn't work at all. Lippa couldn't believe it. Broder was actually contradicting Gallo. He asked him for the data. Broder refused. Broder, in fact, never sent Lippa the data and never explained how he had reached his conclusions.

Lippa appealed to Gallo, but Gallo said he couldn't do anything. It was Broder's lab. It was Broder's test.

Luckily for Lippa, the three-month silence drove him to cover himself. He asked Marc Weksler from Cornell, a member of the company's Scientific Advisory Board, for help in verifying the original positive results. Weksler introduced Lippa to a new junior faculty member, a wunderkind, Jeffrey Laurence. Laurence quickly replicated the Gallo lab's results showing AL

721 worked against the AIDS virus in a test tube. He called Lippa with the good news just a week after Broder reported that AL 721 was a failure.

Years later, Broder would even deny he had ever tested AL 721. "I don't believe it left Prem Sarin's laboratory," he has said.

When confronted with contrary evidence, Broder falls back on a strange excuse—loss of memory: "I don't know if we tested it. I'm not a historian."

His excuses don't stop there. Recovering a bit of his memory, Broder then dismisses AL 721 as a natural compound; it wasn't even a "real" drug: "AL 721 is a complicated situation. It's not a drug in the usual sense of the word. It's a combination of lipidlike things."

Finally, Broder gets closer to the truth. What was needed back in '85 was "to have a demonstrated project, not a theoretical project, not some promissory note, but a product in hand that [showed] you could do something about the AIDS epidemic in people that were infected. We could not serve as the arbiter of what will work and won't work for somebody else."

Actually, Broder did precisely that. He set up his lab and Mitch Mitsuya's assay as *the* arbiter of any and all drugs against the AIDS virus. He went to a dozen pharmaceutical companies, including Burroughs Wellcome, and told them his lab stood ready to use its new technology to test their drugs. But he only made the offer to big companies. Start-ups were not welcome. They didn't have the big bucks. And not all drugs. Just some drugs. Not "lipidlike things." Just "real" drugs such as AZT.

Finally, Broder gets down to the bottom line: "The issue of AL 721 is immaterial. AL 721 is not a product of discovery in *my* laboratory. I'm talking about the efforts of *my* laboratory. Okay?"

Once Arnold Lippa received word from Laurence that the Gallo test results had been replicated, he submitted a paper to the *New England Journal of Medicine.* There are four esoteric biomedical sources the *New York Times* regularly uses. In fact, a good percentage of the *Times* science stories begin as press releases from these four magazines and journals. The *New England Journal of Medicine (NEJM)* is the most scholarly and most prestigious. *Science* is an arm of the American Association for the Advancement of Science, the AMA of science. *Nature* and the *Lancet* are British.

Lippa argued in his paper that the AIDS virus was very rigid due to the large amount of cholesterol in its membrane. When treated with AL 721 in vitro, the amount of cholesterol was reduced. That changed the shape of the outside viral membrane. It was possible, Lippa argued, that once the shape of the AIDS virus changed, it could no longer attach itself to the wall of the host cell. That would end the reproduction of the AIDS virus (it relies on the host cell's genetic material to duplicate itself) and stop the spread of the disease. Lippa argued that the body's immune system would have a chance to recover. People might be saved. If clinical trials on humans showed this to be the case, then AL 721 could be an effective treatment of AIDS.

Lippa knew how to write a scholarly paper for publication. He had written dozens of them over the years. He submitted this one to the *NEJM* in September. Though Lippa wrote the letter, the researchers listed were Sarin, P. S.; Gallo, R. C.; Scheer, D. I.; Crews, F.; and Lippa, A. S. Because of Gallo's prestige at the time, Lippa's letter to the *NEJM* would soon be known by AIDS activists as "the Gallo letter."

The *NEJM* had just instituted a new policy to speed up the publication of articles dealing with AIDS. It promised to get out any article on AIDS within two weeks of acceptance. Furthermore, if the research was presented as a short letter, the editor himself, Arnold Relman, could approve it. Lippa called Relman and told him about the article on AL 721. Relman suggested that he shorten it and submit it as a letter. That would get it out fast. Lippa agreed and sent it in.

Two weeks went by and Lippa heard nothing. Shit, he thought, this feels like Broder all over again. He called. Relman said that he had discussed the letter with a few colleagues and decided to break the new policy and send it out to reviewers. Lippa protested but Relman wouldn't change his mind. He had the letter reviewed by two people and then called Lippa. He told him the research was too controversial and recommended that the *NEJM* hold back publication until further work was done. Lippa blew up, reminding Relman that letters weren't even supposed to be reviewed. Relman said he would send it out to one more reviewer. A month later, Relman called. If Lippa would dramatically tone it down, the *NEJM* would publish the letter. Lippa knew he didn't have much choice and agreed. A watered-down version was published on November 14, 1985, entitled "Effects of a novel compound (AL 721) on HTLV-III infectivity in vitro."

Lippa never found out who had reviewed the letter, but it didn't matter. Lippa knew that nearly everyone in AIDS was into molecular biology or protein biochemistry. No one specialized in lipid biochemistry or membrane engineering. AZT was hot. It fit right in by interfering in the DNA/RNA loop. DNA was where the action was in virology. Certainly not cholesterol, he thought to himself.

John James began the biweekly *AIDS Treatment News* in San Francisco in April 1986. It was a time of despair. People were dying. Nothing was coming out of Washington.

The *ATN* quickly became the voice of the AIDS underground medical movement. As people with AIDS and their local community doctors increasingly took to determining treatment themselves, *ATN* came to reflect the community's choices. It served a critical information and educational function that no one and nothing else did. It spread the word about drugs as they became popular, and it wasn't afraid to say that certain compounds weren't working.

James became one of the country's leading treatment advocates. He was tired of hearing "You have AIDS and six months to live," year after year. In the *ATN*, he exhorted people with AIDS to develop their own, independent medical expertise. He never used the term *empowerment*, but that was his message. Medical empowerment. Power to stay alive.

The *AIDS Treatment News* fought to change the standard operating procedures for drug development held sacred by the tight network of medical scientists and bureaucrats who controlled the NIH, the FDA, and the pharmaceutical companies. James was not a doctor or a scientist. His self-defined job was to report on the community consensus about specific drugs and to examine the public policy and ethical issues surrounding AIDS research.

James wrote fifty issues of the *AIDS Treatment News* between April 1986 and February 1988. During that time he discussed dozens of drug treatments popular within the gay community. They were all promising. All went untested by the government during that time. But AL 721 was *the* drug of choice in the gay community in 1986 and '87, and James's newsletter reflected that. The first issue of the *ATN* focused on AL 721. In fact, thirteen out of the first fifty issues dealt entirely with AL 721. Recipes for bootleg AL 721 were printed regularly. The drug was mentioned in 1988 and '89 as well, although with declining frequency as other drugs came on the scene.

James was thorough from the very first newsletter. He provided a long bibliography of scientific publications about AL 721 and said that trials were taking place in France and Israel. He ended his first issue by saying, "We should continue to watch AL 721, along with the other proposed new treatments for AIDS. It is important that testing and availability not be blocked by bureaucratic inertia and red tape, especially when, as in this case, safety concerns are minimal."

Then James took a swipe at Praxis by saying that "research and treatment for life-threatening illnesses must not be held up to suit the schedule of a handful of researchers or companies."

Intrigue and mystery surrounded AL 721, as it did many other underground anti-AIDS drugs. Stories abound of million-dollar offers for drugs from Hollywood stars, Wall Street investment bankers, and Washington, D.C., politicians. Access to treatment—any kind of treatment—was in such short supply that people were willing to go to any lengths to help their loved ones.

None of these stories, however, compares to this one. On May 5, 1986, a secretary from Ronald Reagan's office called Arnold Lippa at Praxis headquarters in New York City. She said that someone on the White House staff had a son who was infected with AIDS. She hastened to add that he got it through blood transfusions during an operation. She said she had heard that AL 721 was an effective treatment. Could Lippa arrange to send a supply of the drug down to Washington?

Lippa told the woman to call Jacobson in California. Lippa gave her Jacobson's phone number. She said she would call immediately. Like many other AIDS mysteries, nothing else is known about the strange White House request.

It was freezing in New York when the first U.S. clinical trial of AL 721 began. The number of AIDS cases reported to the CDC was soaring. The dimensions of the epidemic were now making themselves clear to doctors, scientists, and politicians. Most important, five years after the first person with AIDS had been diagnosed, the gay community was waking up to the fact that not a single drug had come out of the NIH to treat it, much less cure it.

The publication in the November 1985 *New England Journal of Medi-*

*cine* of the Gallo letter had increased the public awareness of AL 721. People in New York and San Francisco began talking about it.

At the American Medical Foundation in New York, everyone was talking about AL 721. Michael Lange, one of the first doctors in the country to perceive the severity of the AIDS epidemic, was on the Scientific Board of the AMF. Terry Byrne, who later worked for both the American Foundation for AIDS Research (AmFAR) and Senator Edward Kennedy, was at that time also at the AMF.

Byrne made it his business in 1986 to try to get as many potential anti-AIDS drugs out into the gay community as he could. He first heard about AL 721 from Robert Gallo over dinner in Bethesda. Then he read about it in November when the *NEJM* letter came out. Byrne brought it to the attention of Lange, who was the number two person in infectious diseases at St. Luke's–Roosevelt Hospital in New York. Lange was anxious to do a trial on the drug. He talked with his boss, Michael Grieco, who agreed. Lange liked Arnold Lippa. He checked him out and found that Lippa was a reputable scientist.

Lippa had hired an outside firm, Oxford Research in New Jersey, to be Praxis's clinical house. Oxford would write the protocols, deal with the FDA, find clinicians to run human trials of the drug. Since Praxis was basically a six-person operation, everything had to be outsourced, from the production of the drug to the sweet-talking of venture capitalists. Big pharmaceutical companies such as Burroughs Wellcome have all these functions in-house.

Oxford had begun writing the initial Phase I safety protocol in November 1985. It called for testing AL 721 in three sites, each using eleven patients. The application for an IND was sent to Ellen Cooper at the FDA in January of 1986. She was very helpful, and the go-ahead came in thirty days—not as fast as Sam Broder's five but quick by the bureaucratic standards of Washington. At St. Luke's, there were dozens of volunteers. Lange and Grieco were ready in February. But Praxis wasn't.

Lippa and Jacobson couldn't get the drug. Since Praxis didn't have any production facilities, it outsourced the manufacture of AL 721. But the drug was not easy to make, and batch after batch came in either contaminated with yeast or not in the correct 7:2:1 proportion. Quality became a cloud that would hover constantly over the tiny company.

In May, the first clean batch of AL 721 that met FDA specifications arrived. Unfortunately, there was only enough for seven AIDS patients, not the thirty-three originally planned. Grieco and Lange proceeded to give it to seven people who had lymphadenopathy, one of the very earliest symptoms of AIDS. They were given 15 grams twice a day on a special diet that cut out all other lipid intake.

The drug worked. After eight weeks Lange and Grieco could see an antiviral effect in five out of the seven people with AIDS. The level of the AIDS virus dropped 60 percent. The same people also showed weight gain and said they felt better. Their T-4 cell counts didn't reverse themselves and go up, but they did stop falling. There were no toxic side effects. The drug was absolutely safe and showed signs of being effective. Things looked good.

The stock of Praxis took off that summer, jumping from two dollars to a high of five. It was funny, because the results of the St. Luke's trial had not been announced. The Securities and Exchange Commission investigated, but no charges of insider trading or anything else were ever filed.

The first Phase I trial was so promising that Grieco and Lange wanted to continue it. Unfortunately, Praxis couldn't come up with clean AL 721. Six months later, Lippa got a good batch. Grieco and Lange went back to their original seven patients. In the interim, however, one had died, and the others had progressed to show more severe symptoms of the disease. Grieco also changed the diet and started feeding the patients foods with fat in them. This second time around, the trial didn't indicate any efficacy, although the drug was still proven safe.

Lange and Grieco then broke ranks on AL 721. Lange continued to believe in the drug; Grieco didn't. Grieco went on to become a major researcher on AZT and a powerful force in the NIH. Lange remained an outsider.

Lange continued to see patients taking AL 721. He had two patients with fairly advanced AIDS who went to Israel for treatment. One had severe anemia, proof of destruction of his red blood cells at such a rate that he needed three to four units of blood a week to live. When he went on AL 721, his transfusion requirement stopped. It was very dramatic. Eventually, he died of PCP.

After the St. Luke's trial, Arnold Lippa thought that AL 721 had been proven to be safe beyond any reasonable doubt. It had been put into people safely in Israel, France, and the United States. He wanted to move fast to the next step—doing trials to show that the drug worked, that it had efficacy. He asked Oxford Research to write a series of protocols. One called for AL 721 to be tested against AZT. Directly. Another called for a comparison between different doses of AL 721, with no placebo.

Then Lippa called Dr. Donna Mildvan at Beth Israel Medical Center and asked if she'd like to participate. Mildvan knew Michael Lange. She, like Lange, had been involved with AIDS since the early eighties. She knew Michael Grieco also. She was working on AZT with him. Later she would throw her career behind AZT. But at the moment, she was still open to trying new therapies.

Mildvan believed that safety had been proven and wrote up an efficacy protocol for AL 721. This time around, Ellen Cooper at the FDA wasn't helpful. In fact, her decision ultimately proved fatal for AL 721.

Cooper replied that the maximum allowable dosage of AL 721 had not been established at St. Luke's. Instead of 30 grams a day, what if the max were 50? Cooper was simply parroting the cancer chemotherapy line: Test until you got to the maximum allowable dosage. The same procedure was expected for AIDS drugs.

Unfortunately, community doctors were already showing that *reduced* doses of certain drugs were the most effective in the case of AIDS. Years later, the National Institute of Allergy and Infectious Diseases (NIAID) and the FDA would agree. But not this year. Cooper rejected the efficacy protocol. She demanded a dose-ranging trial first to find out how much AL 721 could be put into humans.

Then Cooper recommended that Praxis wait for the new ATEU, or AIDS Treatment Evaluation Units, system that NIAID was building. It would be finished shortly and the government would test out AL 721. For free.

Jacobson and Lippa agreed. Money was getting hard to come by at Praxis. Even though upwards of $5 million had been raised, the half dozen people at Matrix were consuming it fast. And Praxis was living pretty high for a little start-up company. Almost as much creativity was applied to expense accounts as to science. Flying was first-class, hotel rooms were always the best; indeed, they were suites. Leased cars were de rigueur for the officers. Lippa was like a kid in a candy shop. An irresponsible kid.

Lippa was the nexus for a whole series of tremendous scientific breakthroughs. He didn't originate the ideas, but he was the catalyst. Under Lippa, Praxis was responsible for showing that the AIDS virus belonged to a special family, lipid viruses; that a natural, safe compound, AL 721, could change the shape of all cells that had lipid envelopes or membranes; which meant that AL 721 could affect the AIDS virus, as well as normal human body cells distorted through aging and addiction. This was important science. It was what Lippa did best.

What he did worst was manage the process. As president of the company, Lippa was responsible for "QC"—quality control of the product—which was *the* major problem with AL 721. The pure drug was always in short supply. It was difficult to make and had to be carefully and continuously monitored. This was not Lippa's strength. Just as he was not terribly good in the lab, so he was not very proficient in the dull but necessary day-to-day operations of a company.

Neither, apparently, was Jacobson. As the chairman of the board and major shareholder in Praxis, it was Jacobson's duty to make sure the company was running smoothly. He didn't delve deeply enough into the company to guarantee the quality of AL 721.

Worse, Jacobson was indecisive. While he had played the major role in financing the early development of AL 721, Jacobson then backed off and time and again refused to commit.

No one really was in charge of running the company. No one took final responsibility for things that were essential for success. Both Lippa and Jacobson saw themselves as entrepreneurs, but neither one was a proper business manager. But because they saw themselves in that way, they didn't hire an outside businessman to run Praxis. It was a sad song about lost hope that was sung many times over during the eighties by small start-up companies.

And then there was the Broder Doctrine: Only the biggest pharmaceuticals with lots of bucks and clout can realistically get a drug developed. Praxis may have had its internal problems, but there were strong outside forces working against AL 721 as well. Sam Broder, the National Cancer Institute, and the FDA—basically the entire government effort against the AIDS epidemic in 1985—were all biased toward big drug corporations and against little companies. To say that this bias narrowed the development of possible anti-AIDS drugs is to say the least. Should this have been the government's biomedical policy in a public health emergency? Absolutely not. Should it have been the *unstated* biomedical policy? Of course not.

Arnold Lippa and Jake Jacobson were victims of far more than their own inadequacies.

# ..4..
# The Clap Doctor

He was known as the "clap doctor" and he carried the moniker with both pride and shame. Joseph Sonnabend was proud of his practice in the Village—New York's Greenwich Village. Sonnabend saw his practice as the kind that had long ago disappeared from medicine: a doctor with an actual kinship with his patients. They were gay. So was he. They were outsiders. He was a South African expatriate Jew, no less. They suffered from a strange, truly bizarre stream of infectious diseases. He was one of the few who could treat them.

A boyish barrel-chested man, almost shy, he stood with his arms straight down at his sides, head bent. With a heavy salt-and-pepper beard, bushy eyebrows, a full head of curly black hair, and a big nose, his face made him resemble nothing less than a kindly Caliban. Sonnabend had the softest of voices. It drew people toward him, and, once near, they stayed to listen to what he had to say. Yet that same voice had enormous projection in anger or excitement, especially when he was talking about science and its shortcomings. Later it would reverberate with talk of AIDS.

Sonnabend's manner triggered something in his patients that was sometimes described as two steps away from love. Seeing his potbelly hanging over pants that often failed to hide his underwear, they felt a need to protect him from a hostile world. He wore his personal dishevelment as a badge of unyielding, uncompromising principle, but instead it gave him the unmistakable mien of tragedy. To his patients, Joe Sonnabend was the quintessential tragic hero.

Sonnabend wasn't alone in building a special practice. At that time, other doctors in New York, San Francisco, and Los Angeles were building practices with intensely close patient-doctor ties. What they didn't know was that within two or three years, when the AIDS virus presented itself full-blown, these networks would prove lifesaving to the lucky few who belonged to them. They were the foundation for a new, alternative medical system about to arise in reaction to the failures of the government's biomedical establishment.

In the mid-seventies, Sonnabend's office was crowded with people suffering from syphilis and gonorrhea of the penis, the mouth, the anus. Chlamydia was also rampant in the gay community. But there was a lot more than the clap walking through Sonnabend's door. Hepatitis B was almost epidemic, and even tuberculosis was making a comeback. Oral and anal herpes were so common they barely were worth a mention to those infected. Sonnabend thought the gay population, at least the slice of it he was seeing in the Village, was clearly sicker, with stranger diseases, than the populace at large.

In the late seventies, a new wave of disease hit his community—parasites. Amebiasis, giardia lamblia, shigellosis, and cryptosporidium, a parasite that usually inhabits the bowels of sheep. These enteric diseases are caused when certain organisms get into peoples' gastrointestinal tracts. How they were getting there was no mystery. The parasites are present in fecal matter. Anal intercourse increases the chances of the parasites infecting one or both sex partners. But the growing popularity of rimming, or oral-anal intercourse, in the late seventies provided an almost perfect vector for these parasites to enter parts of the body unaccustomed to their presence.

This second wave of sexually transmitted disease terrified Sonnabend. Dozens of patients were coming into his office with infection after infection. His earlier research had shown him how fragile the body's immune system is. He knew that these venereal diseases were putting tremendous stress on the immune systems of his patients. As their immune systems began to break down under the onslaught of one sexually transmitted disease after another, their bodies were exposed to all kinds of horrors. They were becoming defenseless against the common bacteria, viruses, and parasites that normally inhabit our bodies but are kept in check. It was beginning to happen right before his eyes.

Sonnabend had taken a long and tortured personal and professional voyage to get to Greenwich Village. His mother was a physician, his father a university professor. Sonnabend originally related more to his father's academic calling, preferring the realm of theoretical science to the nitty-gritty of dealing with sick people.

While in 1956 he had received an M.D. from the University of Witwatersrand in Johannesburg, South Africa, Sonnabend was more interested in medical research than in medicine. He specialized in infectious diseases at the Royal College of Physicians of Edinburgh, Scotland. In the sixties he did work at the prestigious National Institute for Medical Research in London.

At one point, Sonnabend's father emigrated to Israel. When Sonnabend visited, he always made a point of stopping off at the Weizmann Institute to check up on their latest research.

What he was most interested in was interferon. At the NIMR in London, Sonnabend worked under Alick Isaacs, the man who discovered interferon in 1957. Scientists at the Weizmann were also running experiments on this substance, which occurs naturally in the body.

Sonnabend was good in the lab. Really good. His sloppy demeanor, his hesitant, shy personality and almost muttering personal speaking style disappeared once the man walked into a laboratory. Transformed, Sonnabend became a decisive, commanding force. He was clearly in control among the test tubes, chemicals, and precise machines. Indeed, Sonnabend appeared to take on many of the characteristics of these precise machines.

Interferon has always had a checkered history. Isaacs and his disciples claimed that the substance had powerful qualities. It was said to work against cancer, for example. The scientific establishment was skeptical, unwilling to accept interferon as a legitimate substance appropriate for experimentation. Researchers on interferon have tended to be relegated to the wings of the science stage.

Sonnabend made one of the most important discoveries in the field. While he was at the NIMR, he showed for the first time how interferon had antiviral properties. It worked against viruses. This was the first discovery that proved that interferon was a critical part of the body's immune system. It indicated how the substance might play a significant role against virus-induced diseases. His research gave some weight and importance to interferon, giving it a semblance of legitimacy within the larger scientific community.

In the early seventies, Sonnabend came to the States as an associate professor of microbiology at the Mt. Sinai School of Medicine in New York City. He was on a grant that paid him to continue his work on interferon.

Despite his discovery of interferon's antiviral properties, however, the field continued to be out of the scientific mainstream. Sonnabend's grant was not renewed and he was forced to return to London. Sonnabend liked the United States, or at least New York, and was unhappy at having to leave.

Back in London, morose over losing his grant and angry at the way interferon research was treated by the science establishment, Sonnabend lost hope of ever doing work in the United States again. Then a miracle! He received a fat tax return from the IRS. It was totally unexpected, but it paid for an airplane ticket and another crack at America.

This time he got a job at Downstate Medical Center in Brooklyn, part of Kings County Hospital, a public hospital. It was not a plum appointment. The hospital was overcrowded and dirty. "It was clear that nobody wanted to work in that place," he says.

Downstate didn't pay very much, so Sonnabend moonlighted at the New York City Department of Health. His interest in infectious diseases led him to the Bureau of VD Control. There Sonnabend was "discovered." Because he was not only a doctor but a researcher, in 1978 Sonnabend was made director of medical education for VD control. As director, Sonnabend came into contact with the Centers for Disease Control in Atlanta. He also established ties with New York's gay community by doing volunteer work at a gay clinic for sexually transmitted diseases.

Sonnabend had never really been comfortable in the Kings County department of medicine, surrounded by doctors whose main interest in life appeared to be money and golf. They were all high-income earners interested in the things that money could buy—stocks, real estate investments, Porsches, beach houses in the Hamptons. None of them did volunteer work at public VD clinics.

The medical department chairman who had hired Sonnabend was replaced by a new doctor, and the chemistry between them was not right; in fact, it was poisonous. "He was really like a businessman," says Sonnabend. "For the first time I was in a department of medicine where I really wasn't doing too well." The new chairman didn't renew his contract.

In his forties, Sonnabend was out of work. Without his hospital affiliation, he couldn't continue at the Health Department. He could have returned once more to London to work at the NIMR, but running back twice after failing in America was not appealing. Funding for interferon experiments was hard to come by in the United States, so working solely in a research lab wasn't an option.

There was one thing that Sonnabend hadn't done, one thing for which he was eminently qualified. Being a doctor. A simple community physician. It wouldn't be easy. He had always worked in academic settings where he never had any contact with sick people. Disease had always been dealt with only in slides and experiments.

But Sonnabend was, by this time, one of the world's top experts on sexually transmitted diseases (STDs). There was an epidemic of VD spreading through the gay community, and his work at the gay clinic had given him good community contacts. So in 1978 he rented an office in Greenwich Village, hung out a shingle, and went to work. He didn't know much about colds, flus, or chicken pox, but ask him about treating gonorrhea and Sonnabend knew all the answers.

Until the fall of 1980. That's when Sonnabend ran out of answers. It happened the day Sonnabend suddenly realized that something new and deadly was stalking his patients. He looked down at the young man on his examining table and became profoundly afraid. His patient was the latest in a series of people he had seen in recent weeks with swollen lymph nodes, fevers, and anemia. The man had cytomegalovirus, a herpes virus that was becoming so widespread that it had a nickname—CMV. People were getting CMV in different parts of the body. Many were coming down with CMV retinitis and were going blind.

Sonnabend ran blood tests and found that his patient's immune system was severely suppressed. The T-4 cells, which normally sweep the blood clear of disease invaders, were down to a count of 100 per cubic millimeter of blood. If this man had been healthy, that T-4 count would be in the 800-to-1,200 range.

Earlier, Sonnabend had seen infections with Epstein-Barr virus. It too was associated with a weakened immune system. But now something new was happening. Sonnabend had no idea exactly what was behind this wave of disease, but he suspected it had to do with what he had begun to fear most—that the immune systems of the people in his community were being decimated.

Sonnabend had set up a small research lab at Beth Israel. He worked at the lab in the morning and saw his patients in the afternoon. Sonnabend prescribed antibiotics for his patients with the new diseases, but, unlike those with parasites, bacterial infections, or funguses, few of these people were getting better.

Six months later, in early 1981, Sonnabend saw a patient and for the first time knew he was looking at a separate, as yet undefined entity—a new disease that would come to be called AIDS. The young man had been in his office before with anemia, parasites, and pneumonia. There was fungus on his fingers, and he'd had diarrhea. Sonnabend gave him the usual round of antibiotics. Nothing appeared to work.

Sonnabend saw the young man several times. In one visit he noticed that the patient had an unusual infection. It was *Pneumocystis carinii* pneumonia, usually found in young children with leukemia whose chemotherapy suppressed their immune systems. Adults undergoing organ transplants also got PCP because of the immune-suppressing drugs used to prevent organ rejection. But this young man didn't fit either category. He had PCP and Sonnabend didn't know why.

Sonnabend immediately sent the man to the hospital. In the course of investigating his pneumonia and his anemia, the doctors discovered that the patient had Kaposi's sarcoma inside his stomach. It soon appeared on his skin as well.

This was quite bizarre. KS was a rare skin cancer, even rarer than PCP. First reported in the late nineteenth century, only a few hundred cases had ever been documented, and they all involved Italian or Jewish men in their fifties or sixties. Very few ever died of the flat, purple lesions on their skin. There were a few reports of KS in Africa, among the Bantu. There KS proved to be more widespread and more deadly.

But Sonnabend's patient wasn't an older Italian or Jewish man, nor was he an African. He was a gay man in his early twenties. Sonnabend asked around and discovered that thirty-six cases of this rare cancer had been reported within the past few months. All were men, all were white, and all were gay. Sonnabend's patient was number thirty-seven. He died several days after being admitted to the hospital. He died an agonizing, painful death. The *New York Native,* a newspaper for the gay community, began carrying regular feature stories on "gay cancer."


The first published report on AIDS was on page 2 of a booklet mailed to thousands of hospitals and public health institutions every week. Anybody involved with infectious diseases and public health receives the *Morbidity and Mortality Weekly Report* of the Centers for Disease Control. The *MMWR* dated June 5, 1981, contained a breakdown of the new cases of nearly every infectious disease on a state-by-state basis.

The article signed by Drs. Michael Gottlieb and Joel Weisman, detailed four strange new cases of *Pneumocystis carinii* pneumonia in Los Angeles. It noted the links between PCP and CMV. It read simply, "*Pneumocystis* pneumonia—Los Angeles." There was no reference to gays in the title, perhaps to avoid offending homophobes or gays or both.

The text, however, referred to the fact the patients were homosexual and suggested that the gay lifestyle might play a role in the spread of *Pneumocystis*.

Joe Sonnabend read the *MMWR* and knew that what he had been seeing was not a local phenomenon. Like a few of his patients, the disease was bicoastal.

In October, Sonnabend visited an old friend, Mathilde Krim, in her lab at the Memorial Sloan-Kettering Institute for Cancer Research. Sonnabend had first met Krim thirty years earlier at the Weizmann Institute. Krim was there with her first husband, David Danon, whom she'd met when she was studying biology at the University of Geneva.

Krim was as much a world traveler as Sonnabend. Born in Italy to an Austrian mother and a Swiss father, Krim had moved with her family to Switzerland when she was a child. At the university, she met a group from what was then Palestine. Krim converted to Judaism, joined the militant Zionist underground, the Irgun, and smuggled guns to them. After independence was won she received her Ph.D. and moved to Israel with her husband to work at the Weizmann.

Krim stood out among the scientists at the Weizmann. She was then a young beauty with lustrous blond hair, high cheekbones, and bone-china white skin. She had a low voice and a middle European accent that made her sound like an intellectual Zsa Zsa Gabor.

Even then she had "bad-girl" eyes, mischievous blue-green eyes that challenged authority. They were the only telltale hint of the rebellious nature of this serious scientist from a very bourgeois Swiss family. In those eyes you could see the runaway daughter who left Switzerland after World War II to fight for the Jews in the Middle East. You could see the convert to another religion. It was no accident that Krim gravitated toward research in interferon. She was a scientist who chose to study a subject on the fringe of mainstream science. Sonnabend and Krim talked briefly then, decades ago, in Israel. He would remember it in sharper detail than she.

In 1956, after her first marriage ended, Krim gave a tour of the Weizmann to Arthur B. Krim, founder of Orion Pictures, and soon married him and moved to New York. Arthur Krim moves in powerful political and social circles. He has served as the financial chairman of the Democratic Party and advised Presidents Kennedy, Johnson, and Carter. And, of course, he knows all the big movie stars and movie-business moguls.

Sonnabend and Krim kept in touch over the years through their mutual interest in interferon. They were part of an "interferon mafia" of scientists around the world. She was very impressed with Sonnabend's work on interferon's antiviral properties.

Krim spent the seventies at Sloan-Kettering working to prove that interferon was an effective therapy against cancer. She personally financed a number of international interferon conferences to popularize and legitimize research into the substance and to overcome mainstream opposition. At one point, Krim was known as the "Interferon Queen."

Unfortunately, she was unable to prove at that time that interferon was an effective anticancer treatment. There were many signs that it would work against rare leukemias and other diseases, but nothing definitive.

Krim remembers that October meeting with Sonnabend in her lab at Sloan-Kettering quite clearly. "Joe was the first physician in New York to get seriously alarmed by what appeared to be cases of young people who had suddenly developed a violent immunological reaction to something."

Sonnabend told her that it was strange, but all the people who showed the symptoms were young gay men. "Sonnabend [pronounced Zonnabent in her Swiss-German accent] had no idea what the etiological agent was to which they were responding. Neither did I, of course." But Sonnabend did suggest he might have stumbled across the epidemic of the decade. He told her that this was an irresistible opportunity. Although Sonnabend the doctor realized it was a horror of grotesque proportions, Sonnabend the scientist told Krim that it "was a most wonderful, incredible event." Krim agreed.

Before 1981 was over, Sonnabend and Krim began a series of experiments in her lab at Sloan-Kettering. Both had spent their most productive research years studying interferon. They couldn't give up the idea that the substance played a significant role in disease. They hypothesized that they would find circulating interferon in patients with CMV, Epstein-Barr (EBV), or any number of other infections that were associated with a breakdown in the immune system. It wasn't hard to find. Later, when the AIDS virus was discovered, it turned out that increased levels of interferon were a good prognostic indicator of the disease. But like so much of interferon research, this discovery was ignored by mainstream scientists.

The two were a perfect match—the eccentric genius and the powerful socialite Ph.D. By that time, though, interferon was going nowhere for Krim. AIDS would soon be her cause.

Joe Sonnabend grew increasingly convinced that sexually transmitted diseases were doing tremendous harm to his patients. He set out to prove it in one of the earliest AIDS experiments in the country. He turned to his practice for volunteers. Virtually every patient wanted to participate and help.

Sonnabend then turned to one of his old "interferon mafia" buddies for help in showing the relationship between STDs and body immunity. Dr. David Purtilo at the University of Nebraska was one of the first scientists to do work in human T-4 cell research. He pioneered in the technique of counting T cells and relating the count to immune function. Purtilo showed that as the T-4 count fell, so did the body's immunity.

Sonnabend drew blood from thirty gay patients: ten were in monogamous relationships with their male lovers; ten dated around; and ten were "sluts," according to Michael Callen, one of his patients who participated. "I was one of the sluts," he says. People in this group had many sexual partners, hundreds if not thousands of them. As a result they also had the highest number of sexually transmitted diseases.

Sonnabend sent the blood samples off to Purtilo at the University of Nebraska. Within a month he received the results. Sonnabend was astounded at the closeness of the correlation between STDs and immunity. The people with monogamous relationships had normal T-4 cell counts. All the "sluts" had extremely low counts; they had the most suppressed immune systems.

It was extraordinary research: clear, simple, and the first of its kind. Sonnabend showed that the immune system of an entire community, the gay community, was under severe stress because of constant attack by syphilis, gonorrhea, chlamydia, and other STDs. He showed that these diseases were wearing down an entire group's protection against infection.

Sonnabend published his results in the *Lancet* in early 1982. The last sentence in his piece said that promiscuity was suppressing the immune system. Just before the article came out, he turned to one of his patients and told him: "If you don't stop fucking around, you'll die." Sonnabend told him that he had almost no T-4 cells left. He was dangerously immunosuppressed. Sonnabend said that he had the same blood parameters as his patients who came down with *Pneumocystis carinii* pneumonia and Kaposi's sarcoma.

Then Sonnabend wrote the same warning in the *New York Native.* He said that the fast-lane gay lifestyle was killing people. He said they were going to have to stop being so promiscuous, that having hundreds if not thousands of sex partners was making them very sick and very vulnerable.

It was a message the gay community didn't want to hear at that time. After fighting for the freedom to be themselves, they didn't want to hear about restraint. Indeed, for a large part of the male gay community, freedom was not simply the ability to love other men without legal or social restraint; it was defined in terms of sexual promiscuity. For many, to be young and gay and liberated in New York City meant having anonymous sex with two, three, four partners a night, night after night, year after year, STD after STD.

Sonnabend began to preach to his practice. He told them to stop screwing dozens of men every week; to stop the crazy stuff, the fisting, the rimming, all the oral-anal sexual practices. He advocated condoms long before "safe sex" became fashionable. Condoms would reduce most of the venereal diseases afflicting his patients, both the old-fashioned ones and this new epidemic.

Sonnabend's *Native* article and his personal message to his patients provoked a tremendous storm of protest. He was perceived as agreeing with the most right-wing, religious moralizers of the new Reagan era in America, of blaming this new "gay disease," this "gay cancer," on the gays themselves. The victim was to blame, or at least the victim's lifestyle. In truth, Sonnabend *was* telling them they had some responsibility for this new epidemic.

For his efforts, Sonnabend was denounced by virtually all of the gay community's leaders. He was vilified in the community itself. It seemed that everyone, except perhaps the thirty patients who participated in the "sluts" research, was angry with Sonnabend. He couldn't quite understand it. It was simply logic. He had done an experiment and proved a point. He was trying to save their lives. Not only was the uproar baffling, it caused Sonnabend tremendous pain. His own community was turning on him. It was a betrayal.

Despite the barrage, Sonnabend was still happy about one thing. He was back in the lab doing important research, leading-edge research. This is where he was always the happiest. He showed his data to Mathilde Krim. She told him it was the most important work being done.

When Sonnabend heard that the Centers for Disease Control in Atlanta was sending someone to New York to check out the mysterious new wave of PCP and KS, he grew excited. He had all this new data to show the CDC, this important new information. Sonnabend thought they'd be incredibly impressed.

Jim Curran was in charge of the CDC's venereal disease prevention division. Cases of KS and PCP were appearing with increasing frequency in Los Angeles, San Francisco, and New York. An ad hoc group at the CDC had recently been put together to investigate this disturbing trend. In time it was formalized into the Kaposi's Sarcoma and Opportunistic Infections (KSOI) Task Force; its job was to hunt down any leads about these cases.

It wasn't easy. There were no succinct categories for what was happening around the country. Specialists in virology, venereal disease, immunology, cancer, and toxicology were in the KSOI. After publication of the June 5 article on PCP in the *MMWR* report, calls were coming in about the pneumonia. Interestingly enough, many of the doctors were also seeing several different infections in one patient. In addition to *Pneumocystis carinii*, KS was common, as was CMV, parasites, and often anemia.

Curran decided he had to see some of these patients. He flew to talk with Dr. Alvin Friedman-Kien and Dr. Linda Laubenstein at the cancer institute at New York University. Curran also wanted to talk with local doctors who were treating these patients. That led him to Sonnabend.

Sonnabend talked nonstop when Curran came to his office. He said that several patterns were beginning to emerge from his research, and he described them excitedly to Curran. So far, the only people coming down with KS and PCP were young gay men. But not all young gay men, he explained. It was the homosexuals with a long history of syphilis and gonorrhea, who usually also had had hepatitis B and various parasitic infections, who were getting KS and PCP. Both were usually accompanied by other infections. It was the combination of infections that was important; cumulatively they were weakening the immune system.

Sonnabend also told Curran that there appeared to be a social factor behind all the infections. Only those who lived in the gay fast lane seemed to be coming down with disease. Men who had many sex partners. Moreover, the sex was fairly kinky. Fisting, inserting the hand into another man's anus; and rimming, running the tongue around and into the anus, were common among people who came down with the most venereal diseases, including these new cases of KS and PCP.

Curran listened but seemed somewhat annoyed with Sonnabend. He didn't appear terribly interested, certainly not impressed. In fact, he left the strong impression that Sonnabend's research wasn't very good. After all, he had used patients in his practice, hardly a true scientific sampling of the population. The CDC, on the other hand, knew how to track down diseases.

"Leave it to us," Curran told Sonnabend. "You take care of your patients and we'll sort out this thing."

Curran's condescending attitude infuriated Sonnabend. He was, after all, a scientist by training. More important, Sonnabend felt that *he* was the one in the gay community actually treating these people. It was he who saw the trends. And it was he who did the research. Not the NIH. Not the FDA. Not the CDC. "Curran's comments really got me angry," Sonnabend says. "It was a real put-down, and I've never forgotten that. Absolutely never forgotten that."

It was as if Curran had held Sonnabend and his work to be invisible. Curran's message—the CDC message—was clear. It was not Sonnabend's role to suggest theories about the growing epidemic. It was not Sonnabend's role to hypothesize about the origins of the infections or about the possible treatments. Leave that heavy-duty stuff to the professionals. Neither doctor nor patient was supposed to have the ability to figure out what was behind the epidemic killing the community. Certainly they were not supposed to know how to stop it.

When the National Institutes of Health finally got into the act several years later, America's top research scientists would also hold the community-based doctors and the community itself, the people with AIDS, to be invisible. They would ignore them for many years before a handful of AIDS activists and community doctors forced them to pay attention to the front lines of the epidemic. Unfortunately, in each year of the epidemic, thousands would die as a result of poor research protocols written by well-intentioned academic scientists in ivory tower labs cut off from what was really happening on the ground. These scientists just followed standard operating procedure. AIDS, however, turned out to be anything but a standard infectious disease.

* * *

In late July of 1982, the epidemic finally received its formal name. That happened at a meeting of hemophiliacs, blood industry officials, gay political leaders, and various big shots from the CDC, NIH, and FDA.

Several months earlier it had become clear that the new disease could be spread not only through sexual body fluids but through blood as well. The CDC hoped that from this meeting would come guidelines to prevent the contamination of the nation's blood supply. It wanted to ask people who fit into high-risk groups not to give blood. By this time, Haitians and IV drug users had joined gay men as being the most at risk for the new disease.

The meeting was a disaster. Hemophiliac groups didn't want their blood disorder to be associated with a gay disease. Gay community leaders were fearful that being prevented from donating blood was just the first step in quarantining all gay men. Indeed, right-wingers in Washington were already making noises about sending gays to "camps." The FDA and the CDC fought over turf. Regulation of the blood industry fell under traditional FDA authority. The involvement of the CDC was perceived as a threat. Many FDA doctors didn't even believe that a new disease existed. They thought the CDC was simply stitching together a number of unrelated diseases to boost their budget funding.

No one was willing to agree to anything except to wait and see. There was one accomplishment, however. Different groups on different coasts were calling the new disease by many different names. *Gay-Related Immune Deficiency* was the most popular, but it was clearly untrue since IV drug users and Haitians were shown to be vulnerable. *Gay cancer* was used mostly in New York, but it focused on only one of the many opportunistic infections associated with the disease.

Someone at the meeting suggested *AIDS*—Acquired Immune Deficiency Syndrome. It sounded good. It distinguished this disease from inherited or chemically induced immune deficiencies. It didn't mention the word *gay* or even suggest gender. AIDS. It stuck.


July 27, 1982, the day the CDC adopted AIDS as the official name of the new disease, is the official date of the beginning of the AIDS epidemic. At that point, about five hundred cases of AIDS had already been reported to the CDC, of whom approximately two hundred had died. Cases had been diagnosed in twenty-four states, and the pace of new diagnoses was doubling every month. The CDC started calling the outbreak an epidemic.

By the summer of 1982, Sonnabend was beginning to see an increasing number of *Pneumocystis carinii* pneumonias among his patients. He did what any other professional doctor should do. He did a search of the literature. It wasn't difficult. In the *Index Medicus,* Sonnabend quickly found out that PCP, once a rare infection, had recently become increasingly common. Both cancer therapy and organ transplant procedures produced severe depression of immune function.

Sonnabend discovered that as far back as 1969, doctors were treating PCP with sulfa drugs. In 1977, Dr. Walter Hughes of Tennessee had published an article in the *NEJM*—four years before Gottlieb noted his mysterious cases of PCP in another *NEJM* piece. Hughes had shown that in a placebo-controlled, double-blind trial, a drug called Bactrim prevented *Pneumocystis* in patients with compromised immune systems.

This was an amazing discovery. PCP was a major killer. Now Sonnabend had a treatment. He immediately began to correspond with Hughes. As a result, he started to prescribe Bactrim and a similar drug, Septra, to all his patients with AIDS. That didn't prevent them from coming down with opportunistic infections, but it did save them from the deadly PCP. Sonnabend also called other community doctors with the news. They too began prescribing Bactrim and Septra. The lucky few who had Sonnabend and a handful of other doctors as their personal physicians received treatment for one of AIDS' worst killers. For the rest, there was nothing but prayer.

At no time did anyone from the biomedical research establishment at the NIH in Bethesda, at the FDA in Rockville, or at the CDC in Atlanta make any attempt to contact Sonnabend or any other community doctor to discuss AIDS treatment. The government scientists were totally cut off from the object of their growing efforts, the patients and the doctors treating them on the front lines of the epidemic.

In late 1982, Joe Sonnabend received a call from Mary Ann Liebner, a publisher. She had heard that he was doing research on the new disease AIDS and she wanted to fund a new journal. Liebner asked Sonnabend if he wanted to run it. "Well, yes, of course," he said, trying to control his absolute joy. "It would be a very good idea," he said.

Indeed. Sonnabend launched *AIDS Research.* He called a lot of his buddies who had done work on interferon and who were now doing research on AIDS. Don Armstrong at Memorial Sloan-Kettering in New York joined the board.

The manuscripts that arrived at his office were a little thin at first, but over the next three years Sonnabend was to publish a number of very good scientific articles. The journal covered a wide spectrum of scientific issues. And it kept a very skeptical eye cocked at the etiology of AIDS.

The more research Sonnabend did, the more convinced he became that the breakdown in immunological function was due to simultaneous infection by at least two viruses, CMV and EBV, hitting people already weakened by previous exposure to a series of STDs. Until 1984, when the virus was found that was said to be the cause of AIDS, Sonnabend continued to believe in a multicausal theory for AIDS based on CMV and EBV. Even afterward, he remained convinced that HIV was not the sole cause of AIDS. It needed a cofactor, something else to trigger it off. He published a paper expressing his views in his journal *AIDS Research.* He was very proud of that article. "I've never retracted it," he says. Years later, his point of view would be redeemed by none other than Robert Gallo. The term *cofactors* would become hot on the campus of the NIH nearly eight years after Sonnabend used it.

But in late 1982, Joe Sonnabend had another problem to deal with. He was going bankrupt. He couldn't pay his bills. His debts were big and growing.

Although Sonnabend had a large and growing practice, he wasn't making any money. Part of the problem was that he refused to take any payment from a patient who was included in his research. He said it wasn't right to ask people to pay a doctor who was using him in a study. Unfortunately, since he was such a thorough researcher, practically all his patients were included in his scientific work, so hardly anyone was paying him for visits and treatments.

The biggest drain on Sonnabend's funds, however, was the research itself. He was collecting and storing sera, making detailed records, and shipping the blood samples around the country to colleagues in laboratories. A big percentage of the material was sent to Nebraska for testing. He did the packing himself.

Mathilde Krim remembers saving Styrofoam and cardboard boxes for Sonnabend's shipments through the post office and Federal Express. She saw that he was on the verge of going under and decided to do something about it.

"Mathilde really rescued me," he recalls. "I must say, I was in terrible financial straits. She got me a lawyer. She really cleaned me up."

That was a role that Krim continued to play for many years to come. Krim was a realist. She saw a problem and she sought a solution. It was just as simple as that. Krim knew she had financial, social, and at times even political resources that most people didn't have access to. In the fight against AIDS, Krim used whatever she had. She never flagged.

But Krim also never failed to be pragmatic. She wanted things done, solutions to problems. Whatever it took. Sometimes it took friendship.

Krim figured out that Sonnabend was putting out several thousand dollars a month just mailing his research to laboratories. She literally came over to Sonnabend's lab, added up his expenses, and came up with a budget that would keep him in operation. She was the Mother Teresa of AIDS—a personal saint to Sonnabend.

At first Krim also helped Sonnabend out through her own personal funds. "I took an interest in him as a friend," she says. "And he was also one of the few guys really doing something at that time. . . . We needed to give money to this guy," she says emphatically, almost defiantly. But Krim knew that the only way to really support Sonnabend's work was through a nonprofit organization. Many of his patients said they wanted to give money to help him, but they couldn't give it to him personally.

In late 1982, Krim started putting a nonprofit organization together. There are certain rules and regulations to follow. She needed a three-person board of directors, and Sonnabend couldn't be one of them if he was going to receive any money. So Krim became chairman of the AIDS Medical Foundation, and the lawyers who had been helping her became the trustees. It took until April 1983 for New York's attorney general to grant the nonprofit status and for the first money to flow to Sonnabend. "The AMF bailed me out," says Sonnabend. "It really helped with the work."

With the AMF behind him, Sonnabend's practice began to look more and more like a research center. "I was a scientist put into the role of a practitioner still being a scientist," he says. "So I utilized my practice in a different way."

Other doctors doing research on the growing epidemic heard about the nonprofit organization and applied for funds. Michael Lange, one of the earliest doctors to be involved in the AIDS epidemic, needed funds to keep his research going. He collaborated with Sonnabend, and Sonnabend told him about the AMF. Lange then became the second person to be helped by the nonprofit organization.

But once the AMF became something more than just a foundation to support one individual scientist, Krim had to put into place an IRB, an Institutional Review Board. It was made up of independent doctors and scientists and interested people who analyzed all scientific proposals for research with an eye toward protecting the patients. Safety was their major concern. Krim and Sonnabend proved they could do the legal paperwork correctly, create an IRB, request research proposals, and receive, review, and finance them. Neither one had ever done anything like this before.

But it wasn't all sweetness and light at the AMF. There were tensions, albeit small ones, between Krim and Sonnabend even in the beginning. They always revolved around bureaucratic details. Sonnabend hated them, despised bureaucracies in general. One of Krim's greatest talents was her ability to make organizations work for her, to make institutions focus on her goals and accomplish them. The AMF worked because of her extraordinary talents.

Sonnabend, however, was often obstreperous. When the AMF started expanding and hiring staff, he had trouble with them. At meetings, he shifted restlessly in his seat; he had no patience at all with parliamentary procedure.

Yet Sonnabend remained the paterfamilias of the AMF, the heart and soul of the foundation. The AMF was a true breakthrough in AIDS research. It arranged the financing for the first human trial on anti-AIDS drugs in the United States. Sonnabend ran a trial of isoprinosine, an immune system booster, and showed it had promising properties. Krim provided the contact to Newport Pharmaceuticals, which owned the drug. Newport financed the isoprinosine trial, Sonnabend ran it, and the AMF proved that good research doesn't always have to be done in a fancy lab. In fact, the AMF set a precedent and suggested that, in the case of AIDS, the best chemical research might be done in places outside the NIH and the top academic science centers.

Mathilde Krim believed in fund-raising. It was almost a way of life for her. Not only was she good at it, but it did a tremendous amount of good. Krim had been raising money for causes for years. But now she was financing AIDS research, and it was proving to be the most difficult kind of fund-raising she had ever tried.

In fact, Krim was finding raising private money for AIDS nearly impossible. Some small amounts of cash were coming in, but only from a very small circle of people who were aware of the worsening epidemic. They usually had a friend or lover who was sick.

It was that group of people who attended the AIDS Medical Foundation's first fund-raiser at Studio 54. Steve Rubell organized it and managed to raise several thousand dollars. That was followed by a fashion show at a downtown art gallery. "We collected gifts from the fashion industry and we auctioned them off," Krim remembers. "Mrs. Carter came from Plains to attend our fashion show. She's wonderful. On that occasion, for the first time, we made $100,000 profit, which was a fantastic achievement for us."

But beyond that circle it was nearly impossible to get contributions. Traditional philanthropies turned their noses up at the disease. Krim had been a member of the board of the Rockefeller Foundation, and she approached them with an appeal to help fund Sonnabend and other researchers. The head of the Rockefeller Foundation's health program, Kenneth Warren, was a personal friend. "In 1983 I went to tell him about AIDS. I said this is going to be a worldwide problem. It's going to be a catastrophe, a calamity. It's going to destroy the economy of the Third World. Rockefeller is interested in world health." Warren's reply made Krim very angry. "This is a small local problem," he said. "We deal with *big* questions." Krim felt she could have strangled him then and there. She went over to see Frank Thomas at the Ford Foundation, gave him the same spiel, and got a similar no-thank-you. It was like that at all of the major foundations.

Corporate America wasn't much better. They wouldn't touch it. The only money the AMF received was from individuals, and women at that time were far more generous than men. The men were always complaining that they wanted to help her out but they couldn't put the word "AIDS" on their checks. "What if my secretary sees it or my accountant?" they said. So Krim had to do some fancy maneuvering. She and her husband have a small private foundation, and it was used in a rather unusual way. "I had to route checks through the Krim Foundation. You know, launder the money." Corporate chairmen and CEOs could write a check to the Krim Foundation, but the AIDS Medical Foundation just wasn't socially acceptable.

It wasn't until Rock Hudson died in 1985 that established foundations and corporations began funding AIDS projects. AIDS had been "legitimized" to a certain degree. After all, Rock Hudson had been a personal friend of the president and his wife. Indeed, the president would say the word "AIDS" at a fund-raiser organized by Krim—the first time he uttered the word in the five years of the epidemic. By that point, money was pouring out of Washington. Back when it was desperately needed, the private sector didn't give a dime. When it was safe, it joined the parade.

When the telephone rang in Joe Sonnabend's St. Luke's Hospital laboratory in the middle of 1985, it was bad news. Mary Ann Liebner, the publisher of *AIDS Research,* was calling. She had been talking with Max Essex of Harvard recently, and he had told her that Sonnabend's view of AIDS was outside the mainstream of science. Essex told her that Robert Gallo had proved that AIDS was caused by a single agent and nothing else. He said that there was no scientific evidence to back up Sonnabend's multicausal theory.

So Liebner told Sonnabend that after three years as editor, he was out. His views were not acceptable in the halls of established science. Dani Bolognesi from Duke University was going to take over her journal. It was now *his* journal. Thanks. Goodbye.

Bolognesi did take over within weeks. He fired Sonnabend's entire editorial board and replaced it with an AIDS retrovirus mafia of his own, which included Gallo, Essex, and Luc Montagnier. All of them were big names in AIDS research and all believed that AIDS was caused by a single virus. Adding insult to injury, Bolognesi renamed the journal *AIDS Research and Human Retroviruses.*

This second boot in the face was hard on Sonnabend. "This was a consequence of my heretical views," he says. "Why did these people need a new journal? They could publish anywhere. They just wanted to close me down."

Larry Kramer lived with furies inside him. Every few minutes they rose up, and Kramer spiked into a hot, blistering anger. A calm would then settle on him, only to be replaced with yet another outburst. It went on like this every hour, every day, every week, every year. Larry Kramer was the Vesuvius of anger. He was one of the angriest men on earth. Nothing was successfully camouflaged from his sight. Kramer saw injustice everywhere. It was almost like an affliction.

Luckily for Kramer, his anger was an incredibly fecund pool of molten fury. Out of it streamed books, plays, and movie screenplays. In 1978, he wrote the novel *Faggots*.

*Faggots* was meant as a Waughian ramble through the dark corners of the seventies gay sex scene. The quote at the very beginning, from Evelyn Waugh's *Put out More Flags*, sets the tone: ". . . the ancients located the deeper emotions in the bowels."

The book has hilarious scenes of group gropes in Upper East Side apartments, drug-inspired sexual frenzies in discos, the rimming of gay virgins, fist fucking at the infamous Toilet Bowl bar. It has it all, written playfully with a sense of fun. The protagonist is a Jewish screenwriter-producer clearly patterned after the author. A few years before, Kramer had written the screenplay of D. H. Lawrence's *Women in Love*, which he also produced.

Yet there is a strong moral undertone running through the pages. In *Faggots*, Kramer describes in relentless detail the new life he felt gays were creating for themselves after their liberation. It quickly becomes apparent that the sex is more than fun, it is compulsive; the relationships are less than permanent, indeed they are anonymous. By the end of the book, the freedom that came with liberation—the dark back rooms of bars, the public orgies of the baths, the pissing, the sadism and masochism—becomes a world spinning out of control. A world populated by fickle friendships and lack of commitment. A world without love.

Fred Lemish, the protagonist, cries out in pain and fury, "Why do faggots have to fuck so fucking much?! It's as if we don't have anything else to do. All we do is live in our Ghetto and dance and drug and fuck. There's a whole world out there! As much ours as theirs. I'm tired of being a New York City–Fire Island faggot, I'm tired of using my body as a faceless thing to lure another faceless thing, I want to love a Person! I want to go out and live in the world with that Person, a Person who loves me. We shouldn't *have* to be faithful, we should *want* to be faithful."

Then Fred tells the object of his love, Dinky, that he never sees happy gay couples. He's traveled all over the world and has seen not more than half a dozen couples that appear happy together. Dinky replies: "That should tell you something!" And Fred answers: "Yeah, it tells me something. It tells me no relationship in the world could survive the shit we lay on it. It tells me we're not looking at the reasons why we're doing the things we're doing." Things have to change fast, Fred continues. Lasting relationships built on love have to have a chance. Sooner or later, he tells Dinky,

GOOD INTENTIONS

he is going to have to commit to someone. "Which means making a commitment to yourself. And a commitment to the notion that our shitty beginnings
don't have to cripple us for life."

This has to happen, Fred cries out, "before you fuck yourself to
death." The words, written in 1978, bear an eerie resemblance to those
spoken by Joe Sonnabend years later to his patients who, it turns out, were
quite literally fucking themselves to death.

For his literary effort, Kramer was shunned that summer at the gay
resort of Cherry Grove, the scene of *Faggots'* concluding chapters on Fire
Island. Old friends looked him in the face at the Ice Palace, Fire Island's
hottest gay nightclub, and walked away without saying a word. His best
friend stopped speaking to him. This ostracism went on for years.

In a December 21, 1981, letter sent to the *New York Native*, playwright
Robert Chesley charged Kramer with homophobia and antieroticism. "I
think the concealed meaning in Kramer's emotionalism is the triumph of
guilt; that gay men deserve to die for their promiscuity. In his novel
*Faggots*, Kramer told us that sex is dirty and that we ought not to be doing
what we're doing.

"Read anything by Kramer closely. I think you'll find that the subtext
is always: the wages of gay sin are death."

It wouldn't be until the actual discovery of the AIDS virus in 1984
that criticism of Larry Kramer or Joe Sonnabend by the gay community
would die down. Very few people in the gay community could accept the
idea that the sexual freedoms they had fought so long to obtain were
suspect. Even when doctors such as Sonnabend began warning them in
1981 and 1982, few listened. The idea of sex causing AIDS was anathema
to those who defined their liberation as gay people in terms of having as
much sex with as many people in as many places in as many ways as
possible.

Ironically, in describing his longing for love in gay life, for commitment between two individuals, Kramer was prophetic in his warning about
promiscuity. In 1978, gays were already talking over dinner about the latest
parasites to strike them and the latest medicines their doctors had prescribed. Over Sunday brunch, men were talking about their shingles and
amebiasis. The year before it had been chlamydia and fungus.

They sounded like a group of retired seventy-year-olds in Century
Village down in Florida complaining, over gin rummy, about their hearts
and their operations and how they keep forgetting which pocket their
nitroglycerine is in.

94

# ..5..

# Luck, Classic Coke, and the Love of a Good Man

The fictional world of Larry Kramer's *Faggots* came to life in Joe Sonnabend's medical office. The characters paraded through his doors in the flesh, indifferent to their health, indulgent in their lifestyles.

Michael Callen, one of Joe Sonnabend's first patients, walked into Sonnabend's Greenwich Village office in early 1979, just two weeks after arriving in New York. Callen's case was typical. He was white, middle-class, young, in his twenties, gay. He had grown up in Hamilton, Ohio. His father was an auto worker and his mother a schoolteacher. Callen had graduated from Boston University. Now he lived fast-lane gay life down in the Village, a life that in the late seventies translated to fucking his proverbial brains out.

Callen spent his nights singing in tiny Village dives, cabarets with five or six people sitting around tables the size of a big pizza. His first musical director was the piano player for the great black jazz singer Mabel Mercer, so he was into the music of the thirties and forties. Callen was also into imitating Barbra Streisand.

He loved the fast-lane life—the sex, the drugs, the music. It wasn't unusual for him to be up most of the night, singing at a club then dancing at after-hours joints, having sex with a lot of strangers. He inhaled "poppers," butyl nitrite, to keep him going until dawn. It was sexual liberation time and he was getting as much of it as he could stand.

That meant a monthly visit to Sonnabend's office to take care of that disease-of-the-month. By twenty-seven, Callen guessed he'd had 3,000 sexual partners. He'd had them in bathhouses on St. Marks Place in Manhattan, in the grass and on the sand on Fire Island, on the Hudson River docks, in back rooms of dozens of bars, in apartments of friends and lovers all around Manhattan.

A CDC study of fifty gay men with AIDS in the spring of 1981, the first of its kind, would later show that they had a median number of 1,150 sex partners. They also had a history of sexually transmitted diseases (STDs) to boggle the mind. Callen had the averages beat hands down.

Callen thought he knew the price. He came down with every sexually transmitted disease in the medical book. His body was a walking petri dish. Before the appearance of AIDS, Sonnabend could plot each and every wave of STD that washed through the gay community in the seventies and early eighties through Callen. He had dozens of bouts of syphilis and gonorrhea; nonspecific urethritis; chlamydia; *Candida albicans;* an endless series of episodes with *Entamoeba histolytica; Giardia lamblia;* salmonella; shigella; hepatitis A; hepatitis B; hepatitis non-A and non-B; venereal warts; herpes simplex Types I and II; Epstein-Barr virus; cytomegalovirus infections; disseminated varicella zoster (shingles).

Callen had done it all and had come down with it all. Sonnabend was appalled. He worried about all his patients, but Callen was special. This tall, lanky man with jade green eyes and black hair had a wry wit and a sense of fun about him.

Callen treated Sonnabend as just a clap doctor to visit every month. Sonnabend saw Callen as yet another immature young male who had grown up learning what society taught about gay men—that they were promiscuous, effeminate, lonely, and vaguely criminal. So he was.

AIDS. The word cracked through Michael Callen like a fist through glass. It would all be "after" and "before" for the rest of his life. The fissure line of diagnosis would run through Callen's future as it would through American society.

He'd been sick for most of the winter and spring of 1982. He lost weight week after week. He'd had bloody diarrhea eight or nine or ten times a day. He threw up constantly. He was asleep half the day.

Finally in June, Callen collapsed at home and was taken to a hospital emergency room by Joe Sonnabend's assistant. He had a temperature of 104 degrees. It was to be the first of dozens of trips to the hospital in the years to come.

The doctors told Callen what was wrong. He had cryptosporidiosis, soon to be known by everyone in the gay community as "crypto." It was a parasite usually found in feces. There was no cure. They would keep Callen hydrated and hope for the best.

Despite the illness, it was a wonderful relief to Callen to finally know what exactly was causing all that agony. On the other hand, crypto was one of the diseases that the Centers for Disease Control listed as officially qualifying a person for an AIDS diagnosis. Callen heard his death sentence. The doctors told Callen that if he survived this bout with crypto, he should join one of the new AIDS support groups. He had six to eighteen months to live. It was so incredibly depressing. And he hadn't even *done* anything yet.

Callen later wrote that "AIDS was a gigantic cosmic kick in the ass." It stopped him "dead" in his tracks and he took inventory of his life. What had he been doing? "Well, you moved to the city to make music," he told himself. "Instead, you've been spending a lot of time and money and energy pursuing sex and paying for its aftermath in terms of doctors' appointments and being sick and hanging out in parasitology labs. . . . You're basically very lonely and unhappy and unsatisfied with your life." It was a brutally honest assessment of a young man's shattered life.

Then Callen did two things. He started talking with his doctor, Joe Sonnabend, about AIDS. And he discovered that the so-called experts didn't know a lot about the disease. Outside and inside the gay community there were debates about how to treat it, and there was controversy over its cause.

Sonnabend told him that despite what he was reading in the press or hearing from other doctors, there were a lot of treatments available. People don't die of AIDS, he told Callen. They die of specific infections that they get because their immune system is decimated by the AIDS virus. If a doctor focused on the infections, he could treat them, despite the lack of any drugs for the AIDS virus itself. There was a great deal to do, Sonnabend said. And there was a great deal to learn.

Callen began to see that he didn't have to roll over and wait for Death's cold hand to touch him. He wasn't powerless. Since there was so much unknown about AIDS, he should learn as much as possible about it. That might just keep him alive. It certainly would give him a goal in life beyond the crap he had been doing. It would give him a degree of power over his destiny. Actually, it would give him a destiny.

"Looking back, I realized all my life I'd been waiting for some *force majeure,* something or somebody, to come along and radically alter my life," Callen has said. "I'd win the lottery, or like Barbra Streisand in *Funny Girl,* the ugly duckling would be exposed for the swan that I truly was. I waited and waited for something to happen, frittering my life away. I viewed my life as a rehearsal, awaiting that all-important performance which never came."

Michael Callen gave up his for-now life of gay bacchanalia and moved on to a larger stage. Joe Sonnabend coached from the wings. At twenty-seven, tall, thin, a Sam Shepard look-a-like, Callen discovered that he possessed charisma that hadn't evidenced itself before. He had a great voice for speaking as well as singing, and an ability to write clearly, compassionately, and with wit. Callen had always liked to perform. Now he took center stage in the most important social and medical drama of the decade. Callen, and others, would lead the first social movement born in a doctor's office.

First Callen changed his personal life. He started a rock and roll band. Torch singing was "before" AIDS. It was sweet and soft. Rock was tough, full of energy. Callen hired Keith Avedon as musical director, changed his singing style, and placed an ad in the *Native* for musicians to play in a new band called Lowlife, an apt symbol for how Callen felt at the time. He chose two women and Richard Dworkin, a drummer. Dworkin and Callen became lovers and the depression that came with the AIDS verdict finally lifted.

Callen saw himself as "damaged goods" and had given up any hope of finding love, much less sex, after the diagnosis. Dworkin proved him wrong. After that, Callen made a major point of fixing people up, especially people with AIDS. Matchmaking was life-affirming. When asked years later to what he attributed his longevity—Callen had lived seven years "after" at that point—he said, "Luck, Classic Coke, and the love of a good man."

Michael Callen's first major "after" performance was not singing or rock and roll, but writing an article in the *Native* with Richard Berkowitz and Richard Dworkin. It was a nailed-to-the-church-door-type declaration that attacked the gay lifestyle since liberation.

Entitled "We Know Who We Are: Two Gay Men Declare War on Promiscuity," and dated November 8–12, 1982, the article said:

> Those of us who have lived a life of excessive promiscuity on the urban gay circuit of bathhouses, backrooms, balconies, sex clubs, meat racks and tearooms . . . could continue to deny the overwhelming evidence that the present health crisis is a direct result of the unprece-

dented promiscuity that has occurred since Stonewall [a 1969 riot considered the start of the modern gay movement], but such denial is killing us. Denial will continue to kill us until we begin the difficult task of changing the ways in which we have sex.

What ten years ago was viewed as a healthy reaction to a sex-negative culture now threatens to destroy the very fabric of urban gay male life. . . . We must recognize the self-hating shortsightedness in knowingly, or half-knowingly, infecting our sexual partners with disease, only to have that disease return to us in exponential form.

We can no longer tolerate knee-jerk defensiveness to any discussion of promiscuity as a medical issue. Not everyone who wishes to discuss alternatives to promiscuity is sex-negative or a sexual fascist. To date there has been little rational discussion about the impact of promiscuity on gay male culture; the present health crisis provides the unique opportunity for such a dialogue to begin.

Whether we know it or not, an entire generation of gay men for whom gay life is synonymous with promiscuity is about to make the difficult transition to new, medically safe lifestyles. This transition is sure to have profound personal, social and economic ramifications and will no doubt be painful, difficult, and politically volatile.

For his brutal honesty, Callen was attacked as being a "sexual Carry Nation." The *Native* was filled with furious letters and rebuttals, including one by a Charles Jurist, "In Defense of Promiscuity," which belittled the connection between infection and sex. He said it was "premature to call for an end to sexual freedom in the name of physical health." Ironically, the piece also belittled AIDS by saying that gay men were more likely to be killed by getting hit by a car than by coming down with this new disease. Denial was not the exclusive property of the Reagan administration when it came to AIDS in the eighties.

AIDS was a death sentence. That's what everybody was saying in the gay community. It was driving Michael Callen crazy. He could feel it whenever his friends got together for dinner. Terror was in their eyes, and fatalism. It was all they could talk about. "Jerry has it. Tony has it." And it was all said with such resignation. The message always was: Nothing could be done once you got it. Callen hated that refrain, nothing could be done. He saw people rolling over the moment they saw a purple lesion on their leg. He saw people giving up after their first case of PCP. To Callen, it seemed as if the gay community were actually buying into the Jesse Helms/Moral Majority bullshit that AIDS was a punishment from God. People were behaving as if they believed they somehow deserved to die.

Callen couldn't accept that attitude. *He* was still alive and it was 1983, over a year after first being diagnosed. Some of the doctors back in 1982 had given him six months. Callen was sick a lot, but that didn't make him a sick person. It didn't mean he was inevitably going to die. To Callen, the very fact that he was fighting AIDS increased his chances for survival. Callen found himself telling friends that "the unthinking repetition of the notion that everyone dies from AIDS denies both the reality of—and more importantly the possibility of—survival."

Callen knew there were things to be done to fight the disease. True, nothing was coming out of Washington. The drug companies were silent about treatment. But his own doctor, Joe Sonnabend, was aggressively fighting the disease through his system of close patient management. Sonnabend's goal was to stop the opportunistic infections that actually do the killing in AIDS. When Callen told him of his AIDS diagnosis, Sonnabend immediately put him on Bactrim to prevent PCP. Sonnabend was preventing the pneumonia. To Callen, that was important. It was doing something, not waiting to die.

To Callen, it was a question of victimization. Just when gays were coming out of the closet and were beginning to feel good about themselves, this damn disease made them feel like victims again. Increasingly, all of Callen's friends were becoming "victims" and "patients." Both words implied that people with AIDS were all passive recipients of treatment. The words implied helplessness and dependence. That infuriated Callen. He believed a person with AIDS needed a will to live inside in order to continue living in the world outside. He felt people had to fight against the patient-victim attitude, but very few were. They didn't know how. They didn't think there was anything to do.

Callen believed he was living proof that there was plenty to do. He had warded off the Big P, *Pneumocystis.* Prevention was action. That was how to fight back.

The battle was bicoastal. Bobbi Campbell was building his first AIDS medical guerrilla group in San Francisco just as Michael Callen was making his own transformation to social-medical activist in New York.

In California, it all began with Bobbi Campbell, but it didn't end there.

Campbell was a man of many firsts. He was one of the first persons in San Francisco to be diagnosed with Kaposi's sarcoma. He was the first person to go public as a person with AIDS, a courageous act at the time. He began the first newspaper column on the new disease by writing, "I'm Bobbi Campbell and I have 'gay cancer' " in the *San Francisco Sentinel*. He formed the first support group for people with Kaposi's sarcoma. Finally, Campbell conceived of the notion that would eventually grow into the self-empowerment movement.

Campbell, a native of Tacoma, Washington, was first diagnosed in September of 1981. One day he looked down at his feet as he was taking off his hiking boots and saw purple lesions. They grew larger as the days passed, so Campbell went to Dr. Marcus Conant, who told him he had a rare cancer, Kaposi's sarcoma. In fact, it would turn out that Campbell would be the sixteenth person in San Francisco to be identified as getting KS at that time.

Conant was a dermatologist who worked out of the University of California at San Francisco's Ambulatory Care building. Conant was a herpes specialist and was particularly interested in KS because a herpes virus, cytomegalovirus, had been linked to KS in Africa. To actually show a link between a virus and a cancer would mean a major breakthrough in science. His friend in New York, Dr. Alvin Friedman-Kien at NYU, had also seen new cases of KS. It was on both coasts.

Campbell went for chemotherapy. He was lucky. It didn't kill him. Until the late eighties, medical researchers advised doctors treating AIDS to follow the standard operating procedure pioneered for cancer chemotherapy by the National Cancer Institute at the NIH: prescribe the maximum amount of drug possible. Unfortunately, the SOP didn't work for AIDS. Instead of the maximum, the minimum often worked best in treating AIDS and its symptomatic infections.

When Bobbi Campbell went for treatment for his Kaposi's sarcoma, he received full-bore chemo. Next to him, also receiving chemo, was another person with KS, John. Campbell survived, but many others were seriously hurt by their medical treatment. John and Bobbi set up a support group for other KS people. It was one of the earliest, if not the first, support groups for people with AIDS in the country. But John died shortly thereafter, in 1982, and Campbell was left alone.

Campbell then met Dan Turner, who was diagnosed with AIDS in

February 1982. Both were seeing Marcus Conant, who suggested they get together and talk about their experience. Campbell went to Turner's house in the Castro district of San Francisco, sporting a button that read SURVIVE. He was already feisty, already in a fighting mood. That meeting was the first of many that led to the establishment of the group People With AIDS–San Francisco, the first organization ever set up by persons with AIDS.

But first Campbell and Turner hit the lecture circuit. They became "star cases," brought forward by doctors and the members of the gay community to talk about AIDS. Campbell proclaimed himself "KS Poster Boy" and marched as such in gay parades.

Campbell's behavior brought a lot of attention to KS in San Francisco. While the *New York Native* was full of stories about KS and other diseases striking the gay community, the San Francisco homosexual newspapers basically were ignoring the growing health problem.

At the time, most of the gay community just didn't want to hear about disease. It was too busy having a good time. Gay leaders were also worried about a backlash against gays by the right-wing Neanderthals in the Reagan administration, such as Jesse Helms. Finally—perhaps most importantly—bathhouses were big business in San Francisco. The sex was hot, heavy, nonstop, and anonymous at the baths, and bathhouse owners were big advertisers in gay newspapers. The last thing the newspapers wanted to do was anger a major advertiser with articles on "gay cancer" and how people could catch it sexually.

Like Callen on the East Coast, Campbell felt that PWAs should not be passive recipients of help because they were "victims" of a deadly disease. Campbell saw himself as a PWA—a person with AIDS—actively taking a role in his own treatment. He believed that an AIDS diagnosis was not simply a death sentence to be accepted, or perhaps to be rescinded at the last hour by some faraway scientist in a laboratory or some white-coated doctor with an injection. AIDS had to be fought, tooth and nail, by those it struck. Campbell decided that all service organizations in San Francisco helping people with AIDS should have PWAs in decision-making roles.

Campbell joined the San Francisco KS/AIDS Foundation's national board, and Dan Turner was elected to the KS/AIDS Foundation's local board.

On May 2, 1983, the first candlelight march was organized by Campbell and other PWAs to bring attention to the epidemic. During the march, a banner was unfurled proclaiming what was to become the motto of the self-empowerment movement: FIGHTING FOR OUR LIVES. Three weeks later, People With AIDS–San Francisco met and voted to send Bobbi Campbell and Dan Turner to the upcoming Second National AIDS Forum in Denver. The decision to send two people with AIDS proved to be a spark that ignited New York.

In the gay heart of New York City, Greenwich Village, Larry Kramer lived in a great apartment just across the street from Washington Square Park on Fifth Avenue. He furnished it with the money he had made from *Women in Love* and *Faggots.* From his living room window he could see the fountain where the NYU students and purveyors of various illegal substances gathered. The big arch was so close, it almost appeared to be part of Kramer's kitchen. This apartment would give birth to two of the most important gay organizations in the history of the fight against AIDS.

In the summer of 1981 Kramer had eighty people to his apartment for a fund-raiser. Dr. Friedman-Kien addressed his audience from the center of the living room. The balding doctor said he thought an epidemic was taking place and that the cause was unknown. The one trend that he could see at that time was that the men who had come down with Kaposi's sarcoma had a history of STDs. Then he asked the assembled to please give as much as they could for the research he and Dr. Linda Laubenstein were doing at NYU.

Kramer had just met Alvin Friedman-Kien. He had been reading Dr. Lawrence Mass's stories in the *New York Native* about the appearance of a strange new rare cancer in the gay community. Mass was an old friend and Kramer respected him. Then Kramer read a *New York Times* story on AIDS, its first. The article was buried on an inside page and was headlined RARE CANCER SEEN IN 41 HOMOSEXUALS. Kramer got very scared. He knew that he'd had many if not most of the sexually transmitted diseases shared by the forty-one gay men described in the *Times* piece. He called Larry Mass and asked whom he should see for an examination. Mass told him to call Friedman-Kien at the New York University Medical Center. He was an infectious disease expert who had done work on herpes. Recently Friedman-Kien had reported several cases of the rare Kaposi's sarcoma.

Kramer went to NYU to see Friedman-Kien. Before he told Kramer to go downstairs and get a blood test, he asked him to organize a fund-raiser. He wanted to tell an audience about KS and what they should do to prevent getting it. They had to stop their promiscuous lifestyle. In return, he'd ask them for money to help him continue his research.

Many of those assembled in Kramer's living room didn't like what they heard. Overall, the group hated being lectured to about promiscuity. They felt that Kramer had found an expert to simply repeat what Kramer had written in *Faggots*—screwing around was both wrong and unhealthy. Most of them felt that screwing around was liberation.

Kramer passed the hat for Friedman-Kien's research and came up with $6,635, the only money raised privately in all of 1981 to fight the growing AIDS epidemic. Gays just did not want to hear about cancer or KS or research. They would rather party at the Ice Palace disco and spend their money on drugs to keep them rockin' till the morning. It made Kramer sad and angry. Not much had changed since he had written *Faggots* three years ago.

Six months later Kramer tried again. He invited six friends back to try something different. Kramer wanted to start the first private AIDS organization on the East Coast. He began by being angry. He said Mayor Ed Koch wasn't doing a damn thing about taking care of all the people coming down sick with AIDS. Kramer said that many of them were locked away in their own small apartments, shriveling away alone, dying a miserable death. Furthermore, nobody was telling the gay population what to do. There was plenty of medical information about this disease out there. Some organization had to get the word out.

Kramer said the city government of New York wasn't about to do it. Kramer told the audience that Mayor Koch wouldn't even see any gay leaders, much less listen to them. Kramer had been trying for months to get the mayor to set up a meeting.

Kramer said they had to set up an organization that would care for their own and fight for their rights.

The men listening in his living room agreed. The name they gave to their new organization summed up what they believed they were facing— the Gay Men's Health Crisis, or GMHC.

But while Kramer's anger gave birth to the GMHC, his creation did not resemble his personality in any way. The men in the room—among them Paul Popham, Nathan Fain, Dr. Lawrence Mass, Paul Rapoport, and the writer Edmund White—were very different from Kramer.

When the first board of directors meeting of the GMHC was held, Popham, Mass, Fain, and Kramer were on it, as well as Harry Diaz and Joe

Hernandez, Larry McDevitt, Brad Frandsen, and Joe Paschek. Paul Popham was made the board president.

Popham and Larry Kramer were a study in contrasts. Popham was very West Coast, born in Oregon; Kramer was as New York as you can get. Popham had movie-star good looks; Kramer was short and wiry. Popham was self-assured and calm; Kramer was insecure and volatile. Popham had served in the Green Berets in Vietnam; Kramer had fought against the war. Popham voted Republican, like so many other gays who worked on Wall Street or in Rockefeller Center in New York. Kramer had voted Left his whole life. Popham was in the closet, again like so many gays in New York. Kramer was Kramer. He didn't hide anything.

Within a very short time, the GMHC became an outpost of Ivy League good works. It was well mannered; it cared for the ill and kept out of trouble. It was careful and clean and didn't rock the boat. It wanted to be inside, to become part of the official city care system by proving it was responsible. It didn't attack Mayor Koch. It wasn't, the GMHC voice whispered, anything at all like Larry Kramer.

There were many differences between the New York and San Francisco gay communities, and these differences over the years would pit them against one another over many issues. One significant difference was that a far higher percentage of the gay community in the East was in the closet. They lived in fear of being found out, discovered, and this affected how they viewed the issues and organizations that developed out of the AIDS crisis. The GMHC is a perfect example.

Paul Popham was an executive at McGraw-Hill, working at its corporate headquarters in the new, westernmost section of Rockefeller Center, built in the seventies. Popham believed he could be fired for being gay. As president of the board of directors of the GMHC, Popham instilled a covert culture in the organization. As it grew into the largest private AIDS service organization in the country, indeed in the world, a sense of caution and control and propriety would grow along with it. Confidentiality and individual rights, for example, were more important than education when it came to sex.

By the summer of 1982, the GMHC had three hundred volunteers enlisted to help people with AIDS get by. A "buddy" program was set up to send men into apartments where the sick were wasting away alone. Support groups were set up for the friends and lovers of people who had come down with the disease. The GMHC was doing the caring, the nursing, the helping that the city administration refused to do. What the GMHC wouldn't do was the fighting, the lobbying, the politicking necessary to change the system. That began to drive Larry Kramer's furies wild.

Within weeks, battles began to break out every time the GMHC board met. It was Kramer against all the rest over the very nature of the organization. Kramer wanted more direct political action to pressure the city into giving services to the gay community. The board wanted to provide those services itself and not confront the mayor. Let's raise the money and help where we can, it said every time it met.

Kramer also split with the board on sex. He wanted the GMHC to come out in support of what nearly every community doctor with a gay practice was telling his patients: Promiscuous sex is killing you. People should either stop having sex or at least use condoms. He wanted the organization to fight for the closing of the bathhouses. It should educate the community in what's right and wrong for this epidemic.

The board members wouldn't hear of it. They supported those who lived life in the fast lane, doing the disco-bar scene in Manhattan and Fire Island. It represented their liberation from years of finger pointing by parents, teachers, priests—everybody. The GMHC's job should be to provide the latest medical information to its members, they felt. No more. Kramer came across as a prude in his book *Faggots.* They weren't. Everyone should make his own choice on sexual matters. It was his right. They were not going to be the Sex Police.

In the loud, screaming board fights, Popham came across as the handsome, popular one, the leader. He clearly had the board on his side. Kramer felt like the New York loudmouth, the outsider, the pariah.

Then Mayor Koch finally agreed to meet with representatives of several AIDS organizations, the Gay Men's Health Crisis included. Kramer had been fighting for this for almost three years and was ecstatic at the news. He figured that he and Paul Popham would go to the meeting for the GMHC, but Kramer was wrong.

Popham chose Mel Rosen, the executive director. Actually, Popham didn't trust Kramer not to shoot his mouth off at the mayor and get Koch so angry he wouldn't do anything for them. He didn't want Kramer in the same room as Koch.

An incensed Kramer told Popham that *he* was the one who had fought so hard to set up this meeting with the mayor. *He* had founded the GMHC, and he should go. If he didn't go, Kramer threatened to quit the board of directors. Popham said that was okay by him. He'd polled the board already and it was unanimous. They all wanted Rosen to go and Kramer to leave. They were sick and tired of his angry outbursts, his bullying, his sanctimonious, holier-than-thou attitude.

Kramer was stunned. He was being cast out by the people he loved, by the family he had created. He was being rejected by those closest to him. Didn't they understand that he got so angry *because* he loved them and wanted them to do the right thing and save lives that would otherwise be lost?

Kramer had put so much into the GMHC. In the end, he felt it betrayed him.

Kramer wasn't the only one. Michael Callen and a group of younger gay men with AIDS sat through meeting after meeting at the GMHC, listening patiently to doctors, nurses, lawyers, and insurance experts tell them what it was like to have AIDS. They felt helpless and angry. Who knew more about their disease than they? Callen wondered, Why wasn't anyone asking *them* what was going on? After all, Callen's own doctor, Joseph Sonnabend, was offering him treatments that many of these doctors didn't even know about.

In November 1982, Callen and Richard Berkowitz formed the first New York people with AIDS group. It was called Gay Men With AIDS and "dealt primarily with AIDS and sexual addiction problems." It didn't survive very long. Callen blamed the GMHC. "They refused to acknowledge its existence and undermined it," he says.

Callen and Berkowitz then joined the New York AIDS Network, a group that met each Thursday morning at eight in the East Village, where the younger, hipper gays were starting to live. The network had been set up by Virginia Apuzzo, Hal Kooden, and Dr. Roger Enlow. It was more politically oriented than the others. Larry Kramer, already in constant disagreement with the board of the GMHC, started showing up.

At this time, New York PWAs were becoming aware of Bobbi Campbell and what he was doing on the West Coast. Most couldn't believe this guy had the courage to "out" himself—to publicly declare himself as a gay man, much less a gay man with AIDS. They followed what was happening in San Francisco by occasionally picking up the latest *Sentinel* at the Oscar Wilde Bookshop in Greenwich Village.

In the spring of 1983, at a meeting of the AIDS Network, a decision was made to attend the Second National AIDS Forum in Denver. Callen and

Kramer learned that Bobbi Campbell was telling AIDS service organizations to send one or more gay men with AIDS to the conference. PWAs should make decisions about their own lives, Campbell was saying.

This idea of PWAs representing themselves grabbed Callen and the small rebel band at the AIDS Network. That was what was bothering them about the GMHC! People with AIDS were not playing any role in their own lives anymore. They were being taken care of, as if they were children.

The feminists and lesbians in the AIDS Network had been talking to Callen about the women's health movement of the seventies, but he didn't quite understand it. He had been out playing in the seventies. Callen couldn't connect it to himself until that moment. One of the key issues in the women's movement was the arrogance and condescension of male doctors toward female patients. Doctors saw themselves as deities and were treated as gods by the older generation. Women, however, wanted to take responsibility for their own health. They began demanding information from their doctors, treatment options to choose from, and finally, respect as individuals. *Our Bodies, Ourselves* was only one of many books to come out reflecting this dramatic shift in the relationship between patient and doctor. This notion of self-empowerment, borrowed from the women's movement, began to play itself out in the gay community. Callen and other New York PWAs wanted to go to Denver to join Bobbi Campbell and his California colleagues. The GMHC refused to finance their trip, but one individual, Alan Long, came up with enough money to send Callen, Berkowitz, and one other New York PWA to the conference. Others paid their own way.

The Denver conference was organized by the San Francisco contingent. Helen Shietinger, a nurse, set aside a hospitality suite for PWAs to meet in. About a dozen PWAs found themselves in a room. It was immediately electric. They went round-robin, as in an Alcoholics Anonymous meeting, telling their stories of AIDS. They discovered that each of them was being treated in the same way, as a passive victim. After hours of bitch sessions, they came to a general consensus. Two people, one representing East Coast interests, the other West Coast concerns, were chosen to come up with a list of principles. The Denver Principles.

"Bobbi Campbell and I emerged as the two control queens," says Callen. "We wrote the Denver Principles. Tremendous power was delegated to us by the other PWAs and we took it very seriously."

The discussion between Campbell and Callen quickly transformed itself into a negotiation between the West Coast and East Coast. There was a lot of hard bargaining. The West Coast wanted to insist that PWAs have the right to have sex. The East Coast fought to include the idea that "people with AIDS have an ethical responsibility to inform their potential sexual partners of their health status." Callen later said, "That's the one that always gets dropped." Callen felt strongly about including a phrase addressed to doctors and other health care professionals to "always clearly identify and discuss the theory they favor as to the cause of AIDS, since this bias affects the treatments and advice they give." Joe Sonnabend was his model for that one.

Campbell insisted, absolutely insisted, that right on top of the page they had to print: "We condemn attempts to label us as 'victims,' a term which implies defeat, and we are only occasionally 'patients,' a term which implies passivity, helplessness, and dependence upon the care of others. We are 'People With AIDS.'"

Callen thought the whole sentence was tedious and not terribly important. "I was wrong on that, wasn't I?" he said later, with a self-mocking smile.

Their finished project in hand, Callen and Campbell went back to the small PWA group in the hospitality suite to get their approval. It came quickly. They all decided to storm the closing session and present their demands to the entire conference. Each PWA took a turn reading out one of the points until the whole list of recommendations and responsibilities was aired. Then with great flair the San Francisco contingent unfurled their banner: FIGHTING FOR OUR LIVES.

There were seventeen Denver Principles, all promoting the idea of self-empowerment. They were grouped under two headings. Among the "Recommendations for People With AIDS" were the following: PWAs should (1) form caucuses to choose their own representatives, to deal with the media, to choose their own agenda, and to plan their own strategies; (2) be involved at every level of decision making and specifically serve on the boards of directors of provider organizations; (3) be included in all AIDS forums with equal credibility as other participants, to share their experiences and knowledge; (4) substitute low-risk sexual behaviors for those which could endanger themselves and their partners and . . . inform their potential sex partners of their health status.

Then there were the "Rights of People With AIDS," including: "(1) to as full and satisfying sexual and emotional lives as everyone else; (2) to quality medical treatment and quality social service provision without discrimination of any form including sexual orientation, gender, diagnosis, economic status, or race; (3) to full explanations of all medical procedures and risks, to choose or refuse their treatment modalities, to refuse to participate in research without jeopardizing their treatment; and to make informed decisions about their lives; (4) to privacy, to confidentiality of medical records, to human respect, and to choose who their significant others are; (5) to die—and to *live*—in dignity."

On the way back to New York, in the smoking section of the plane, Bobbi Campbell, Michael Callen, Richard Berkowitz, and Artie Felson plotted. Campbell and Felson in particular talked about setting up a National Association of People With AIDS.

Infused with energy from Denver, Callen and Berkowitz placed an ad in several gay newspapers asking people to join a new political organization, PWA–New York. It too was killed by the GMHC. As one of its first activities, Callen thought they should have a public forum on the importance of AIDS in sexual behavior and invite Gloria Steinem to speak. PWA–New York suggested putting on a joint forum with the GMHC, and several members went over to discuss it. In the end, "they stole the idea from us," says Callen.

The GMHC even refused to have any PWA associated with the presentation. Then it relented but insisted on its own PWA, not Callen or any of the more "radical" people with AIDS.

PWA–New York also designed, wrote, and distributed the first poster for bathhouses warning about AIDS and urging safe sex. GMHC promised to pay for them but then refused, according to Callen. It attacked the poster, saying it wasn't scientific enough. "That gave the bathhouse owners an excuse for taking them down, and nothing was done in bathhouses for another year and a half," Callen explains. During that time, of course, multipartner sex was spreading the AIDS virus throughout New York.

Both the open theft of the idea for a public forum on sex and the reneging on the safe-sex posters demoralized PWA–New York. The quick death of many of its founders hurt deeply as well. While PWA–San Francisco thrived, PWA–New York collapsed.

Six months after the Denver meeting, Bobbi Campbell was dead. Before that, however, he took one last poke at his disease at the annual San Francisco Gay Freedom Day Parade. With the crowd breaking into a cheer as the FIGHTING FOR OUR LIVES banner went by, he walked down the street after it wearing a lavender T-shirt that read AIDS POSTER BOY.

\* \* \*

He was a smuggler, a swashbuckling adventurer, a modern-day Robin Hood. He braved the border guards and the Feds to bring in drugs to help people with AIDS. James Corti, a registered nurse in Los Angeles, was the "Dex Kid," named after the dextran sulfate he smuggled in from Mexico.

In the early eighties, with friends and lovers dying around them and no hint of treatment or cure in sight, people with AIDS began to treat themselves. It was a quiet act but no less revolutionary for its silence. It was the first positive action taken by the gay community and it would eventually lead to the creation of an alternative, underground medical movement.

A few at first, mostly on the West Coast but growing in number, defied their own doctors and refused to accept their diagnoses: "You have AIDS and three to six months to live." It was an act of arrogance, an attitude of defiance. A finger in the eye of the powers that be.

Beginning in 1983, picking up steam in 1984, and going very strong by 1985, people were breaking the law on a large scale. The search for power to live rather than accepting the inevitability of dying meant defying both politics and the law. It mean circumventing the FDA's rules and regulations on importing drugs from foreign sources to treat diseases.

This was the heyday of the Dex Kid. Dextran sulfate had been available over the counter in Japan for decades to treat cancer. Over a dozen Japanese companies made it, although one, Ueno, was the chief manufacturer of the compound.

Word was out in L.A. and San Francisco that dextran sulfate helped stop the advance of AIDS. People were streaming down to Mexico to get it on their own. But many were too weak or afraid to risk the trip. The Dex Kid brought back kilos of the stuff. He was a hero.

Then he disappeared. Not much was heard from him until 1989, when he was called out of "retirement." Years after penetrating the border of Mexico, the Dex Kid would secretly enter China and return to San Francisco from Shanghai with a purified extract of a Chinese cucumber. It was called Compound Q.

A few people knew who the Dex Kid really was, but not many and they didn't talk. Yet his Robin Hood life is the perfect metaphor for the growing medical underground.

\* \* \*

Access to drugs, access to treatment, quickly became the rallying cry of the AIDS activists. Their life-threatening disease meant that access *equaled* treatment, access even to experimental, unapproved drugs. By the mid-eighties, people with AIDS everywhere were talking about access.

Access to AZT became an issue. Sam Broder was broadcasting the success of his Phase I safety trial, and it was clear by early 1986 that a big Phase II efficacy trial was about to begin. For the first time in six years, an experimental drug was suddenly available from the government.

But there were no clear rules on which PWAs would be selected to enter the trial. Who would decide? What were the criteria? The government wasn't talking and neither was Burroughs Wellcome. Ugly things began to happen.

Congressman Henry Waxman (D.-Calif.) sent Senator Lowell Weicker (R.-Conn.) a letter in the summer of '86. In it Waxman said he was receiving frequent requests from "constituents, friends and total strangers for help in admission to NIH research projects involving possible therapies for AIDS." He said many members of Congress were getting similar requests. It was simple logic. The NIH was a government organization. So hundreds were calling up trying to gain access to treatment. They were trying to save their lives by getting special political favors.

Waxman told Weicker that the issues raised by these requests were "some of the most personally troubling of any issue I have ever worked on." He asked how the NIH would choose the one thousand people needed for testing AZT from the ten thousand living people with AIDS.

Waxman told Weicker that after a great deal of personal struggle, he had concluded that the ethically and medically correct answer was to give the researchers at the NIH free rein without any interference. He had therefore declined all requests to exercise his influence in the selection of patients for the trials.

But it bothered the hell out of him. All one thousand of the slots for the AZT trial had already been filled. Waxman wrote that "everyone that I will tell to work within the system will be told that the system now has no room for them."

Waxman went on to ask Weicker for $7 million in added appropriations to increase the test slots. He also asked Weicker for $40 million to set up a "satellite" trial system that would include all living persons with AIDS.

Weicker came through on both requests, as he did virtually each and every time with funding for AIDS during his tenure in the Senate. The money for the satellite system was appropriated, but being "fungible," it disappeared later into NIAID.

The summer of 1986 was a crucial time in the development of an AIDS underground medical movement. From the very beginning of the government effort to find treatments for AIDS, it was clear that only a small percentage of those with AIDS would have access to trials. It was also clear that the scientists and doctors and government bureaucrats made all their decisions on who had access by themselves, using their own criteria. They felt no need to talk with the people who actually had AIDS.

In addition, there was no felt need to publicize the trials and give people affected the information necessary for them to make choices. This was all done within the club. The patient and the patient's doctor were not in that club.

Access became one of the major issues for AIDS activists. They pressed for new rules that would make more information available on open trials. They hammered home the message that access to research meant treatment for people with AIDS and that without treatment, they would die. Access was the only hope. Later, they would go further and set up their own research trials in an attempt to increase access to new drugs for more PWAs. They would pick up on Waxman's "satellite" trials idea and call for a "parallel track" system.

Project Inform was born out of an underground medical trial. By the time Martin Delaney decided to start a new organization devoted to informing people with AIDS about new treatments, ribavirin and isoprinosine were already hot. People were streaming down to Mexico to buy both the antiviral drug, ribavirin, and the immune booster, isoprinosine.

Many people, often with the help of their doctors, were combining the two as treatment. The NIH wasn't testing out either drug at this time. If it had, it wouldn't have combined two drugs anyhow. That procedure was considered unorthodox by the medical establishment, which preferred to do one drug at a time, to keep the data "clean."

Delaney thought combination therapy made sense. One of the first projects for Project Inform was to organize a research study of the effects of using ribavirin and isoprinosine together. Both drugs were smuggled across the Mexican border. Not much is known about the Dex Kid except for one fact—he was a close buddy to Martin Delaney.

A number of people with AIDS took the drug combination. They were asked to fill out questionnaires. ICN Pharmaceuticals, the manufacturer of ribavirin, paid for the analysis.

A few months later, several of the participants in the study set up BARIG, the Bay Area Ribavirin Interest Group, which put together monthly trips to Mexico to buy ribavirin. ICN also gave Project Inform money to finish the analysis of the ribavirin questionnaires. It was an early example of a drug company financing the medical underground that was to grow as the years passed.

Delaney began sending out information on ribavirin and isoprinosine to dozens of doctors and people with AIDS around the Bay Area. Physicians got a more detailed information packet, including a huge bibliography of ribavirin dating back to the early seventies.

Martin Delaney started Project Inform in 1985—five years after he was supposed to die.

Delaney left California in 1980 with chronic hepatitis that was destroying his liver. He then signed up for six months of experimental drug treatment at Stanford University. The two drugs Delaney took stopped the deterioration of his liver but left him with a severe neuropathy that caused terrible pains in his feet. Delaney had to take methadone daily to subdue the pain.

His experimental trial was stopped in 1982 and the drugs Delaney was on were never marketed. Five members of Delaney's support group for people with hepatitis died after they stopped receiving treatment. None of them was given any choice in the matter. It was all decided in secret by scientists, doctors, and Washington bureaucrats. It was a lesson Delaney didn't forget.

For the next three years, Delaney built up a successful consulting business. He was comfortable moving in the corporate world, comfortable moving among people with power. Delaney was a quiet person, a behind-the-scenes person. His consulting work was accomplished one on one, in person, discussing options, recommending tactics.

Two years later, in 1985, Delaney closed up shop and took his skills with him to set up a new organization, Project Inform. His major goal was to gather information about treatments for AIDS and to increase access to those treatments. With his earlier experience with hepatitis in mind, Delaney wanted to penetrate, circumvent, and defeat the bureaucracy of the biomedical world. That translated into Washington bureaucrats; physicians working out of big medical schools and hospitals, such as San Francisco

General Hospital; NIH researchers with their heads in ivory towers; and, finally, greedy drug companies.

Delaney used his skills as a persuader and negotiator, central to the consulting business, to generate change. He was to become the quintessential behind-the-scenes man in Washington, the first person among all AIDS activists to break the ice with FDA Commissioner Frank Young and NIAID director Tony Fauci.

In the summer of 1986, Delaney made his first contact with the FDA. He called and talked to Ellen Cooper and to her boss, Dr. Paul Parkman. They set up a meeting. Cooper remembers what Delaney was like at that meeting: "He came in and talked to us about ribavirin. Calmly."

It was the first of dozens of contacts between Delaney and his Project Inform and the FDA, and it reflected Delaney's style. He pushed for dramatic change but almost always through normal channels. As Cooper puts it, "Martin made demands but through letters, telephone calls, things like that. Not shouting." Many of these contacts were made directly at the commissioner's level. Frank Young and Delaney were to become fairly close until Young was asked to resign in 1989.

From the beginning in 1985, Delaney and Project Inform took a firm position in favor of early HIV testing and early, aggressive treatment even before symptomatic infections appeared. The pro-testing position put him at odds with most of the New York organizations at the time, including the Gay Men's Health Crisis, which were more concerned with the issue of confidentiality. There was a great fear of discrimination if names somehow leaked out, particularly among the large contingent of gays still in the closet in New York. When it came to medical practice, however, Joe Sonnabend and other New York City community doctors agreed completely with Delaney and "the Coast" on the need for early treatment.

Delaney, like Michael Callen and Bobbi Campbell, believed the AIDS patients had to take a very active role in their treatment. Doing nothing was unacceptable. Doing nothing meant death.

Delaney was to play the key role on the West Coast in fighting for access to treatment, for PWA rights, and for changes in the way drugs are developed in America. He was one of three or four AIDS movement "heavies" in the eighties, not nearly as visible as some, more quietly influential than most. He was to lead the first social movement born in a doctor's office.

# PART TWO

## FIGHTING FOR THEIR LIVES

There was an all-star cast at the meeting. The dapper Dr. Anthony Fauci, Tony to friends and enemies alike, three years into his directorship of the National Institute of Allergy and Infectious Diseases (NIAID), had organized the lineup of scientists and bureaucrats. And Fauci had asked the "Ice Queen," Ellen Cooper, to hop the red line and represent the FDA at this meeting; he also asked Henry Masur to attend. Masur was chairman of the Clinical Center, the big NIH hospital, and a key member of the NIAID drug selection committee, which was, by the spring of 1987, the key gatekeeper to all anti-AIDS drugs tested by the government. In all, Fauci had about fifteen of his colleagues sitting around a huge table facing the five AIDS activists who had requested this meeting. It was the first time top NIH officials had sat down to talk with leaders of the community of people with AIDS since the epidemic had begun. It was incredible but true.

The arrogance was simply part of the NIH culture. No one thought that people with AIDS and their local doctors had anything to recommend in terms of their own treatment. The same was true of people with cancer. They were all "patients" or "victims" to be pitied and helped by the white-coated scientist-heroes.

Michael Callen came with four allies: Larry Kramer, Nathan Kolodner, and Dr. Barry Gingell of the GMHC, and Tim Westmoreland, assistant to Congressman Henry Waxman. Westmoreland had arranged the meeting at Callen's request. Fauci couldn't refuse.

The angry five faced the nervous fifteen.

Callen started it off by saying that AL 721 was the preeminent drug of choice among PWAs. He told Fauci that everybody was talking about it. He said that everybody wanted it. Bootleg AL 721 was being sold on both coasts. "God, we were up to our tits in lipids at that time," Callen remembers.

Despite the AIDS community's clear preference for the drug, AL 721 had not moved forward for testing and approval. Why not? asked Callen. With a disgusted look on his face, Fauci replied, "There's no evidence that lipids do anything." It was almost as if Fauci couldn't even bring himself to discuss the sticky egg compound. His body motion, his entire manner, was dismissive.

Masur jumped in, hot with emotion. He was spoiling for a fight. "There's not a shred of evidence that AL 721 has any effect on AIDS," he said. Just months before, NIAID had given AL 721 the next-to-lowest priority rating. It had grudgingly recommended that the drug be tested at all only because of the immense political pressure put on NIH by AIDS activists and Congress. No one on the committee believed AL 721 worked. If it had been up to Masur, he would have canned the drug entirely.

"Wait a minute," said Callen, taking out the 1985 letter to the *NEJM* signed by Robert Gallo, saying that AL 721 was "promising." "AIDS groups are screaming for help, and this says AL 721 is promising." Callen tried to hand the article to Fauci. Without taking it from Callen, Fauci said, "Oh, that. Look, we tried those experiments and we couldn't duplicate them. The lipids didn't stop HIV replication in the test tube."

"We" meant Sam Broder at the NCI.

NIAID never tested AL 721 against live AIDS virus. Robert Gallo did. Jeffrey Laurence did. Both found it *was* active against AIDS. Fauci simply picked the one lab and one assay out of the three that showed negative results.

The more emotional Fauci got, the more "New Yawk" his speech became. Fauci was from the Brooklyn streets and used the stigmatized speech of the lower middle class in Brooklyn. He dropped his *r*'s, and "organism" became "awganism," as in "awful" or "caught." Whereas Sam Broder had left his Detroit street accent behind in his climb to success, Fauci's stuck like a piece of wet gum.

Fauci changed tactics when Callen reminded him that outside Broder's lab, AL 721 had been shown to work. "I could put oregano in a test tube and it would probably stop the AIDS virus," Fauci said. "Does that mean I should do clinical trials of oregano?" "Well, yes," said Callen. "Oregano is probably not toxic."

Then Fauci jumped to a third reason why AL 721 was not yet in trials. He blamed Praxis. "Look, what can you do to put pressure on a company to test a drug it owns?" he asked. "I don't know what to think about a company that doesn't do as well as it should." None of this made sense. Lippa was dying to test out AL 721 against AIDS. Praxis was privately financing its own small-scale trial. It was the NIH that was dragging its feet!

But no matter. When the subject was AL 721, emotions ran very high at the NIH, and logic went out the window.

It got very uncomfortable in the conference room in Building 31. People were almost yelling at one another. Discouraged over AL 721, Callen then brought up another drug, aerosol pentamidine. He took a deep breath and said, "Look, Dr. Fauci, I have a proposition to make to you. I'd like you to just issue guidelines to doctors to consider using PCP prophylaxis."

Joe Sonnabend had told Callen the week before that in cancer research, the NIH would sometimes convene a "consensus group" meeting to discuss possible treatment. It brought together experts and practitioners for a kind of clinical consult. The goal was to come up with a consensus on how to treat a specific condition. It had been done with breast cancer surgery and had resulted in many surgeons' switching from radical procedures to simple lumpectomy surgery.

Callen told Fauci that there was plenty of evidence from community doctors that it was possible to prevent the onset of *Pneumocystis carinii* pneumonia by prophylaxing with a new drug, aerosol pentamidine, or with an older drug, sold as Bactrim or Septra.

Fauci nearly shouted, "I can't do that. I can't issue these kinds of guidelines and I can't convene a consensus conference." "Why not?" shot back Callen. "There's no data," Fauci practically screamed.

Callen was dumbstruck. No data? What the hell was Fauci talking about? There was data all over New York. Joe Sonnabend, Nathaniel Pier, and Barbara Starrett were all using Bactrim and aerosol pentamidine with their patients. No one had died from PCP in New York in months. There was no data? Callen was furious. There was plenty of data, if only Fauci and the rest of NIH were willing to look at real people in real communities instead of the endless bottoms of their test tubes.

"Please, I *beg you*," Callen said. "Just tell doctors to simply consider it." Fauci dismissed the idea with a quick shake of his head. "I can't do that," he said. Callen was simply horrified at what was happening. He couldn't believe it.

Fauci then gave Kramer, Kolodner, Gingell, Westmoreland, and Callen a lecture. "In the history of science, people have thought they've observed things and then it later turned out to be not so," he said. By implication, he, Dr. Anthony Fauci, was not about to let that happen to him. He would not take that risk. He would not be humiliated. Not even, thought Callen, if Fauci's decision cost the lives of tens of thousands of people with AIDS.

Fauci ended the meeting by saying that three trials were planned for aerosol pentamidine. After that, *then* we will have some real data, he said.

When the meeting was over, Fauci worried that he had antagonized the AIDS activists in the room. He turned to Larry Kramer and asked how he thought the meeting had gone. Kramer told him, "Everyone thought you were real cute."

Later, when Kramer was furious at Fauci for not using all the hundreds of millions of dollars AIDS lobbyists had squeezed out of Congress, he would say: "The main reason that Fauci has gotten away with so much is that he's attractive and handsome and dapper and extremely well spoken and he never answers your question."

Two years later, almost to the day, Michael Callen was back in Washington pleading for the exact same thing—aerosol pentamidine to prevent PCP. That day in Tony Fauci's conference room had haunted Callen.

Nothing, of course, had come of the NIH trials of aerosol pentamidine. Fauci still lacked "proof." Callen was reliving a nightmare.

There was one difference, however, since his last meeting with Fauci, in 1987: 16,929 people had died from AIDS-related PCP. This wasn't just some made-up number. Callen had asked a CDC statistician to do the math. How many AIDS-related deaths from PCP had occurred between May 1987 and February 20, 1989, the last date for which the numbers were available? Had Fauci two years ago agreed to issue guidelines for doctors, just advising them that aerosol pentamidine might be a good prophylaxis for the number one killer of people with AIDS, nearly 17,000 people might have lived longer.

That thought made Callen very tired. His body slumped with the weight of Fauci's refusal. The prospect of being turned down a second time made Callen slowly close his eyes. Had anyone walked into the room at that moment, they would have sworn that Michael Callen was silently praying, not for himself perhaps but for others.

Callen began his testimony in front of the FDA by saying that "I have witnessed firsthand the tremendous, unnecessary suffering caused by PCP: people with AIDS gasping for breath, twitching on respirators, unable to speak."

Callen then told the gathered doyens of AIDS research before him his Fauci story. "In May of 1987, I and other AIDS activists met with Dr. Anthony Fauci—the closest person we have to an AIDS czar. We asked him—no, we *begged* him—to issue interim guidelines urging physicians to prophylax those patients deemed at high risk for PCP. Although it would not have cost the government much to have done so, he steadfastly refused to issue such guidelines. His reason: no data. So the Catch-22 was complete and many people died of PCP who didn't have to."

Callen went on to say that the AIDS community was finally forced to do the kind of scientific experimentation that would prove to the scientific establishment what dozens of community doctors and thousands of PWAs already knew: that aerosol pentamidine prevented PCP. Just a few months ago, local groups in New York and San Francisco presented data to the FDA in support of aerosol pentamidine. The data had not been generated out of Tony Fauci's multimillion-dollar drug-testing system, said Callen. That system has not been able to enroll a single person in its trials of aerosol pentamidine. The data presented today, Callen went on, was generated in the community itself and paid for by a private company, LyphoMed. "The community has rolled up its sleeves and done an end run around federal incompetence and indifference." It was a comment that Dr. Anthony Fauci would never forget.

# ..6..
# Empire Building

Rock Hudson changed everything by getting AIDS. For the first time, President Ronald Reagan and his wife Nancy knew personally someone with the disease; he was even a Republican. Five years into the epidemic, the Reagan administration dropped its opposition to funding AIDS research.

On July 19, 1985, the Reagan administration sent Congress a new budget. It was three days before Congressman Henry Waxman was scheduled to hold yet another hearing on AIDS. Waxman was planning to subpoena HHS Secretary Margaret Heckler. He was determined to find out what the true requests for money had been from the different agency heads fighting AIDS. Waxman knew the administration hid those requests from Congress. The NIH and the CDC had to go through the Office of Management and Budget (OMB) before going before Congress. The OMB, in effect, was trying to run the nation's biomedical research, including the fight against AIDS.

The Friday evening before the hearing, the White House requested a 47 percent increase for AIDS in the fiscal '86 budget, boosting its appropriation from $40 million to approximately $60 million.

Congress had been doubling whatever the White House ended up spending on AIDS. It was a tradition by now, dating back to the first year Ronald Reagan came to Washington. This time Congress appropriated $234 million for fiscal 1986, up from $108 million the year before. At long last big money was starting to flow into AIDS research.

To Dr. Anthony Fauci the money spelled *opportunity* with a capital

*O.* Fauci had taken over as director of the NIAID on November 2, 1984, from Dr. Richard Krause. The orange-haired, shrill Krause had a reputation at the NIH as a relatively unambitious and passive manager of one of the campus's smaller institutes. Krause was content enough to live as a bachelor in one of the stone buildings the NIH offered its institute directors.

Krause had shied away from involving the NIAID in the growing AIDS epidemic. Nearly all of the AIDS research taking place on the NIH campus was at the NCI. Larry Kramer and many other AIDS activists would later compare Krause's inaction with New York Mayor Ed Koch's inactivity during the early years of the crisis.

Tony Fauci was as different from Richard Krause as shark is from goldfish. Fauci looked as if he had just stepped out of a limousine. Trim and athletic, Fauci's tailored suits, cuff-linked shirts, and aviator glasses set him far apart from the rest of the scientists and administrators at the NIH. Old jeans, Nikes, and threadbare dress shirts under long, white lab coats were de rigueur inside most labs. At the managerial echelons, off-the-rack black and gray suits were the uniform of the day. Fauci, however, stood out in sartorial splendor, even if he was a bit short.

Fauci's raciness also extended to his cars. He would soon have a sleek two-door maroon Toyota Celica parked in front of DIRECTOR, NIAID, just four slots down from Sam Broder's plain Honda Civic sedan.

Fauci had come a long way from Brooklyn. He'd gotten his M.D. from the Cornell University Medical College in 1966. Two years later he finished his internship and residency at the Cornell Medical Center in New York City. In 1968, as the war raged on in Vietnam, Fauci donned the white uniform of the Commissioned Corps of the Public Health Service at the NIH. His first job was as a clinical associate at the National Institute of Allergy and Infectious Diseases. By 1977 he was deputy clinical director of NIAID. Fauci did competent, if unremarkable, research on immunology. Where he really excelled was in administration.

Fauci was an aggressive administrator from the start but he wasn't a details man. In fact, Fauci hated details. That was small stuff to be delegated. Fauci thrived on the hard-driving, must-do leadership role. He was, as one high-ranking NIAID official puts it, "a hit-the-front-page-every-day kind of guy." A big-picture kind of guy.

Fauci saw AIDS as a dreaded disease—and an opportunity for NIAID to grow into a much bigger, more powerful institute. AIDS was his big chance. He wasn't well known as a brilliant scientist, and he had little

Empire Building

background in managing a big bureaucracy; but Fauci did have ambition and drive to spare. This lackluster scientist was about to find his true vocation—empire building.

To transform NIAID from an institutional weakling into an NIH powerhouse, Fauci had to fight for a bigger piece of the AIDS research pie. When Congress began to appropriate big money in 1985, Fauci went about securing a large portion of those funds for his own institute. He started the most important bureaucratic battle in the history of the fight against AIDS. The outcome of this single fight had enormous consequences for the lives of thousands of people. Had it turned out otherwise, many people who died might have lived.

Fauci took on Dr. Vincent DeVita, head of the NCI. In the winter months of 1985, a series of meetings took place that determined the future of government AIDS research. The most important meetings were just between Fauci and DeVita. Occasionally, James Wyngaarden, head of the NIH, sat in. Most meetings took place in Building 31, where all of the institute directors had their offices. A few meetings occurred over drinks and dinner in D.C. area restaurants. The NIH campus, as big a rumor mill as any large university or corporation, was soon abuzz over the tug-of-war between the two men. Lab chiefs describing what was taking place in their little world were suddenly making references to the old *Godfather* movies, with cracks about "Don" DeVita and the new challenger, Fauci.

The meetings were always polite, but they were always tough. Both DeVita and Fauci knew that the National Cancer Institute had the jump on NIAID. Bob Gallo was the American credited with discovering the AIDS virus and he was at the NCI. The blood test for the AIDS antibody had come out of the NCI. Research on Kaposi's sarcoma, one of the first diseases associated with AIDS, originated at the NCI. Sam Broder's lab was responsible for all anti-AIDS drug screening. That's what DeVita brought to the table.

What did Fauci have? Not much. Except that his institute was named the National Institute of Allergy and Infectious Diseases, and AIDS was certainly an infectious disease. Bureaucratically, at the NIH, AIDS "belonged" to NIAID. The NIH was nothing if not extremely sensitive to bureaucratic turf. At the bottom of the chain, lab chiefs fought for their territory and the territory of their postdocs. At the top, institute directors had their elbows out all the time, Richard Krause being the exception rather than the rule.

So theoretically, Fauci could claim that the NCI should ship all of its facilities over to NIAID to allow his institute to do its proper job. Fauci could have argued that they were entering a second stage in the scientific search for a treatment of and cure for AIDS. The NCI had done a terrific job at Stage I. Thanks a lot. Now NIAID was going to spearhead Stage II.

Instead, the negotiations over research turf started with the small stuff as Bulldog DeVita and Tony Fauci studied each other and probed for weakness. There weren't many research bucks in preclinical testing, the experiments done on animals and in test tubes in the lab, so they began slowly with that.

NIAID didn't have its own preclinical program for testing promising anti-AIDS drugs, and Fauci wanted one. It was a matter of prestige. If NIAID was to be a real player in AIDS research, it needed one.

DeVita reminded Fauci, ever so smoothly, that the NCI already had a preclinical screening program up and running for both cancer and AIDS. Wouldn't it be wasteful to duplicate it? he asked Fauci, with responsibility written all over his face.

Of course that would be wasteful, Fauci replied. But what if NIAID began to do targeted drug development and testing? NIAID would try to develop new compounds specifically made to treat AIDS. This way, *both* institutes could do preclinical drug testing. "Vince and I agreed that they would do the screening and we would do the targeted drug development because AIDS was an infectious disease," Fauci later reported. Brilliant. It was an I-win-but-you-don't-lose move by Fauci. DeVita was impressed. This guy was a worthy opponent, an impressive bureaucratic tactician.

This first round of talks on whose turf was whose wasn't easy, according to NCI and NIAID officials who were near the negotiations at the time. Each day Fauci and DeVita would return to their respective institutes following talks and call satellite sessions to discuss strategy for the next day's struggle. "Let me just say that it wasn't all that smooth," says one high-ranking official. "It took a lot of discussion, *a lot* of discussion." But the early talks were just warmup.

The most important battle between Fauci and DeVita was over which institute was going to run the big clinical trials with hundreds of patients. That's where $20 million appropriated by Congress was going to be spent that year. Government-sponsored clinical trials were held at the major medical school hospitals around the country. Whoever controlled the money for those trials had real clout. The very best and brightest researchers in

America would have to go to *them* to request funding. It was a position of special power in the nation's scientific establishment.

DeVita, of course, wanted his NCI to run the clinical trials for AIDS drugs. He told Fauci that only the NCI had the experience. It had been running clinical trials for cancer drugs for nearly two decades. Chemotherapy treatments had slowly but steadily evolved through these trials. He reminded Fauci that he, DeVita, had been a pioneer in chemo and had participated in the trials. The NCI knew exactly how to get them up and running. He didn't want to be blunt, DeVita said, but the facts spoke for themselves, didn't they? What had NIAID ever done? DeVita didn't say it, but the real question was in the air: What had *Fauci* ever done when it came to big clinical trials? Where was *his* experience? What was *he* pioneer of?

Fauci conceded that NIAID's trials had been mostly small-scale. They had led to the generation of data for scientific journals, not for FDA approval of new drugs. But none of that mattered and both Fauci and DeVita knew it. Fauci pulled out his big gun and told DeVita that AIDS was due to a virus and the National Institute of Allergy and Infectious Diseases was the place for research on such a disease. The NCI had entered the AIDS picture only because one of the earliest opportunistic diseases had been Kaposi's sarcoma, a cancer. Now that everyone knew that AIDS was a virus, it belonged to NIAID, he said.

DeVita knew the bargaining was over. Fauci had the bureaucrat's trump card—the name of his institute. It was all he needed to claim turf rights to AIDS and the research dollars behind it.

So the deal was cut. The NCI, through Sam Broder's shop, would continue to screen new drugs for possible effectiveness against AIDS. The NCI would continue to run Phase I safety trials on those drugs in the NIH hospital. Bob Gallo would continue to do his thing, which had evolved by that time into looking for an AIDS vaccine. DeVita had defended his people. He had done his job.

NIAID would then come in and do the big clinical multicenter trials that would show drug efficacy. Fauci would build himself an entirely new trial system. Then he would learn how to run it. Of course, that would take time, the one thing people with AIDS didn't have.

A growing budget for AIDS research, like a rising tide, lifted Tony Fauci's profile considerably on the NIH campus. In 1982, NIAID received $297,000 in AIDS funding. In 1986, it received $63 million. In 1987, the sum reached $146 million. By 1990, NIAID's annual AIDS funding was pushing half a billion dollars. Tony Fauci's ship had come in.

When Dr. Maureen Myers left Tony Fauci's office on an early fall evening in 1985 she was excited as hell. The tall scientist sometimes told jokes to friends about the difference in height between her boss and herself, but she wasn't laughing tonight. Fauci had just asked her to build an entirely new, huge, multicenter, multiprotocol trial system, NIAID's first. He told her that the money was finally there from Congress and that NIAID, not the NCI, was going to run the clinical trials. "Are you willing to take this on?" he asked, meaning ninety-hour weeks, few free weekends, and lots of pressure from the outside.

Myers rushed home that night with her head buzzing with lists of things to do. Of course she would take the job. What an incredible opportunity, she thought. They had nothing! Absolutely no staff working on this kind of AIDS research. It all had to be created from scratch. She couldn't stop making mental lists: How many components to the program would they need? What would be the topic areas? Whom can we get to cover them? How much would it cost? And on and on and on through the night.

And where would she find the time? Myers was already working full-time at NIAID's antiviral substances program. In fact, she *was* the antiviral person, responsible for all antiviral compounds, especially drugs to treat severe herpes infections. Fauci hadn't mentioned anything about hiring someone to help her out.

Myers's background in herpes was a pretty good bridge to AIDS. She was already in contact with a whole bunch of principal investigators—top scientists who ran research trials on drugs at the nation's leading medical schools and hospitals. These PIs were the critical scientific players in all off-campus, extramural research. Every disease had its PI. In the case of herpes and AIDS, they were clinical virologists specializing in testing antiviral drugs.

The PI is the building block of American science. A relatively small number of these scientists actually do most of the scientific experiments run each year. An even smaller number, several hundred, determine the nature and direction of virtually all biomedical research, not only for the United States but for most of the world.

Each field of science has its PIs; sometimes as few as one, sometimes two dozen individuals dominate each discipline. They are the main players who sit on the "gateway" committees for journals and funding, receive much of the grant money themselves, and determine the paradigm within which scientists in a given field generally work.

"Investigator-initiated research" was the mantra for American science. It was repeated with religious fervor, cradled with loving care, and brought forth to ward off any perceived interference into the scientists' domain by "outsiders," especially regulators or politicians. "Scientists do science," went the slogan. "Researchers must be free."

This pool of investigators and their mode of operation had been nurtured by the NIH for decades. Through its Extramural Grants Program, the NIH funneled billions of dollars into the hands of PIs. In fact, the NIH was founded after the Second World War on the principle of investigator-initiated research. At that time it found itself with surplus funds and sent out letters to the deans of medical schools asking for proposals. A thousand came in, $10 million of grant money poured forth, and the NIH was in business as the premier biomedical research unit of the government. In 1987, the NIH budget was $6.1 billion, and $4.6 billion went for grants to individual investigators off campus. In 1990 the budget rose to $7.6 billion, with over $5 billion going to twenty thousand PIs in thirteen hundred institutions around the country.

While the National Security Agency, which was housed at Fort Meade, Maryland, not far from the NIH campus at Bethesda, was secretly created by the executive branch of the government after the war, the NIH was Congress's baby. Key congressmen have been the driving force behind the NIH from the beginning. They learned early on that their constituents believed in spending dollars on science. Science gave them longer lives.

In every year since the early fifties, Congress appropriated more for the NIH than was requested by the White House. It didn't matter whether he was a Democrat or a Republican, the president would send in his budget request and Congress would hike it. There was never enough money for the NIH.

Congress was also fond of creating more institutes. By the mid-seventies there were sixteen, including a National Institute on Aging, a National Institute on Deafness, and a National Institute on Drug Abuse.

Congress was also responsible for a second track in providing research funds. It differed dramatically from investigator-initiated research. In 1955, Congress put pressure on the National Cancer Institute to put more resources into the then-new field of chemotherapy. The NCI used contracts to speed up the work. The institute determined priorities and assumed initiatives and then parceled out the work. It didn't wait for the PIs to send in grant ideas. Contracts were very effective in expanding the use of chemotherapy.

Yet they were never popular. PIs resisted them as infringements on their freedom of scientific investigation. It was almost as if they felt contracts impinged on their Bill of Rights. PIs in the field were supposed to control the scientific process start to finish, from conceiving the ideas to sending in the grant requests to sitting on the NIH's "study sections," which peer-reviewed applications. PIs wanted to control each step along the way. Ninety percent of the time, they did.

The independence of PIs, however, was circumscribed by one factor—money. While the NIH became a major source of funding for their research, drug companies were even more important to many of them. The amount of money drug companies spent on research each year dwarfed the sum put out by the NIH. PIs gravitated toward that money. They would basically hire themselves and their clinics out to do testing for a private company.

Over time, each drug company built up a network of PIs whom it paid to test its new drugs. Companies such as Burroughs Wellcome, Merck, Schering-Plough, and Bristol-Myers contracted with the medical school and/or teaching hospital to pay certain sums for trials. Often it was a per-patient fee, ranging from $5,000 to $10,000 per patient in a drug trial. A good half, sometimes two-thirds of that money went to academic "overhead," and was used by the institution for general support. Other monies went to support the PI's assistants and lab. Ways were also found, through honoraria and speaking engagements or first-class tickets to foreign conferences, to compensate the investigator directly as well.

Over time, PIs tended to cluster around one drug firm or another and generally test that firm's drug on their patients. These doctors and the patients they had access to were used over the years in trial after trial. For example, PIs who had done work for Burroughs Wellcome would not be inclined to test a Squibb drug. As one researcher who was not part of either the Wellcome or government clinical trials network puts it: "Clinical testing is all about money. Burroughs Wellcome, for example, controls clinicians [investigators] by paying them money. If you work for Wellcome, then you're going to test AZT and Wellcome drugs. You're not going to test other companies' drugs because you're not being paid by other people."

PIs, however, felt free to take government money, and many of the Wellcome PIs came to dominate NIAID's clinical trial system. They formed a web linking Wellcome, the drug AZT, and the NIH. They came to sit on the institute's key drug selection committee, and they voted on whether to give high or low priority to the testing of each anti-AIDS drug, including those that might possibly compete with AZT in the marketplace. The PIs were a power unto themselves. They were, in fact, out of control.

The first order of the day for Maureen Myers was to write an RFP, a Request For Proposals in government science-speak. This RFP was sent out to leading clinical virologists to enlist them and their medical institutions in NIAID's fight against AIDS. At this time Myers was working under the assumption that for the first year at least, all trials in the new NIAID system would be small Phase I trials for safety. The likelihood of having any drug ready for a large-scale efficacy trial she considered extremely remote. In fact, it never really occurred to her that one might be required—not for years, anyhow. It didn't occur to her boss Tony Fauci, either.

Officially, Myers worked under John LaMontagne, who was director of the newly constituted NIAID AIDS Program. But LaMontagne was a laid-back, low-key kind of guy. Although he had an excellent reputation as a scientist and was considered very bright, he wasn't a leader. He preferred quiet persuasion behind the scenes to visible take-charge leadership. Myers immediately became the driving force in the operation.

So in December 1985 Myers put the $20 million Congress had coughed up for a new clinical trial system into "solicitation." At this stage, all she was trying to do was put into place a network of medical institutions that could do collaborative trials in the future. Myers just wanted to get them to have their resources in place for future testing, when drugs would be coming out of the NCI-NIAID pipeline. So her first RFPs merely asked for a description of capabilities and an example of a written protocol. It was a simple test to see if the hospital or medical center could even write a protocol, or do basic research.

The real key to winning in this competition, however, was access to AIDS patients. That was the number one worry at NIAID. Without a substantial number of people with AIDS, the institute couldn't do the testing. Control over the sick either desperate enough or brave enough or both by PIs was their major source of power. This was true in all diseases, not just AIDS. Any threat to undermine that control over patients hit directly at the status of PIs in American biomedical research. In the end, the PIs who won out in the "solicitation" and received NIAID funding were those who could demonstrate that they had access to lots of AIDS patients.

Myers was the only one writing the RFPs and reading the proposals as they came in, all the while continuing to do her old job. Unfortunately, Myers followed standard operating procedure and required the investigators at each medical institution to submit an enormous amount of paperwork. Thousands and thousands of sheets of paper flooded into her office. In addition, the RFPs were extremely vague. They were asking for "potential capabilities," which left the investigators both unclear as to what she meant and free to write as much bureaucratic bull as they thought necessary to win one of the awards. It took months for Myers just to read them. Fauci was nowhere to be seen.

So it wasn't until May of 1986 that fourteen awards were finally made and fourteen institutions were signed up. It took another month, until June, before Myers got around to announcing them. The testing sites were called the AIDS Treatment Evaluation Units, or ATEUs. Unfortunately, it didn't do any good to create a network of PIs on call if there wasn't any coordinating body around to collect and analyze their data. With Myers busy with the RFPs and doing two jobs at once, she couldn't find the time to write an additional RFP for a data coordination company to link up all the institutions. She began writing it only after she finished getting the fourteen PIs on board. The award of that contract for a Clinical Trials Coordinating Center, or CTCC, went to the Research Triangle Institute of Research Triangle Park, North Carolina, just a stone's throw away from Burroughs Wellcome's headquarters. It wasn't until September 1986 that any kind of drug evaluation system was in place, a full year after Tony Fauci was given the authorization to set up the government's one and only clinical trial system. Vincent DeVita and Sam Broder didn't say so publicly, but there were a lot of I-told-you-sos around the NCI.

Then it all fell apart. On September 19, 1986, Myers got a call from the Data and Safety Monitoring Board for Burroughs Wellcome's big Phase II clinical trial testing the efficacy of AZT. The board had decided to break the code on the AZT experiment. AZT had shown efficacy against the AIDS virus. It worked. A drug had been found to work against AIDS.

Myers was dumbfounded. She wasn't prepared for this. No one had warned her. All the protocols written for the fourteen institutions were now obsolete. They were all small studies checking the safety of certain drugs. If AZT was effective, then each and every antiviral drug had to be tested against AZT. And if AZT really worked against AIDS, then practically all trials should involve AZT. The logic and the ethics of the situation were clear. NIAID had to gear up immediately for large-scale trials. It wasn't years away. It was now.

An entire year in the government's fight against AIDS went down the toilet with that one phone call. Strange as it seemed, no one at NIAID appeared to be monitoring the AZT Phase II trial. At least no one at NIAID was preparing for the possibility that the Burroughs Wellcome drug might work.

Where was Tony Fauci at this time? Nowhere. Myers, at least, had the excuse of being overworked. She was doing all the work in building Tony Fauci's new clinical trial network. Fauci had simply delegated it to this one woman and walked away. He wasn't, after all, a "details" man. He was busy being a "hit-the-front-pages-every-day" kind of guy.

There was a bittersweet irony to the good-news phone call Myers received. Burroughs Wellcome had taken only a couple of months to set up its own network of investigators and medical institutions for the Phase II AZT trial. By February of 1986, they'd been ready to go.

By May, while Myers was just finishing lining up her investigators on paper, the Wellcome investigators were practically finished enrolling all their patients. When Myers announced her list of investigators in June, Wellcome's David Barry saw that seven out of the twelve PIs in his AZT trial were among the fourteen that Myers had selected for her ATEUs. The same investigators were involved.

It was all rather unbelievable—predictable, but unbelievable. Nevertheless, only a handful of PIs came to dominate both the private and the public efforts against AIDS.

Sam Broder had finished his Phase I safety trial at the Clinical Center in December of 1985, just a month after Congress allocated its first big chunk of taxpayer money to set up the NIAID clinical testing network. By early fall, however, David Barry had already hit the phones to round up his usual PI suspects, people he had the greatest respect for because they really knew the drug development game—what was needed, what was not, to get through the FDA.

It was an old-boy network in the truest sense of the term (though because this was the eighties, some of the old boys were women). They were all clinical virologists in infectious diseases. They worked at the best medical institutions in the United States. They were an elite, among the best principal investigators in the country. They knew each other and each other's reputations. What's more, most of them had worked with Burroughs Wellcome in the past, being paid to run Wellcome drugs in their patients. Many, such as Dr. Donna Mildvan at Beth Israel Medical Center in New York City and Dr. Martin Hirsch at Harvard and the Massachusetts General Hospital, had worked on trials for acyclovir, the antiherpes drug from Wellcome. Others had been involved in interferon when it was being tested for activity against Kaposi's sarcoma. These included Dr. Margaret Fischl at the University of Miami and Dr. Michael Grieco at St. Luke's–Roosevelt—the same Grieco who worked on AL 721. Also, in Boston, Jerome Groopman signed up, while Paul Volberding, John Leedom, and Douglas Richman on the West Coast were happy to join in the Phase II study of AZT.

Margaret Fischl especially liked the project. She was an up-and-comer in the field, well respected and well connected. Fischl was also one of seven Wellcome PIs who were picked by Maureen Myers to join the NIAID's nascent ATEU network. Michael Grieco was on both lists, as were Martin Hirsch and others. When the ATEU system was expanded, all twelve of the Wellcome PIs became NIAID PIs. They bridged both worlds with one thing in common—their careers were bound up with the success of AZT.

These PIs saw no conflict of interest in their behavior. Their arrogance blinded them to the obvious—that their professional careers were bound up with Burroughs Wellcome and AZT even as they took control of the NIAID clinical trial system and voted on possibly competing alternative drugs. In most things, the PIs were accountable only to themselves. Peer review dominated science, including AIDS drug research, and they became the peers for this particular disease. For a profession that insisted on double-blind experiments to ensure that neither doctor nor patient, consciously or unconsciously, let emotions color findings, this system seemed questionable; and the results were not always beneficial.

In late June and early July of 1986, Barry spoke with both Myers and Tony Fauci. He said that his AZT Phase II was staggeringly expensive, and told them Wellcome was doing all kinds of virology and other types of tests that the government ordinarily should have done. Then Barry cautiously reminded them that the new NIAID program had gotten some criticism for being slow out of the gate. He suggested that NIAID pick up the costs of the seven PIs and seven trial sites they both shared. That way, Barry argued, if the Phase II trial turned out to be successful, Fauci, Myers, and NIAID would get some of the credit; Wellcome wouldn't mind because it would be relieved of some of the cost.

Myers couldn't or wouldn't commit. She said, "Talk to Tony." At that time, during the summer of 1986, congressional hearings were under way criticizing the use of placebos in the AZT trial. Mathilde Krim and others were arguing that people facing death shouldn't be given sugar pills. Barry was testifying at one of those hearings when he saw Fauci, who was also scheduled to speak. Barry turned to Fauci and said, "What do you say, is it a deal?" According to Barry, Fauci replied, "It sounds okay to me." Since this was the second or third time Barry had talked with Fauci about the plan to share expenses on those seven centers, he thought he had a deal.

Come the end of July and August, the monthly bills rolled into Burroughs Wellcome. Barry asked Dannie King, the AZT project director, to call NIAID and ask where to send the bills for the seven sites. "Well . . . let's check on that," came the reply. It didn't sound good—and it wasn't. In the end, NIAID told Wellcome that it would not be able to give them any money, despite what Dr. Fauci had said earlier. When Barry checked later at the highest levels, it was clear that Fauci had felt that government rules and regulations prevented him from coming through on the handshake deal.

The no from NIAID came just two weeks before the code was broken on the Phase II trial. No guts, no glory for Fauci, Myers, or NIAID on this one. So far, Fauci and Myers had done nothing right, not even covering their butts.

Pressure from gay activist groups was enormous at this point. It had been building as year after year the government came out with no effective treatments against AIDS. Congress had taken four years from the official start of the epidemic just to appropriate enough money to begin the research. It took another whole year until the fourteen awards were finally given out to medical institutions to start trials. Even then NIAID wasn't ready because it hadn't awarded a data contract. Then the whole system fell apart when the AZT results were announced. Community leaders were furious. They had pressured Congress for millions for the NIH. Where were the NIH's drugs for AIDS?

The day after the Data and Safety Monitoring Board broke the code for AZT, Myers flew all the principal investigators to Washington to have the results personally presented to them. Then they broke into smaller working groups and started designing entirely new protocols. Everything that had been written since June was garbage.

The atmosphere within NIAID was explosive. "Everyone just had to get going, real, real fast," says one person who played a leading role in the institute at that time. "Speed of response became the byword." Fauci had been pushing Myers to hurry things up throughout the year. He wanted a thousand patients enrolled in trials by the end of twelve months. They had zip.

Then came the PI revolt. It had been brewing all year long, ever since Myers decided to use the contract award system in handing out NIAID money. In the contracting process, the government simply says, "I want a product, this is what I want, and you're going to give it to me." The government has strict control over the research and is the ultimate authority in the trial process.

Contracting was rarely used because PIs hated it. The whole idea of science to them, the same idea on which the NIH was founded and funded by Congress, was to have the PIs decide what kind of research should be done. Only the best scientific ideas should get grants, and the only way to do that was through peer review, not government dictate.

Myers decided to use the contract system because it seemed the most efficient way to get things going in a hurry. Everyone around her was shouting, *"Hey, there's an epidemic! Do something fast!"* So Myers decided on contracting. Hers was an exercise in good will and naive thinking. Never having put together a multicenter trial system, Myers didn't realize she was cramming a noxious dose of government control down the throats of hitherto independent scientists. She thought the government *should* be playing the central role in setting priorities. They couldn't sit around and debate the nuances until the cows came home; that would be intellectual masturbation. She needed to get studies finalized, out and active. Besides, her boss, Tony Fauci, agreed with her. Or at least he didn't tell Myers he disagreed.

The PIs had another agenda. They saw the NIAID contracts as forced labor, pushing them to do boring, exhausting clinical trials testing drugs that offered them nothing professionally. Where were the all-important academic rewards in this? Where was the independent research that led to medical journal articles with their names on them? With contracts, they ended up being simply anonymous participants. With their own research, they could become well-known in their field, exercise their intellectual imagination, break the bounds of known science, and go for the Nobel. Where was the Nobel in the contract system?

The revolt of the PIs took Myers totally by surprise. She hadn't anticipated it and no one had warned her. This was the second time Myers was blindsided. Here she was, trying to do her best in a difficult situation and then getting blasted by the very people she was giving money to. Myers didn't really know what to do when the investigators began to moan and groan publicly. None of the PIs was happy with anyone else in the program. There was no sense of community, no acceptance of common goals, so necessary to pull together a big project like this one. No one wanted to sit down and conceptualize where they were going, and no one wanted to talk to anyone else.

To say that the situation quickly overwhelmed Myers is a vast under-statement. By September 1986, things were beginning to crack all over NIAID. The PIs were pissed off; calls were flooding in from the press, from drug companies, and increasingly from gay community groups demanding to know what the hell was going on. Tony Fauci had neglected to gear up NIAID's public relations office to handle the heavy load, and most of it landed on Myers's desk. She didn't get any new staff either and found herself moving furniture, photo copying, and stuffing envelopes for Federal Express well into the night. It was all unraveling, one year into the game. The game Tony Fauci had fought so hard to take away from Vincent DeVita, director of the National Cancer Institute, an institute that had years of experience doing what Fauci was supposed to be doing now.

In time, the clinical trials network Fauci set up would come to be known as the "HUD of the nineties." Money was spent, but trials went underenrolled, drug treatments never seemed to emerge, and people with AIDS continued to get sick and die.


Nothing's happening, thought Mathilde Krim. After all our effort to get those guys money from Congress to get going on AIDS research, nothing's happening.

It was summer 1986, nine months after the Reagan administration finally gave in and allowed Congress to really open the money spigots for AIDS. But there was no word from the NIH. Krim knew that a sum of $20 million had been appropriated and sent over to NIAID to establish a network of testing facilities for AIDS drugs. The very first step in testing a drug is the writing of a protocol outlining the approach. Not one protocol had yet appeared, much less one actual experiment.

Krim flew down to Bethesda to confront Fauci. "What the hell is happening in your shop?"

Fauci looked down and said quietly, "Mathilde, we have to first write the protocols. That's a lot of work. You know it's very difficult."

Krim was incredulous. She couldn't believe Fauci was actually telling her this. "In a shop like yours, it's difficult to write protocols? I mean, who writes the protocols here?"

Fauci looked grim and said, "Maureen Myers. She's the only one who's available to write protocols. But she has other jobs too, so she hasn't had much time to do the protocols."

Krim just shook her head. She knew Maureen Myers and would later say, "She is not a genius, I assure you." It was not a careless description. Krim had been a bench scientist for many years, a serious laboratory scientist. She had many contacts in the world of science, including at the NIH. She knew from them and from the culture she had spent so many years in, the culture of science, that the best scientists do not become administrators. The best scientists do not become coordinators of programs for other scientists in medical schools around the country. The best scientists stay in the labs, they don't push paper. To Krim, Sam Broder was a *real* scientist. He was always in his lab at the NCI. "Broder is a good scientist," she said again and again.

So Krim asked Fauci, "Well, what do you need in addition to Maureen Myers?" Fauci replied, "I need positions. I need more people to do this work." It was a devastating admission. For years Krim, Congressmen Henry Waxman and Theodore Weiss, and Senator Lowell Weicker had led the battle against David Stockman's OMB for the resources necessary to get AIDS research off the ground. By the end of 1985, after nearly five long years of grueling combat, they had won, or so they thought. The big money was supposed to be available. Now Krim was hearing from the man in charge of testing AIDS drugs that money alone wasn't enough. Money, it seemed, couldn't buy people. People were in a separate budget, Fauci told Krim, who wondered why Fauci hadn't mentioned this months ago. Krim couldn't understand why this man didn't make his needs known so that Congress could try to get the right kind of resources for him. Krim even wondered if Fauci, in fact, even knew what he needed, much less how to get it.

As these questions buzzed in the air, Krim turned to Fauci and said, simply, "Fine." On the plane home she plotted strategy. Krim knew that Weicker, the liberal Republican senator from Connecticut, was the key in any bid for new resources to help AIDS research. He could add an amendment to the appropriations bill. If anybody knew anything about this position business it was Weicker.

But Krim did not know Weicker that well personally. She needed a go-between and she knew just the person, a friend of hers. Richmond Crinkley was a Broadway producer, with *Elephant Man* to his credit. He was a southerner and a deeply conservative Republican. A hawk on defense and foreign policy, Crinkley wrote for the conservative *National Review*. He was able to move in both the conservative and liberal Republican worlds of Washington and he knew just about everybody.

Crinkley's conservatism allowed him to understand the Reagan era far better than nearly all gay advocates. The gay lobbyists assumed from the beginning of the AIDS epidemic that homophobia lay behind the Reagan administration's tremendous reluctance to provide new funds to fight the disease.

Crinkley, however, knew that another prejudice was at work, a bias even more powerful than hating gays: hating big government. Crinkley understood that the OMB was the instrument of Ronald Reagan's promise to cut back all forms of government bureaucracy in the lives of the American people. The health system, with its enormous waste and constantly rising costs, was just a part of the overall bureaucratic system the administration was out to trim. Homophobia took second place in the motivation to make sure health care costs were capped.

In part, Crinkley understood what was really going on in Washington because he believed in the administration's anti-big-government goals. But he also understood the internal workings of the capital city. He listened when others were shouting. He was a quick study, and he got the details right. Crinkley also knew which levers to pull. He moved quietly behind the scenes.

He learned that there was one budget for research money and a separate budget for FTEs, Full-Time Equivalent job positions. He knew that lobbing dollars over to the NIH would not produce the lab assistants or protocol writers needed to actually use the facilities the research money bought. No one else realized that.

Krim called Crinkley and told him the situation with Fauci at NIAID.

She asked if he would intercede with Weicker. He agreed and went over to the senator's office and asked for help. Weicker said he would try but getting FTEs was really tough. And why hadn't Fauci spoken up before about his need for more staff? In the end, Weicker was able to shoehorn in five more FTEs for Fauci. It wasn't very many, but it was better than just one person writing all the protocols.

Weicker's same supplemental bill contained one other piece of Crinkley's handiwork. During the spring of 1986, Maureen Myers was trying to line up sites for the new NIAID clinical network. By late spring, she had preselected twenty-five qualified medical institutions. But NIAID could not fund all of them. If Myers had more money, she could get more institutions to join in and thereby get AIDS drug testing off the ground that much faster. Krim heard about this problem and turned to Crinkley again to intervene with Weicker. The senator came through, getting the additional money that made it possible to pick all twenty-five qualified testing sites.

After this flurry of lobbying, Krim relaxed and waited for results. After all, Fauci now had more money and more people, but it would take time. Before giving the preselected sites new drugs to test, NIAID had to come up with the drugs. As a result of Fauci and DeVita's 1985 concordat that divided AIDS research between NIAID and the NCI, the initial in vitro testing of nearly all compounds first had to go through Sam Broder's lab. Those drugs that Broder deemed promising were then sent on to NIAID. NIAID then had its own committee, the AIDS Clinical Drug Development Committee (ACDDC), make recommendations of its own on what it considered promising.

Once the ACDDC made its choices, applications for Investigational New Drugs, or INDs, from the FDA would have to be filed. That took time because the FDA had been hit hard by the Reagan administration cuts and was chronically understaffed.

Krim knew the process well and was patient. But by the beginning of 1987, she became worried once again. There was still nothing coming out of the new trial system. So she called up Fauci and said, "What the hell is happening now? Didn't you hire those five guys that you were authorized to get?" Fauci said, "I couldn't. I now have the FTEs, but I don't have the space, the desks, where to put them." Fauci complained to Krim that his institute, NIAID, was different from the NCI. NIAID didn't have the authorization to rent, build, or remodel space or even to buy desks. Furnishing, he went on, is part of yet another budget.

Krim couldn't believe her ears. Not only was the Byzantine Washington authorization process unbelievable, but Fauci's inability or unwillingness to tell anyone what he needed was inexcusable. People with AIDS were dying every day while this new program stagnated because there was no desk space!

Fauci's bad news wasn't over, either. He admitted to Krim that "Maureen and I were so busy that we didn't have time to interview candidates for those new jobs," the five FTEs that Krim, Crinkley, and Weicker had squeezed out of the OMB. Years later Krim would grow incensed just remembering these events. There was such an atmosphere of unreality and disbelief to what Fauci did and didn't do at that time that Krim would have to punctuate her recounting of the tale with a steady stream of "Ya. That was real. That really happened, you know." Two years later, in 1988, Fauci would be forced to admit to all of this in public hearings that set off a fire storm in the gay community.

Tony Fauci needed help fast. His first big effort as NIAID director was going nowhere. After spending an entire year building a multicenter drug-testing network from the ground up, it was clear to him and to the growing chorus of critics outside the NIH that NIAID's attempt was in shambles. The PIs were furious about the tight control NIAID had put on their research. Protocol writing was an incoherent mess. Sometimes Maureen Myers wrote them, sometimes the investigators wrote them. No one knew who should write them.

When they did write the protocols, PIs had to wait months before hearing back from NIAID. Several complained that they never received a response. Communication between the field and the control center, between line and staff, were tattered at best. Congressmen Waxman and Weiss were getting increasingly angry at the ineffective way the money they had fought long and hard for was being spent. Worst of all, not a single drug to treat AIDS had come out of the government system.

In a preemptive move to salvage his reputation as an administrator, Fauci turned to the organization he had fought with for the privilege of setting up a clinical trials network in the first place—Vincent DeVita's National Cancer Institute. The irony was not lost in the corridors of the NIH.

With DeVita's consent, and Sam Broder's enthusiastic encouragement,

Fauci asked Dan Hoth, an NCI administrator who was familiar with its large extramural clinical drug trial program, to come over to NIAID. His job was to put together an advisory committee to analyze the NIAID system and recommend changes. Fauci was also secretly talking with Hoth at this time about changing institutes permanently and taking over the entire AIDS Program at NIAID. That meant replacing John LaMontagne with Hoth. Neither LaMontagne nor Maureen Myers knew this.

Hoth was very different from LaMontagne. He thrived on crisis management. He was hard-driving, tough, and commanding. He had already proved himself as a successful administrator of big, complex clinical trials at the NCI. He was also involved with AZT.

In Hoth's dynamism and success as a manager, Fauci found what he hoped was a clear reflection of his own personality. With his reputation cresting like a wave before him, Hoth washed ashore at NIAID to take charge. He set up the Ad Hoc Advisory Group for the AIDS Clinical Trials Program of the Treatment Branch of NIAID's AIDS Program. Among the very first members he appointed to this group were the PIs who were complaining the loudest against the contract system.

That included Dr. Thomas Merigan, principal investigator at the Stanford University School of Medicine, who was one of the earliest and most vocal critics of the contract system. It also included Dr. Jerome Groopman, a PI from the Harvard Medical School. Groopman was part of an even larger Boston grouping of four institutions doing AIDS research headed by Martin Hirsch. Groopman, however, rarely came to the meetings. Also included in the Ad Hoc Advisory Group were the following doctors, most of whom were also PIs: Robert Couch, chairman of the Baylor College of Medicine in Houston, Texas; James Bilstad of the FDA; Charles Carpenter of Brown University in Providence, Rhode Island; Thomas Fleming of the Fred Hutchinson Cancer Research Center in Seattle, Washington; William Friedewald of the NIH; Stephen Sherwin from Genentech, Inc., in South San Francisco; and Richard Whitley of the University of Alabama, Birmingham School of Medicine, in Birmingham, Alabama. Three special consultants joined the group to do on-site examinations of the NIAID system: Judith O'Fallon of the Mayo Clinic in Rochester, Minnesota; Brent Blumenstein of the Fred Hutchinson Cancer Research Center; and Anastasias Tsiatis of the Dana-Farber Cancer Institute in Boston.

Hoth really liked the PIs out in the field. He respected them and they reciprocated the admiration. At the NCI, Hoth felt that great progress had

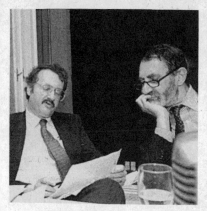

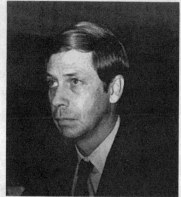

"Mr. AZT," Dr. Samuel Broder (left), director of the National Cancer Institute, persuaded Burroughs Wellcome it could profit from AIDS. Dr. Joseph Sonnabend pioneered community-based medical research; he hated AZT. (© Jane Rosett)

The "Puppet Master," the suave and sophisticated Dr. David Barry, played the drug-development game perfectly for Burroughs Wellcome; he made all the right behind-the-scenes deals with the FDA for AZT. (© Jane Rosett)

Known locally as the "spaceship," the corporate headquarters and research laboratories of Burroughs Wellcome sit conspicuously in the green rolling hills of North Carolina near Raleigh and Durham. It is a U.S. subsidiary of a British charitable foundation that recently sold twenty-five percent of its stock to the public.

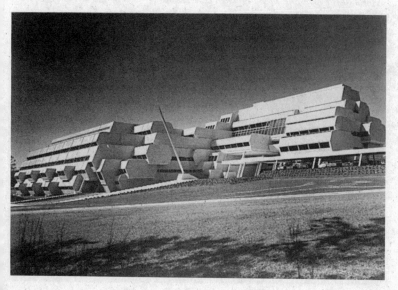

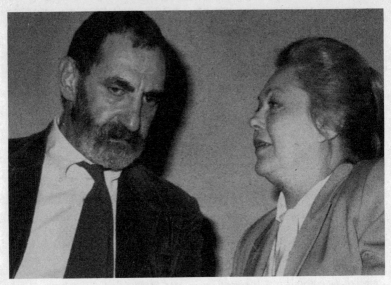

*Joe Sonnabend and Mathilde Krim: the eccentric genius and the powerful socialite PhD. They were a perfect match for a new disease, AIDS. She dumped him for Elizabeth Taylor and Hollywood millions for AIDS research.* (© Jane Rosett)

*Left to right: Marty Delaney of Project Inform in San Francisco fought for major reform at the FDA and then launched a secret test of "Compound Q"; Dr. Barry Gingell put out the word on alternative drugs for PWAs at the Gay Men's Health Crisis; John James launched the* Aids Treatment News, *the Farmer's Almanac of the underground drug movement.* (© Jane Rosett)

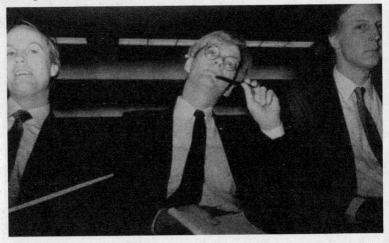

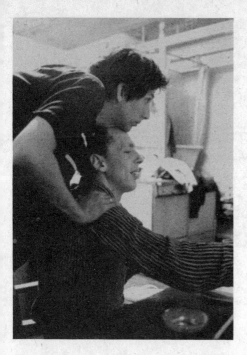

*Michael Callen fought the NIH and AIDS at the same time for the same reason — to survive. Diagnosed with AIDS in 1982, Callen was given six months to live. Callen has never used AZT and is a long-term survivor. Richard Dworkin (seated) is Callen's co-author and lover.* (© Jane Rosett)

*One of the first doctors to detect AIDS in 1981, Donald Abrams helped set up the County Community Consortium in San Francisco, which, along with the Community Research Initiative in New York, successfully tested the anti-pneumonia drug aerosol pentamidine.* (© Jane Rosett)

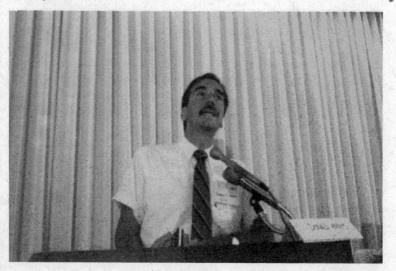

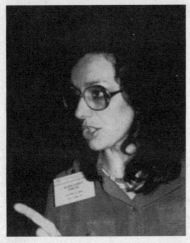

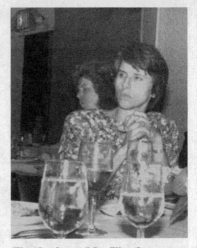

Dr. Margaret Fischl is a key member of the "Old Boy's Club" of principal investigators who dominate AIDS research: she was the chief PI on the Phase II clinical trial of AZT and chaired the NIH committee that refused government funding for the CRI. (© Jane Rosett)

The "Ice Queen," Dr. Ellen Cooper, was the youngest head of the FDA's Division of Antiviral Drug Products. The scientific method was her religion but she was willing to cut pragmatic deals on AZT with Wellcome's David Barry. (© Jane Rosett)

*Left to right: Sam Broder was the consummate eighties AIDS scientist — it was his career-making disease; Joe Sonnabend never valued Broder and his fascination with AZT; Dr. Anthony Fauci spent $1 billion of the taxpayers' money and didn't produce a single new anti-AIDS drug. (© Jane Rosett)*

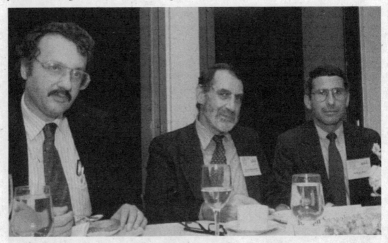

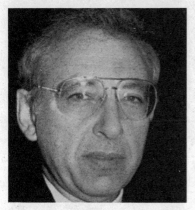

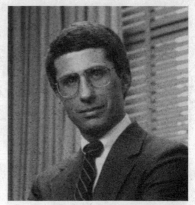

The sneering and dismissive Dr. Robert Gallo discovered the first human retrovirus and may or may not have found the AIDS virus; the NIH is investigating charges that the French discovered the AIDS virus first. While some scientists at the NIH refused to cooperate with Gallo, Sam Broder made it his business to help the powerful figure. (© Jane Rosett)

Tony Fauci wrestled AIDS research away from the huge National Cancer Institute for his small National Institute for Allergies and Infectious Diseases. He wasn't a details man. Fauci was more of a "hit the front pages every day" kind of guy, according to the people who worked for him.

Brought in by Tony Fauci to rescue his flagging AIDS program, Dan Hoth turned it over to the principal investigators, especially those scientists connected with Burroughs Wellcome's AZT.

Maureen Myers single-handedly tried to put together the government's first AIDS clinical trial network without much resource support from her boss, Tony Fauci. In the end, her efforts failed, Dan Hoth took over, and a year of anti-AIDS research work went down the drain. (© Brooks)

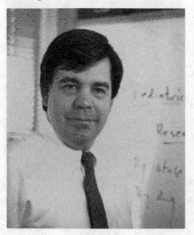

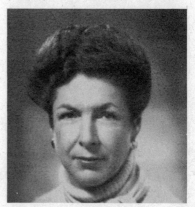

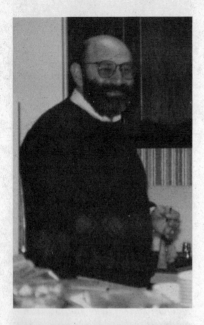

*Left: The brilliant Arnold Lippa was a man whose scientific visions were unmatched by managerial excellence. He got AL 721 tested to show it was safe. He persuaded the famous Robert Gallo to test the drug and show it was effective against AIDS in the test tube. But Lippa wasn't "wired" into the FDA-NIH establishment, and in the end AL 721 fell by the wayside, unproven as an antiviral.*

*Below left: Dr. Bernard Bihari gave AL 721 to a New York City politician with AIDS who then improved; Bihari now runs the Community Research Initiative in New York.* (© Jane Rosett)

*The AIDS drug underground, based on a nationwide network of buyers clubs, began with bootleg AL 721.* (© Jane Rosett)

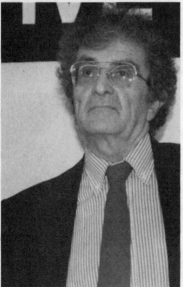

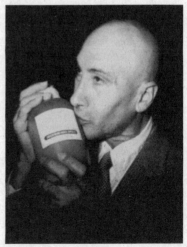

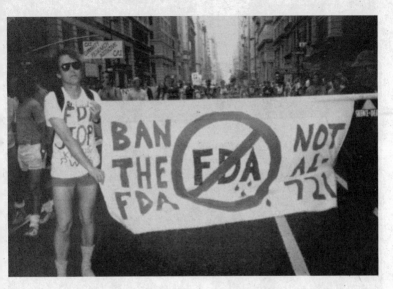

*A People With AIDS protest against the FDA during the 1988 Gay Pride Parade in New York.* (© Jane Rosett)

*A 1987 ACT UP demonstration against Memorial Sloan-Kettering Cancer Institute protests the failure to test drugs that fight the opportunistic infections killing people with AIDS.* (© Jane Rosett)

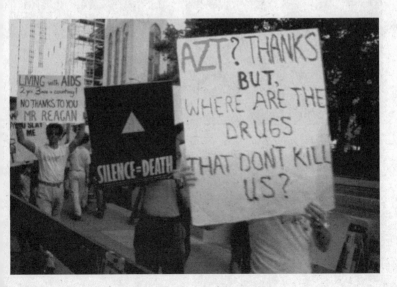

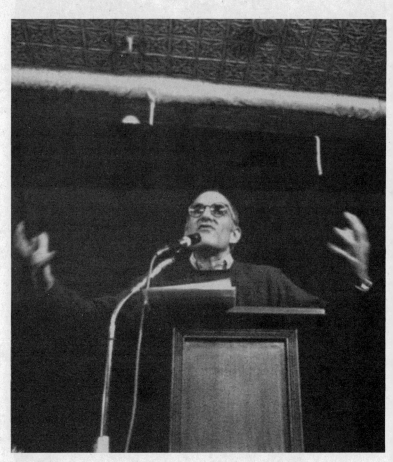

*Larry Kramer, his furies in full force, blasts the NIH and the FDA in a 1987 speech that led to the creation of ACT UP.* (© Jane Rosett)

been made against cancer using the traditional NIH approach of financing investigator-initiated research. The decentralized method, which put the investigators in control, had led to healthy competition and the creation of dozens of new chemotherapies over the years. To Hoth, it was an approach that worked.

The first meeting of the Ad Hoc Advisory Group took place in room 4A48 of Building 31 on July 7, 1987. It discussed the background and current status of the NIAID AIDS Program, including relations with pharmaceutical companies, selection of drugs to test, and the institute's control of clinical trial efforts. This later discussion included a talk titled "Directive vs. Laissez-Faire Approach" and was a critique of Myers's contract system.

As if to emphasize that point, a second discussion, called "Public Health vs. Academic Priorities," was also held. It highlighted the paradox that the two are not synonymous. Right after the third meeting, held on September 11, Hoth officially replaced LaMontagne as director of NIAID's AIDS Program. Maureen Myers had a new boss.

Nearly all of the information about problems in the NIAID trial system had come from Myers. She briefed Hoth and the five or six other members who regularly attended the meetings. After receiving a full blast of wrath from PIs around the country, Myers was anxious to put the contract system behind her. On paper it may have been the fastest, most efficient method of getting AIDS drugs tested, but the reality, she had learned, was very different. Without the support of the investigators in the field, nothing could be done.

Hoth couldn't agree more. Official publication of the "Report of the AIDS Clinical Trials Advisory Group" came in December 1987, but its recommendations to NIAID were known by early November. One of the first was that "the Program should effect the transition from contract-oriented individual institutions to a Cooperative Group," which would be a network of "highly interactive, collaborating investigators and institutions." It would be this new group of PIs that would set priorities and evaluate which were the most promising drug therapies for AIDS. Protocols would be developed by this group of PIs, with input from the NIAID staff.

In effect, Hoth shifted the basis of financing and control from NIAID to the PIs in the field. The contract system was replaced by a form of grant process. A cooperative agreement made NIAID a partner, a junior partner at that, with the investigators. The institute was no longer in a position to tell the PIs what to do. They were calling the shots, as they were used to in the past. Now the investigators would be able to do the kind of research on AIDS that would help them with their own careers. They would be able to do the type of science that led to papers that could be published under their own names in prestigious journals, the type of science that made reputations as well as drugs, the type of science that won Nobel Prizes.

To make the point succinctly clear, the report states that "most ideas for trials should be investigator-initiated. The investigators should develop a scientific agenda, set priorities for trials, initiate development of protocols and make most decisions regarding the ongoing conduct of studies." This was the kind of research the PIs could buy into, could support. Hoth had brought them back, their support was now assured, and NIAID had an operating AIDS Program again. Along the way, Tony Fauci's reputation was saved by this expatriate from the NCI. But Tony Fauci's managerial incompetence had exacted a staggering cost. By 1987, more than a million Americans were infected by the AIDS virus. Not a single drug treatment had come out of the government's enormous biomedical research system. In the end, Fauci barely survived by handing over control of the government's only AIDS drug trial program to a handful of PIs with close ties to Burroughs Wellcome and AZT.

Dan Hoth knew exactly what he had to do. First he renamed the NIAID trial network the ACTG, or AIDS Clinical Trials Group, to show everyone that things had changed as a result of his arrival. The new name also emphasized the "Group," or cooperative/grant, approach over the old contract system. Second, he asked for a lot more people to help Maureen Myers out and for a lot more space to do it in. But he did it the Reagan administration way—through renting, not hiring, people and space.

Hoth pushed NIAID to make a contract with a local Bethesda company to provide operations office support. This outside firm, Social and Scientific Systems Inc., helped out by providing people who were protocol specialists. They worked with the investigators in the field and the administrators at NIAID to make sure everything kept moving along. They typed the protocols, distributed copies, made conference calls, and kept minutes of meetings. The company also provided regulatory support. It also had responsibility for giving lots of logistical support to the ACDDC, the AIDS Clinical Drug Development Committee, the gateway for all new drugs entering the ACTG system, including those that came out of Sam Broder's lab over at the NCI. That committee needed enormous support in keeping files on companies, drugs, reviews, everything.

What was especially nice about Social and Scientific Systems was that it was practically next door to the new office space Hoth had rented for the NIAID AIDS Program, two miles off the NIH campus in an older Control Data building on Executive Boulevard. The physical distance made Tony Fauci's isolation from the AIDS Program practically complete. The AIDS Program that was basically re-created by Dan Hoth was now virtually run by Dan Hoth.

The extra logistical support from the consulting firm was a "present" that Hoth gave to the PIs. "We made a lot of promises to the field," says one NIAID official present at that time. "We promised them protocol specialists who were about to come to their rescue. None of them were hired yet. None of them trained. But it sounded great. We sold this idea hook, line, and sinker to the investigators. It was obviously Dan's official entrance into the group, and I think it was very effectively handled."


Tony Fauci never appeared to have much interest in running NIAID's clinical trial system. After its collapse and rescue by Dan Hoth, Fauci had almost no involvement in it at all. He was only too happy to hand the AIDS Program over if it meant saving his directorship. The management of the government's entire drug-testing system was dropped in Hoth's lap.

When Hoth was finished, the principal investigators were in firm control. Hoth used the scientists in the field to establish his own regime at NIAID, and they had used him to take virtual control of the government's AIDS drug evaluation program.

That happened quickly. Dr. Thomas Merigan, out of Stanford, led the way. He was warmly welcomed by another non-NIAID outsider, Dan Hoth. The real power in the NIAID trial network devolved to the committee system, controlled by the PIs. The committees met every three months. Once most of the trials had been set up, the ACTG then met once every four months. The number of hospital evaluation sites for AIDS drugs grew through 1987 and '88 until it reached a total of thirty-six, each with its own PI.

The PIs and their staffs flew in to Bethesda, Maryland, from all the major teaching hospitals and biomedical centers around the country. By the middle of 1989, that meant over eight hundred people gathering every quarter. The meetings were never open to the public or the press.

After leading the PI revolt, Tom Merigan became chair of the Primary Infection Committee, the core committee of the ACTG. All the drug trials that received priority at NIAID came up through Primary Infection. Merigan, according to the other PIs in the Primary Infection Committee, was a masterful politician. "You have to keep your eyes open when you deal with Tom," says one. The other PIs on the thirty-five member committee included Donna Mildvan, Martin Hirsch, Douglas Richman, Michael Grieco, and Margaret Fischl.

Fischl, Hirsch, Grieco, Richman, and Mildvan were also among the many PIs that were part of the Burroughs Wellcome clinical trials network for AZT. They were, of course, compensated to do the trials. In the end, all of Wellcome's AZT principal investigators joined the ACTG clinical trials network. The PIs that had run the AZT trials under Wellcome also began running trials, mostly using AZT, for the ACTG.

They soon began to run the ACTG. Fischl, Hirsch, and Paul Volberding from San Francisco General Hospital were on the ACTG Executive Committee, overseeing the entire committee system. Fischl was on a total of four committees, including Oncology, Opportunistic Infection, and Primary Infection. Michael Grieco was on three committees—Primary Infection, Neurology, and Virology.

Martin Hirsch served on the Primary Committee as well as the ACDDC, the AIDS Clinical Drug Development Committee that determined which drugs would get tested in the ACTG system. When AL 721 came up for review on February 26, 1987, PIs who had run trials on AZT, whose entire careers were wrapped up in AZT, would vote low priority for AL 721—in effect, no trial for the drug. When Tony Fauci insisted that a small trial be done just to "debunk" the drug and refute the tens of thousands of PWAs using lipids as treatment, Donna Mildvan did it. No one saw any problem with conflict of interest. They were, after all, scientists, and how could scientists have a conflict of interest? They were interested only in the Truth.

Practically all the trials to emanate from the Primary Infection Committee that received priority involved AZT or other nucleoside analogs. The most important were trials 016 and 019. Trial 016 measured AZT against patients with ARC, the earliest and weakest symptoms of AIDS, to see if the drug slowed progression to full-blown AIDS. But the most important trial was clearly 019, the one designed to see whether AZT curbed the progression of the disease in people who were infected with the AIDS virus but were asymptomatic. They were all still healthy. This was the big one; several thousand people were going to be enrolled in it.

The Opportunistic Infection Committee, or OI, was fated to have few trials in general, fewer priority trials, and a general history of not doing very much. The PIs were simply not interested in doing research on *Pneumocystis,* or CMV, or any of the actual diseases that killed people with AIDS. These infections didn't have the glamour of viral research. They were mundane. No Nobels were to be won running tests on these infections, even if they were the most important tests to be run from the point of view of the PWAs and their doctors.

Power within Dan Hoth's ACTG system resided in PIs who ran AZT trials, especially those who had run the original Burroughs Wellcome AZT Phase II study. They were a cohesive group, and they rode AZT to fame. They linked the private pharmaceutical industry to the government. They worked for both, were tied to both, and had tremendous influence in both. Yet they were, in effect, accountable to no one except themselves. They were invisible to the public eye. And they had a lock on the most important decision-making gateways in the government's fight against AIDS. The group may have included several powerful "girls," but it was a proverbial old-boy network.

Where was Tony in all of this? Two miles down the road, trying to be a "hit-the-front-pages" kind of guy.

It was 1988 by the time Dan Hoth and the PIs established their reign. And still *nothing* was coming out of the government to treat AIDS.

By this time, several hundred million tax dollars had somehow disappeared into the nation's biomedical establishment and not one new drug had been produced. Where did it all go? Who benefited? Certainly not the tens of thousands of people with AIDS who grew angrier and angrier with each wasted, passing day.

# ..7..
# An Old-Boy Network

The word went out that the Gang of Twelve was riding again. Burroughs Wellcome was assembling a team of tried-and-true veterans of the drug development wars. A big Phase II trial of a new anti-AIDS drug, AZT, was about to be launched. It was meal-ticket time in the world of biomedical research.

David Barry handled the roundup. He worked the phones, calling a small band of clinical virologists around the country. They were all known to Barry from earlier Wellcome or NIH drug trials. They were the best PIs money could buy.

It took Barry two weeks in early 1986 to put together Wellcome's entire clinical trials system for testing AZT. While Maureen Myers was struggling to launch the government effort, Barry cornered twelve PIs and their hospital sites.

The first person with AIDS to take AZT in the Phase II trial swallowed his pill in early February of 1986. By mid-May, all the trial participants were enrolled. Barry and Wellcome were old pros at this game, in total contrast to Tony Fauci and NIAID.

Originally, 260 people were scheduled to be enrolled. But Sam Broder's Phase I trial at the NIH and Duke taught them that there might be a large attrition as patients dropped out. In the end, 282 patients were enrolled, 145 on AZT and 137 on placebo. There were about 20 patients per medical site.

Wellcome structured the study very rigidly. A dose of AZT consisting of a 250-milligram capsule was administered every four hours, even through the night. There was a lot of discussion between Barry and Broder over which dose to pick. They didn't pick the highest dose given to people in the Phase I safety trial, but it was near the top. That was standard operating procedure for chemotherapy—go for the max to kill the cancer.

Wellcome decided to pick the sickest AIDS patients to test the drug. To be admitted to the trial, one was required to have a T-4 cell count of less than 500 and one recent bout with *Pneumocystis carinii* pneumonia, PCP.

The Phase II was scheduled to end in December of 1986. A Data and Safety Monitoring Board was set up to watch out for the safety of the patients, who were monitored every week for the first month and then every other week.

Since this was a double-blind, placebo-controlled trial, each patient received a code, noting whether he was getting the drug or the placebo. The code was kept secret from both doctors and patients. The entire point of using double-blind trials was to prevent patients from receiving different treatment from doctors, treatment that might affect the outcome of the trial and confuse the results of the test on the drug. Double-blind trials were the heart and soul of science, the proven means for true objectivity, the method for blocking any conscious or unconscious special patient management by the PIs.

Yet within the first month, it became clear to all the investigators which patients were receiving the AZT and which were getting the placebo. People with AIDS began coming down with severe anemias within the first month of the trial, according to Ellen Cooper. It later turned out that nearly half of all AIDS patients receiving AZT required blood transfusions, while only about 5 percent of those on placebo needed them. Many if not most of those being transfused required multiple transfusions. Many had to be taken off AZT for a period of time. A number had to be taken off the drug entirely.

A move to stop the trial began immediately. The toxicity of AZT was proving to be extremely high, much higher than indicated by Sam Broder's previous safety trials. PIs began to worry that AZT was killing bone marrow cells so fast that patients would quickly come down with aplastic anemia, a murderous disease. This was terrifying to many PIs. "There was enormous pressure to stop," recalls Broder. "People said, 'My god, what's going on, we're getting these anemias, what's going on?' We never saw this level of anemia before."

By month number two, Margaret Fischl, the trial's head PI hand-picked by David Barry, came under direct pressure to stop the study. But she resisted. "I think that Margaret and Doug Richman and a few other people were profound heroes of this thing," says Broder, who faced the potential ignominy of being known on the NIH campus as Mr. Suramin, Mr. AZT, and Mr. Anything Else if the Phase II AZT trial failed.

The study became unblinded after just a few weeks, simply because of the transfusions. The doctors were giving the people on AZT more treatment and different treatment than the patients on placebo. Ellen Cooper stands on a technicality in this issue but concedes that "the fact that patients received transfusions, that's something that was clearly known from the management of the patient. That would make an investigator more likely to guess that, well, this patient's more likely to be on AZT than placebo. But it's technically not breaking the blind."

There was also a second source of unblinding. A laboratory result showed who was getting AZT and who was being issued sugar pills. For some reason, the MCV values of the blood taken from patients were not whited out on the forms.

The mean corpuscular volume measures the size of the red blood cell count. People with AIDS, of course, have relatively low MCVs to begin with since the disease attacks the immune system, including the bone marrow that produces red blood cells. Investigators seeing anemias in their transfusion patients were able to go to the MCV counts to track what was happening. By looking at the red blood cell levels directly, the PIs were able to double-check their hunches about who was on placebo and who was on AZT.

Ellen Cooper says that the whiting out of MCV counts was "not routinely done." Sam Broder says it "doesn't matter. Unless what you're saying is that we watched the people who had high MCV and we gave them better treatment. Or that we . . . kept [them] in the study and those with a low MCV we said, 'Get out of the study.' That's an *accusation of fraud,* not bad scientific design. There was no fraud in the study."

Fraud, no. There is no evidence of deliberate fraud in the Wellcome Phase II trial of AZT. Yet the whole purpose of blinding was to keep patient management identical, so that people taking the drug and people taking the placebo would be treated the same. Clearly, knowing the MCV counts reinforced logical hunches drawn by investigators from the sudden and early jump in anemias and transfusions among patients taking AZT. The transfusions themselves produced different patient management.

Was it naive to assume that reading MCV values of patients did not in some way affect PI behavior toward the patients? Or was it naive to think not?

Interestingly enough, when Joe Sonnabend did a research project back in early 1984, he found himself in hot water with the FDA over the very issue of not whiting out figures. The drug being tested, isoprinosine, raises the level of certain blood values. Both Sonnabend and Mathilde Krim, who was the coordinator, believed at that time that whiting out the specific levels was required by the FDA to blind trials properly. Whenever Krim received blood samples from the lab, she obscured the specific levels, photocopied them, and returned them to Sonnabend. He never saw the numbers.

Except for one mistake. The FDA came by and did an audit of what was then an unusual community-based research trial. They audited all of the doctors involved, including Sonnabend. When he received his criticism from the federal drug regulators, they told him that there was a "slip-up in one patient and one value which escaped Dr. Krim," according to Sonnabend. "So the offending thing came to me. The FDA noted it and told me." After that, Sonnabend made sure all the blood values were properly whited out. Presumably the FDA had another set of standards for the AZT test.

While Phase II was progressing, Barry and the FDA's Ellen Cooper began a repeat performance of their earlier tête-à-tête in Atlanta. This time the negotiations revolved around what minimum scientific data would be needed for Wellcome to get an NDA, a New Drug Application, from the FDA. While an IND merely permits a company to test a drug in humans for safety, an NDA allows it to sell the drug on the commercial market for a profit.

Barry knew the trick was to show a decent "risk/benefit ratio." The company and the regulator had to establish that AZT worked to some degree, but without generating a level of toxicity that would harm people. David Barry and Ellen Cooper hunkered down to haggle.

The Phase II trial of AZT was scheduled to last until December, but the mortality figures changed that.

In early August, there were only two deaths, both patients receiving the placebo. By the end of the month, seven people were dead, all on placebo. By September 5, nine people with AIDS receiving placebo pills had died.

On September 10, 1986, Sam Broder was attending a Cold Spring Harbor Symposium on Long Island. He remembers it because it was a critical conference in the history of AIDS. The Cold Spring Harbor Laboratory itself had a grand scientific tradition and was run at the time by none other than James Watson, renowned for breaking the code of the double helix, the structure of DNA.

Tony Fauci was supposed to give a speech at the symposium, but he didn't show up. Broder asked around and found out that Fauci had been summoned back to Washington. "I thought, what issue could be summoning Tony home?" Broder recalls. "Something was brewing. One possibility was that the study was being stopped because of toxicity."

How wrong he was. On September 10, the Data and Safety Monitoring Board met. It was a very unusual meeting. FDA Commissioner Frank E. Young attended. No one could remember ever seeing an FDA commissioner at one of these things.

Young served at the pleasure of the president; he was an appointed member of the FDA. Young's immediate boss was Robert Windom, assistant secretary for health and head of the Public Health Service, to which the FDA and the NIH both belonged. Windom was a political appointee of the White House.

Young's presence immediately politicized the entire proceedings. AIDS activists were boiling over with anger at the Reagan administration's failure to help them. The pressure was on. Young's presence registered a subtle pressure on the people there to vote for early termination of the AZT trial, releasing the drug to the public. Young never actually requested it, but he didn't really have to.

By that time, eleven people, all receiving the placebo, were dead. In contrast, only one person getting AZT had died. The numbers were a shock to the members of the board. *Nothing* could be that good. Something had to be wrong. They decided to take another poll in about a week and told Burroughs Wellcome to check over all the details of the trial to make sure nothing was amiss. Commissioner Young, however, was delighted with the numbers.

On September 18, the board met for the second time. Commissioner Young went to this meeting also. By this time, sixteen patients getting the placebo were dead. The data was even more positive. The board voted that the study be stopped and AZT be given to all those patients currently on placebo. The next day, September 19, 1986, with three more placebo patients dead, the board broke the code to show the doctors which patients had been getting the drug and which had been receiving the placebo. By that time, of course, the doctors already knew that information. The Phase II trial of AZT was officially terminated early after only sixteen weeks instead of the original target of twenty-four.

The Reagan administration then stepped in to grease the regulatory wheels for Burroughs Wellcome and AZT. It was an extraordinary effort never to be repeated for any other anti-AIDS drug.

On September 18, it was clear to David Barry, Sam Broder, Tony Fauci, Ellen Cooper, and the PIs that the trial was going to be stopped. Now they were going to be under enormous pressure to get AZT out to everyone with AIDS: "People were dying," Barry explains. "By the hundreds. Per month."

FDA Commissioner Young took an active part in the discussions that day. All of the participants met to talk about getting the drug out as fast as possible. They agreed that the way to go was to get a Treatment IND, a conditional release, from the FDA. Barry had worked at the FDA long enough to know that it would take months for Wellcome to gather the trial data and negotiate terms for an NDA, permitting him to sell AZT on the open market. In the interim, they had to do something fast to get the drug out. He quietly asked Ellen Cooper whether a Treatment IND would be possible. She quietly said yes.

While an IND authorizes safety tests in a small number of human beings, a Treatment IND permits the widespread use of drugs that have been proven safe and possibly effective but not yet fully approved by the FDA.

Commissioner Young said he was very much in favor of doing anything to get AZT out fast. Granting a Treatment IND for AZT was a great idea. Young said he would make all of his staff available at any time to get it through the FDA as fast as possible. No HHS commissioner had ever personally committed himself to doing that kind of thing before. It was clear to everyone that Young was going to ease the way for Wellcome to get through the regulatory process. It was also clear that Young was acting for the Reagan administration. Barry knew this. He knew it was very unusual for a commissioner to behave in this manner. "It was because he wanted to make sure personally that there was no bureaucratic impediment to reviewing the AZT data," says Barry.

Frank Young was a very happy man at this point. Finally, he could get the White House off the hook by providing proof for the American public that the government was actually doing something about the AIDS epidemic. People with the disease didn't have to fly off to Paris anymore to receive treatment with HPA-23. Ever since Rock Hudson went to the Pasteur Institute for treatment, it had been a constant humiliation to the Reagan administration that America couldn't even treat its own people. Now things were different. The United States had its own drug: AZT. Young had delivered, both scientifically and politically.

So on September 19, Robert Windom, assistant secretary for health, stepped in front of a room packed with press at the Department of Health and Human Services and announced the "exciting" results of the AZT tests. He said that "treatment with azidothymidine prolongs survival of persons with AIDS." It holds "great promise for prolonging life for certain patients with AIDS."

It was a great political show. Everyone there believed it was significant that the press conference didn't occur at Burroughs Wellcome's headquarters down in North Carolina or over at the NIH in Bethesda. The government was determined to show that *it* was responsible for a treatment for AIDS. The platform was packed with so many politicos from the Reagan administration that at one time it looked as if the scientists wouldn't be able to get up on stage.

Windom then said he had personally asked the Food and Drug Administration to speed up the regulatory approval for commercial sale of the drug. He wasn't making it a secret that the White House wanted the FDA to cut corners to get AZT out.

Windom said that a toll-free hotline had been set up to provide information to patients and doctors about getting AZT. Burroughs Wellcome promised to provide the drug free to all people with AIDS who had suffered at least one bout of PCP. This would last until the FDA reviewed the data on AZT and gave Wellcome permission to sell the drug. Within days, that hotline, open seven days a week, from 8:00 A.M. to midnight, was handling fifty phone calls an hour.

But first there was a technicality. Wellcome had to officially request and receive its Treatment IND. The trouble was, no one could remember ever dealing with a Treatment IND. It was on the books but rarely if ever used. The FDA bureaucracy was infamous for taking years to grant drug approvals, not speeding them up. No one knew how.

At that time, Sam Broder stepped forward and told Barry, "Look, I've got a guy here at the NCI who's been very good at distributing Schedule C drugs, which is sort of like distributing drugs under Treatment IND. His name is Dan Hoth."

This was right before Hoth took over Tony Fauci's faltering AIDS Program and saved Fauci's skin. At that time Hoth was in charge of the NCI program that gave out cancer drugs proved safe and probably effective but not yet fully approved by the FDA. "Let me send this guy over to you and see if he can be of help," said Broder.

Hoth dropped by and, like Broder, turned out to be a terribly enthusiastic person. Barry and a group from Wellcome had already had one meeting with the FDA on getting a Treatment IND and said they would like any help they could get. Barry and his crew flew up for a second meeting and stayed at the Hyatt Regency in Bethesda, close to the NIH and the FDA. There were ten of them that morning. Just as they moved up to the desk to register, Dan Hoth arrived. "We literally started working while we were waiting on line to check in," says Barry.

Barry broke the people into several groups. Hoth went with Barry, Dannie King, and a few others "so that we could work out the chapter-and-verse details on how a Treatment IND would work," says Barry. Hoth proceeded to tell Barry how Wellcome could set up a phone board within twenty-four hours to receive calls from doctors asking for AZT. He suggested that Wellcome hire moonlighting NIH physicians to staff the phones. Hoth had done this before at the NCI and knew which doctors needed the money.

Taking Barry aside, Hoth told him that he knew a private contractor, Biospherics, that could set up the whole thing, the entire infrastructure required by the FDA. "We stayed up a good part of that night working out the details," recalls Barry. "By the next day, we had it worked out."

Then it very nearly collapsed because of Ronald Reagan. Barry presented the proposal worked out the night before to Ellen Cooper and Frank Young. Unbeknownst to him, Young, the good soldier, passed it on to Robert Windom who passed it on up to Dr. Otis Bowen, secretary of the Department of Health and Human Services. Bowen was a pure political appointee straight from the White House. He passed the idea on to the president's domestic advisers.

Cooper liked the proposal. Young loved the proposal. So it was okay with the FDA. But the day before the Treatment IND was supposed to be announced, Barry was told that "senior staff" didn't like the plan, because it put the government—the Reagan administration to be exact—in the position of making life-and-death decisions. Since only a limited amount of AZT would be available at first, only the sickest people would get it. Yet there were already many people calling around Congress and the White House asking for favors, asking for access to AZT. There was tremendous political pressure on the administration. Reagan's staff didn't want the president to get blamed for anyone's dying for lack of the drug. "The government just didn't want to be in a position of denying AZT to someone who might need it," says Barry. "They didn't want all of the political fallout that might ensue."

It took twenty-four hours to turn the White House around. Not until an hour before the scheduled press announcement was the Treatment IND cleared by Reagan's staff. Nothing was changed; it was the same Treatment IND plan agreed upon by Hoth and Barry and the FDA. It was just that someone upstairs, perhaps domestic policy adviser Gary Bauer, had found the courage to sign off.

Everyone was jubilant. There was AIDS treatment at last. There was hope. The gay community was ecstatic. The politicians waxed eloquent. Lowell T. Harmison, deputy assistant secretary for health at the HHS, said: "The interaction between industry and public health agencies had produced a drug." It was "the way the capitalist system is supposed to work."

Wellcome's David Barry was prompted to remember what George Hitchings, one of the greats in science, a Wellcome employee and a soon-to-be Nobel Prize winner, had once said: "Work on what is scientifically and medically important. What is profitable often is in the hands of the gods." Indeed.

Sam Broder piped up with nice words for Burroughs Wellcome: "People should appreciate the risk they took. If the drug had harmed people, Burroughs would have been criticized. It was a risk. But they understood that when dealing with a fatal disease, you must take a risk because the ultimate risk is doing nothing."

Forgotten in all the hoopla were the mortality rates. It took a week to organize the movement of all the placebo patients off the sugar pills and onto AZT. In that week, four more people taking the placebo died. But two patients taking AZT also died. It was a dramatic change that would be lost in the shuffle. The statistics on mortality had begun to change.

When the trial was officially terminated on September 19, only one patient taking AZT and nineteen on placebo were dead. A week later, three people on AZT had died versus twenty-three on placebo. The ratio of 19 to 1 had become 23 to 3. Had the trial continued for another week or month, the numbers might have turned out to show something very different from what was announced. The new figures just might have suggested that AZT's effectiveness against the AIDS virus would begin to decline after only three months in severely ill patients taking 1,200–1,500 milligrams a day. Perhaps as researchers would later suggest, resistance to AZT might develop in just a few months.

But this was not the time to consider these facts in the gay community. As might be expected, there was almost a Mardi Gras atmosphere. After seven long years of waiting, there was at least promise of life. After watching so many loved ones die, a drug was now available.

But what kind of drug? Lost in the frenzy of joy was the fact that nearly half the patients taking AZT in the trial had to receive blood transfusions because of damage to their bone marrow and immune systems. Many simply had to stop taking the drug, for a time or permanently. It was unclear how long the benefit conferred by AZT lasted; unsettling questions about a short efficacy period were ignored. Only the most severely ill AIDS patients appeared to benefit. Finally, AZT was not a cure. It didn't kill the AIDS virus in the body. It was only a modest treatment, at best. In fact, AZT was actually a mediocre drug all dressed up by the White House, by the NIH, by the PIs, and, of course, by Burroughs Wellcome as a "miracle drug."

Later Jeff Levi, executive director of the National Gay and Lesbian Task Force, a major gay lobbying effort in Washington, would caution people that "this drug shouldn't be oversold. It's not a cure. We are concerned because people are very nervous, panicked, and they may pressure their physicians into prescribing this drug when it's not appropriate."

But Levi's words were lost in the euphoria. No one asked the basic question: How much time did AZT buy for people with AIDS? Was it a cure? No. Did it keep people with AIDS alive five years longer, ten years, five months, ten months? And what about all those blood transfusions, all those PWAs who couldn't stand being on AZT because of its toxicity?

David Barry flew up to Washington to talk with Ellen Cooper many times over the next six months. When he wasn't on an airplane, he was on the phone.

After the breaking of the code in September and the granting of the

Treatment IND, Wellcome still had to submit yet another series of forms to the FDA for a New Drug Application that would allow the company to sell AZT commercially.

A lot more data was required for the NDA than was needed to get the IND for Sam Broder's small safety trial, but the process was essentially the same. Barry negotiated with Cooper over the minimum kinds of data and the categories of data that she would allow under the circumstances. This time, FDA Commissioner Frank Young sat in on a number of meetings. His purpose was made very clear. He wanted his staff to do everything possible to speed up approval of the NDA. Ellen Cooper, of course, realized this as she negotiated with Barry through the long fall and winter months.

In the end, a deal was made between the FDA and Burroughs Wellcome. Barry would send data to Cooper piecemeal as the company gathered the information from the twelve AZT trial sites, collated it, and analyzed it. This was just like the earlier deal and was designed to speed up approval.

Most important of all, Barry was able to negotiate a lower amount of required data. This was critical. Barry played hardball on the data and he knew he was negotiating from strength. Both Cooper and Young wanted AZT to succeed so much that they agreed to lower standards. "There's no question that the amount of data we had for this New Drug Application was *less* than the amount of data for most New Drug Applications," says Barry. "We had only one clinical study. We had a lot of unanswered questions about such subtleties as lower doses, etc."

Commissioner Young and Cooper had one final hurdle. They had to get the deal for diminished data through the FDA's Anti-Infective Drugs Advisory Committee that rules on drugs such as AZT. This committee is made up of independent scientists, peers, who analyze the data presented on a drug and vote to recommend or veto approval of an NDA. Cooper, as medical officer in the Division of Anti-Infective Drug Products, chaired the meeting but didn't have a vote. Only the independent scientists brought together to review the information had that power. They could ruin everything if they weren't handled just right.

It was the most important scientific meeting held in the AIDS crisis— and the most bizarre one Dr. Itzhak Brook had ever chaired. He had been head of the FDA's Anti-Infective Drugs Advisory Committee for the past two years and he still had another twelve months to go on his term. In all that time, he would see nothing that compared to what happened in rooms G and H, the Parklawn Building, 5600 Fishers Lane, Rockville, Maryland, beginning at 8:30 on the cold winter morning of January 16, 1987.

They were all there. On one side of a long, long table sat the consultants, the cardinals of the AIDS scientific establishment. Most were principal investigators for the Phase II AZT trial. Margaret Fischl was up from Miami. In many ways, the entire Phase II was now associated with her name. Marty Hirsch was down from Boston and Massachusetts General Hospital. Paul Volberding flew in from San Francisco. Sam Broder, of course, took the train over from the nearby NCI.

On the other side of the table sat the infectious disease experts, who were not "AIDS people." The consultants did not have the vote but these eleven "ID" scientists did. They held the power that day. That morning they were going to vote on whether to allow the widespread commercialization of AZT.

Burroughs Wellcome fielded nine people for this meeting. They were led by David Barry and included Dr. Dannie King, the project director for AZT, and Dr. Sandra Nusinoff-Lehrman. Nusinoff-Lehrman, an aging Holly Hunter look-alike, had an amazing facility with numbers.

Brook walked into the meeting upbeat. He expected everything to turn out all right. It usually did when things reached this stage. The pharmaceutical companies almost always did their homework, came up with the proper data, and received a yes vote from his committee. The FDA then took the committee's advice and gave the company permission to market the new compound. It was pretty smooth. So smooth that the day before, Brook had called up the media relations department of the FDA and asked them to prepare a statement for him to read after the meeting that would announce the approval of AZT by his committee. Brook had it in hand when he sat down that morning.

Michael Lange was less sanguine. He had flown down from New York to appear as an expert witness, an AIDS consultant. He'd been treating the disease since 1981 at St. Luke's and had run the AL 721 trial with Michael Grieco before Grieco became an AZT hotshot. Lange didn't like the political undercurrents to this meeting. Gay community activists were putting tremendous pressure on Congress to get something, *anything,* out to treat their disease. The White House was pushing hard to show that America, not France, was in the forefront of fighting AIDS. Sam Broder had been broadcasting to the world about AZT for months. The trial itself had been

161

cut short. Strange currents were in the air. AIDS was the most politicized disease Lange had ever seen. This meeting made him very nervous. Another scientist, deeply involved in AIDS research, would call what happened on that January morning evidence that "science really is nothing but a trashy soap opera."

The hearing started on time. Dr. Brook welcomed the participants, told them that the morning was dedicated to hearing the Wellcome people present their data, and asked everyone to keep their questions to themselves until this was accomplished. He told everyone they had one day to hear the data, to make their arguments, and to vote. Period.

Brook then turned to Joe Price from the Office of Scientific Advisers and Consultants, who had a statement for the record. He read: "To preclude any possibility of even the appearance of a conflict of interest, the relationship between Burroughs Wellcome and all the FDA-sponsored participants at this meeting has been carefully scrutinized. Where necessary, the Agency has granted full waivers permitting total participation of those members and consultants serving under appointments as special government employees. Specific waiver statements with respect to Drs. Lemon, Straus, Mildvan, Hirsch and Richman may be reviewed in the Public Documents room. Statements concerning their relationship with studies of AZT have also been filed by Drs. Redfield, Fischl, Lane and Broder. Thank you very much."

All this was very strange. In the world of Big Science, one of the major rules was that a scientist who had received money from a drug company to run tests on its drugs would generally not be permitted to sit on a committee reviewing that company.

There was a game in their world, and everyone who was a player knew the rules. A person who worked in a government or university lab could do certain things to augment his or her paltry salary—paltry, at least, in comparison to what was paid to scientists working in the pharmaceutical industry. The person could receive honoraria for attending drug company seminars, updating the company's scientists on the visiting researcher's lab work. The government scientist could also be a PI in a drug company trial, testing its new compounds either in vitro or in humans. That, in particular, paid well. Many scientists at the NIH and in academic hospitals around the country added 10 to 20 percent to their annual salary by doing this kind of work. They also strengthened their labs by doing this private work, which supported their staff. Most of all, they made their institutions happy because the institutions could take 40, 50, even 60 percent off the top for "overhead." Running trials for drug companies was good for all concerned.

This practice was accepted as standard operating procedure. In return, scientists were supposed to absent themselves from any review or regulatory action concerning those drug companies they had worked for. This didn't happen when it came to AZT. Two of the eleven members of the voting committee received special waivers—a Band-Aid remedy at the FDA for such problems. Dr. Stanley Lemon was associate professor in the Department of Medicine at the University of North Carolina School of Medicine, Chapel Hill, just down the road from Burroughs Wellcome's headquarters. Stephen E. Straus was a doctor who worked in the Clinical Center of the NIH. All in all it was a peculiar way to begin.

Ellen Cooper then got up to speak. She said she had been involved with AZT since Wellcome brought it to the attention of the FDA in April 1985. "A remarkable story in drug development followed," she said, "as most of you are aware, and today we are meeting barely a year and a half after the first patient received AZT to discuss whether or not it should be approved for general use, a rapid pace indeed." This was hardly a neutral statement from the main referee and implied that Brook's optimism was not misplaced. Cooper, of course, had spent months in negotiation with Wellcome to make sure that what was presented on this date would warrant approval.

Technically, the committee was ruling on Wellcome's application for an NDA, which would allow it to sell AZT for a profit at whatever price it set. But this was not the only option open to the committee. It could recommend, for example, that Wellcome be compensated in some other way for its drug development.

The issue of money and compensation to Wellcome came up immediately and reverberated as subtext throughout all the scientific talk about test results. Within the first five minutes of her talk Cooper said: "The pending action has major financial implications for the sponsor and for the total costs of caring for patients with AIDS." In the afternoon, Sam Broder raised the money issue by reminding everyone in the room that the Phase II trial "was done at considerable cost." David Barry emphasized money as well.

So many times was the issue of compensating Wellcome for its time and effort mentioned that Dr. Calvin Kunin, professor of medicine at Ohio State University and a voting member, finally lost his patience at the end of the day and declared: "I just want to refresh our memories about the charge of this committee and of the Food and Drug Administration, as I understand it. I certainly don't want to sound like a lawyer but it seems to me that the issue of cost is not under the purview of the FDA. The only issue is safety and efficacy. The company can charge one dollar or one hundred million; it has no effect whatsoever on the safety and efficacy issue in regard to the charge of the Food and Drug Administration. So all this talk about compensation is really irrelevant. . . . I think we ought to simply table it."

Spoken like a true scientist, but one who is naive about the nature of drug development. Sam Broder was always saying that very few scientists actually knew how to *really* develop new drugs. They knew nothing about the need for strong private company support and making sure that company got a reasonable return on its investment.

After raising the issue of compensation, Cooper returned to her basic charge, which was analyzing the data on AZT presented to the FDA by Wellcome. She was not happy about it, she said. Cooper summarized the strengths of the drug in about a minute. She said that there was "a highly significant difference in mortality between the two treatment groups." In addition, there was also a significant difference in how soon opportunistic infections appeared in the two groups. Finally, Cooper said that the efficacy of the drug was supported by data on weight gain, mood changes, and "some immunological parameters."

In the transcript of the meeting, Cooper's positive description of AZT takes up a single paragraph. The criticism that followed takes up twelve pages. Cooper launched into a direct attack on the trial. She noted that only a single Phase II controlled study had been done. Until this particular meeting, she said, the FDA had required a minimum of two controlled studies or one very large multicenter test, far bigger than the 282 patients enrolled for AZT. This was necessary, she went on, to ensure that the studies were "adequate," and she had doubts about the AZT trial's adequacy. Cooper said that "there certainly has not been a lack of patients interested in participating in clinical trials" for AZT. So why didn't Wellcome use a larger number of patients?

Then there was a question about the data itself. Cooper complained that the committee now had to analyze data on a trial that was stopped long before completion. In fact, Cooper said, the data on the trial, which had ended September 19, was not sent over to the FDA until December 2, two months later. The committee members barely had time to review it. Furthermore, a whole new series of data had been collected on patients who had been on placebo but who were then given AZT after the code was broken. That material was extremely important, but the committee received it just four days before the hearing, on January 12. Again, there was hardly any time to review the information.

Cooper dug in. Furthermore, she said, there was no proof on just how the drug actually worked. What was the true mechanism of action? "For approval of an anti-infective agent, we normally require in vivo evidence of specific anti-infective activity." Wellcome couldn't show how AZT actually worked. It didn't know.

Cooper also wondered about the long-term effects of taking AZT, and its effect on people who weren't yet very ill. Once Wellcome got the go-ahead to sell the drug, the FDA would not be able to control it. With AZT on the market, doctors could prescribe it for virtually anyone they wanted; less ill people with AIDS, indeed, even people who had the virus but who were asymptomatic, would almost certainly begin taking the drug. They would probably take it for years. But the study had included only the very sick, and it lasted for only sixteen weeks. Wellcome couldn't know how AZT would affect them in the long run.

Cooper appeared relentless in her criticism. In reference to reports of widespread cheating by patients during the trial, she said there was proof that "a substantial number of patients received other drugs for the treatment of non-life-threatening conditions at the same time they were receiving AZT, despite a general prohibition against concurrent therapy." How were they to know whether the test results were "clean"? Perhaps those other drugs boosted AZT. Perhaps they weakened it. Certainly they affected its interaction with the AIDS virus.

Cooper went on to criticize sloppiness in the AZT research. She said the precise cause of death from opportunistic infections, such as PCP, "were not always documented in the case report forms." The diagnosis was frequently not there either. She said it was much better "to have reasonable proof that important events were accurately reported, particularly in a situation where there is only one study."

Cooper lambasted the preclinical studies conducted by Wellcome. She said the animal studies normally required for approval of an NDA "have not been completed." The longest toxicology studies formally submitted to the FDA were the three-month studies in rats and monkeys. Six-month studies had just been completed, very late, she said, but the results had not yet been given to the FDA. In addition, twelve-month chronic toxicology studies hadn't even been started, nor had the tests to see whether AZT was carcinogenic.

Cooper finished her presentation with this: "Although we are all aware of the need for rapid clinical development of drugs to treat AIDS, the approval of a potentially toxic drug for marketing, particularly when it is anticipated that many less ill individuals will take it on a chronic basis, would represent a significant and potentially dangerous departure from our usual toxicology requirements. This fact should also be taken into consideration in the final recommendation of the committee."

Cooper wasn't being subtle here. It was clear from her remarks that under normal circumstances, Wellcome would never ever have gotten a hearing of the FDA advisory committee.

The chairman of the committee, Brook, began to get anxious as he listened to Cooper's criticisms. Maybe things would not go so smoothly after all. Michael Lange was simply dumbfounded. How in the world did Burroughs Wellcome manage to get the FDA to hold a meeting given this kind of criticism? It didn't make any sense to him.

What Brook and Lange didn't know was that Ellen Cooper's long critique was theatre. It was all prearranged. Cooper, and indeed FDA Commissioner Young, had known all along what kind of data David Barry was bringing to the meeting because they had been in constant negotiations with Barry since the Phase II trial ended at the end of September. The two sides had worked out just what Wellcome was responsible for and what it would present to the committee. Cooper's diatribe was for the public record.

Cooper knew all along that there was no question that the amount of data Wellcome had for AZT was less than the amount normally required for an NDA. She knew that there were a lot of unanswered questions—especially about optimum doses, which may have been lower than the rather high one used in the trial. "The FDA had to say that you do not have these things," says Barry. "What she [Cooper] was saying was that the rules say you should have all these things and you don't. Okay? But that doesn't mean she was against approval."

Unfortunately, none of the voting members of the committee knew that Cooper was putting on a show for the record. They didn't know that Wellcome had worked everything out with the FDA before stepping inside the room that morning.

\* \* \*

The Wellcome team took center stage after Cooper to present their data for AZT. The team discussed the structure of the preclinical animal tests, the Phase I safety trial, and the Phase II multicenter efficacy trial. It was a very technical discussion, defining categories, measurements, conditions, and finally results.

The numbers spilled forth from Dr. Sandra Nusinoff-Lehrman in particular. She got up to speak three times and each time was extremely articulate, sometimes even funny, in her presentation. Nusinoff-Lehrman was the head of the infectious disease laboratory at Wellcome and provided the analysis of the basic virology. Dr. Phil Furman also presented. He was well known to most of the people in the room as the man who helped develop acyclovir. Bob Blum presented data on the pharmacokinetics of AZT, how the body dealt with the drug in terms of absorption, metabolism, distribution, etc. Mary Maha talked about the safety of the drug. Dannie King spoke about the overall efficacy of AZT. Finally, Ken Ayers, senior toxicologist for Wellcome, explained the course of the data after all the patients on placebo had been given AZT.

Beneath the statistical rat-a-tat-tat of the presentations that morning, a disquieting tremor began to run through the meeting. The numbers being described by the Wellcome scientists were not all the same figures as those originally presented for the trial ending on September 19. The speakers were including updated figures going beyond September to December, figures on the once-placeboed, now AZT-ed patients. It quickly became terribly confusing. Worse, the purview of the committee extended only to the Phase II data from the original trial. This new information was both puzzling and confounding.

The critical mortality numbers, on which proof of the efficacy of AZT was based, were particularly confusing. As of September 19, the official termination date of Phase II, there had been one death of a patient taking AZT and nineteen of those on placebo. These mortality figures were the reason they were all here. They were the strongest evidence that AZT worked against the AIDS virus.

But the new numbers showed something different. It took a week to get all the placebo patients onto AZT. During that week, four more people on placebo died. But two patients on AZT also died. By the end of September, twenty-three people on placebo and three on AZT were dead. Statistically, this was beginning to look very different from a ratio of 19 to 1. Several committee members began to wonder what would have happened over the *next* week. Would the ratio have shifted even less in AZT's favor?

Was AZT losing its effectiveness in a very short period of time? The numbers were clearly implying just that.

The Wellcome people went on to say that when the placebo patients were put on AZT, they were given 200 milligrams of the drug every four hours, not the 250 milligrams the original patients were taking. The company didn't give a reason for changing the trial design. This divided the population taking AZT into two and was disturbing to committee members and consultants.

When Dannie King got up, things got worse. His numbers on efficacy completely confused the committee members. King said that, since the time when all the placebo patients were put on AZT, thirty-two people had died on placebo and eight on AZT. Here was yet another set of mortality figures. People were literally scratching their heads and looking at one another, shaking their heads in confusion.

There was more talk of survival rates at certain T-4 cell levels, and then Sandra Nusinoff-Lehrman returned to discuss bone marrow suppression, toxicity, and the sharp rise of anemia in patients taking AZT. But the mortality figures hung in the air throughout her speech.

By the time lunch approached, the committee members were visibly upset. Things had not gone as smoothly as anticipated. People were worried. "As the company presented the data, it became clear that a lot of things were missing," Brook remembers. "They answered, 'I don't know,' or 'We'll have to get back to you on that,' to a lot of questions. There were questions about toxicity, even about efficacy." Brook and other members of the committee had looked closely at the mortality numbers. It appeared to them that the placebo patients put on AZT were not as dramatically improved as the early AZT patients. "Even the initial patients were beginning to die," says Brook. Slowly it dawned on the committee that AZT did not prevent death in AIDS. Just what did it do?

Over lunch, the committee members couldn't stop talking about their growing worry about giving the NDA. There was just so much missing. Lange spoke to two consultants, both prominent in AIDS research, as he ate. They conceded that the research was incomplete. There were loopholes everywhere. The actual mean time patients had been on AZT was really only seventeen weeks, not the six months that the trial originally called for. Lange told them that at seventeen weeks, no serious conclusions could be made, certainly not about toxicology. They all agreed that AZT was *not* ready for commercialization.

Brook had the same conversation with the people sitting near him. Everyone was astounded at the inadequacy of the data Wellcome had brought in. Brook had chaired this committee for two years and had never seen anything like this. He was so worried that over lunch he talked with the FDA media person who had drawn up his press release announcing the committee's approval. Brook said, "Look, we should start thinking of making up another press release in case the drug is not approved. There is a good chance it might not be approved."

At lunch, both the FDA and the Wellcome people felt the anxiety in the air. They knew the meeting was not going right. Nothing was going right. Barry and Cooper huddled, and Cooper disappeared for a time.

After lunch was the time to question David Barry and the other presenters from Burroughs Wellcome. The committee members couldn't help asking a few questions earlier in the morning, but they had kept it short. Now they unleashed a torrent of questions.

A Dr. O'Neil started it off by complaining that the committee hadn't had time to analyze the new mortality numbers and he was confused. "I have several points for clarification that I would like the sponsors to address." O'Neil couldn't understand how Wellcome had come up with thirty-two placebo deaths and eight AZT deaths. "My calculations tell me that there are actually nineteen deaths in people who were switched over to AZT. I think it needs to be discussed. It is not clear to me whether the thirty-two deaths should be attributed to the placebo. The data that were presented to us this morning group everybody who was ever initially on placebo and did not break out what happened to those people subsequent to their administration with AZT."

Committee chairman Brook spoke to a very chilling point. "I was struck by the fact that AZT does not stop deaths," he said. "Even those who were switched to AZT still kept dying." The key mortality figures just did not add up.

David Barry and Dannie King then got up to try to clear up the confusion over mortality. Again there was a rattling off of numbers and a flashing of slides, but in the end O'Neil and others only shook their heads again. There was no consistency in the numbers. Where did the thirty-two placebo deaths come from? How did it compare with the original nineteen deaths on placebo? Why weren't the two categories broken out for display and discussion today, this most-important day when the committee had to advise the FDA on AZT?

On that note, the advisory committee began an open discussion of the data. The chairman, Brook, started this way: "This is really a difficult issue for us, because it is an unusual type of decision that we have to make. We have to, on the one hand, deal with a disease that is very devastating and spreading worldwide. This is actually the first drug that seems to have an effect on modifying some of the mortality. However, because of the rushed nature in which medicine and industry are trying to cope with it, we are having to discuss a drug that may not have been studied as adequately or as thoroughly as the FDA is used to having drugs studied."

Lange raised his hand and Brook recognized him. His criticism went to the heart of the Phase II trial. Basically, Lange argued that the protocol was structured in such a way that AZT was really tested against one thing—treating PCP. *Pneumocystis carinii* pneumonia was the key symptomatic measure of AIDS and whether the drug was working against it. The study did show that AZT acted against PCP within certain, very proscribed, parameters. But, Lange argued, there are better drugs to treat PCP, and these weren't tested against AZT's performance. Looking back on it, Lange remembers that "the study was set up in such a way that we were very rigidly controlled about not using any other medication while the AZT was being given. Dapsone, Fansidar, as well as trimethoprim/sulfamethoxazole [Bactrim or Septra] if it is tolerated, are fairly good chemoprophylaxes to prevent *Pneumocystis* from coming back."

Lange argues that because the test was stopped so soon, it was impossible to tell whether AZT had any real long-term effect at all. The trial, in essence, was "a little bit of this, a little bit of that. The art of medicine can come in, and we can almost sort of create a clinical remission I think in many patients. But we all know that the disease always relapses." For Lange, there was a decent chance that AZT wouldn't work at all over time. Only a scientific test running for eighteen months could really tell. To him, the Burroughs Wellcome data didn't prove a thing.

Lange wasn't alone in his concern that AZT might be, at best, an antipneumonia drug rather than an anti-AIDS treatment. Two members of the voting committee voiced their concern during the day. Walter Hughes, a specialist on PCP, asked for more data on the different opportunistic infections to show that AZT worked against them as well as PCP. AZT "is, after all, an antibacterial drug which could influence some of these infections," he said. Wellcome's Barry said that many kinds of infections were observed in the trial, including cryptococcal meningitis, cerebral toxoplasmosis, atypical mycobacteria, and severe genital herpes. That didn't satisfy Hughes, however. "I would like to know how many occurred in each group. I know the list, but what was the distribution between the placebo and the drug-related group?" Barry said he had a hard copy of some data that would address Hughes's concerns. "Could we defer answering that question until we have had a chance to reproduce that?" Hughes said yes and the question was never raised again in the meeting.

Another issue never raised that day, but one that was an object of discussion by Lange and others over lunch, was blood transfusions. Wellcome's data showed that an incredible 46 percent of all patients taking AZT had to receive transfusions to combat the anemia caused by the drug. Most of those patients getting transfusions had to get more than one. The data wasn't broken out, only the term "multiple" was used. Lange and the other clinicians at the meeting who had treated AIDS patients knew that the simple act of giving fresh blood raised T-4 cell counts and white blood cell counts. The blood contained them! There was no mystery there. And patients always felt better after receiving blood. But the Phase II trial didn't control for transfusions. There was no way to separate the rise in T-4 cells due to taking AZT from the rise due to receiving new blood.

By this time, the afternoon was nearly over and the time for voting was getting near. Chairman Brook and the Wellcome people wanted to stop the talk and get down to business. That was literally true: the last two hours of the committee meeting were devoted mostly to a discussion of money and the proper compensation for Wellcome. The discussion was couched within a scientific concern that itself had merit, but the real talk was about profits.

Many of the voting members and consultants were worried that AZT had been proven to be a treatment against a very narrowly defined patient group—those severely ill AIDS patients with T-cell counts at 100 who were recovering from PCP. Beyond that, there was no proof that AZT worked. But everyone at the meeting knew that if the FDA were to give Burroughs Wellcome permission to sell AZT commercially, virtually anyone with AIDS would be able to get it. Even people with no symptoms of the disease. The FDA had no way of policing the sale of drugs by physicians.

One way to restrict access to the drug would be to continue the

Treatment IND Wellcome already had from the FDA and not grant an NDA to permit commercial sales. The Treatment IND allows a company to offer a drug to patients only through physicians who must apply for each dose in writing. In this manner, the company controls who receives the drug.

The downside, however, is that under a Treatment IND, a drug company can't make any profit. Wellcome was determined to fight that all the way.

Martin Hirsch asked: "Is there a mechanism to compensate Burroughs Wellcome for a continuation or an expansion of the present mechanism of drug delivery, without making it available for every physician in the country to use for whomever it wants?" Edward Tabor, Ellen Cooper's boss at the FDA, got up and said, "If there is such a mechanism available, it is outside the purview of the Food and Drug Administration. It is really an issue of permitting cost recovery under an Investigational New Drug application. That is not something that is normally done." In short, no.

Paul Volberding then asked Barry: "Do you have a sense of what this drug would cost if some system like that were to be put in place, some reasonable compensation for the research and development?"

Wellcome's Barry then dropped the bomb. The cost of developing AZT was enormously high. Barry said, "I don't know how to answer you. I know that we have invested more than $80 million, in direct costs, in the program so far, a great deal of that in drug costs, but also a great deal in basic laboratory research and clinical research." Barry was covering his butt. If all Burroughs Wellcome could get from the committee was a Treatment IND, then it was prepared to show that its costs had been extremely high and it would cost the government a lot of money in compensation. The $80 million figure was a beauty, and drawn up ahead of this FDA meeting. Clearly Barry and Wellcome were very worried that after all their effort, they would be stuck with a Treatment IND from the FDA and that would prevent the company from making any profit.

Barry then moved to kill the whole idea of retaining the Treatment IND. "The point of whether this whole problem can be solved merely by continuing or slightly modifying the present IND we look at with great chagrin," he said. "Burroughs Wellcome and the government have worked together very closely and very well on this IND, and we are appreciative of all the help. But I can tell you, it has been a tremendous burden to *them*, and *they wish very strongly for us to take over all costs* [emphasis added]. It has been a tremendous burden to us. But more importantly, it has been a very difficult burden for many patients and physicians, because it is a complicated process. We try to comply with all the regulations, but the paperwork surrounding three thousand or more patients, I can tell you, is staggering, and the delay and frustration for both the patients and physicians are very great. We would definitely prefer not to continue that program as it is for any significant period of time."

Sam Broder then got up to defend Wellcome. He argued that the trial "was done at considerable cost, from any number of perspectives, including a variety of resources, emotional costs, whatever you want."

It went on for some time, the debate over whether Burroughs Wellcome should get an NDA or stay with some kind of Treatment IND. The company's scientists promised they could keep the drug under control by using warning labels and packaging it in a special way.

Then up stood someone who was not listed on the schedule of speakers; his name wasn't even on the transcript of the meeting. "I am Dr. Parkman. I am acting director of the Center for Drugs and Biologics [of the FDA]. I think we have quite clearly gotten the message from the discussion that has gone on here about the concerns of the committee, which I think are our concerns. We have heard the company present a preliminary view of a way in which they might do exactly what you want done—that is, to distribute the drug in a reasonable way, but try and restrict it in a way that people who should not be getting it are not. I think we can also look at the matter in the FDA. We will obviously be having discussions with the company about it. I think we can probably arrive at a plan that will satisfy people here."

Parkman's statement ended all debate. Everything stopped. In all of Brook's years as chairman, he had never seen anything like it. Never had a high FDA official made such a statement at one of these hearings. When Parkman spoke to the committee, Brook turned to Edward Tabor, the director of the Division of Anti-Infective Drug Products, who worked for Parkman, and said, "Did you hear that? He's telling us to approve it."

You could almost see the request in Parkman's face, according to Brook: "By the way he put it, you could see that there was pressure on him. The FDA was under pressure from the public to get the drug out. It would have looked terrible if it didn't."

Before Parkman spoke, Brook was convinced that "the tide was against approval." Afterward, the tide turned again. It could be felt in the room.

Brook thought something had happened at lunch. He didn't remember seeing Parkman at all in the morning session. Brook thought that maybe when he talked to the FDA media person about readying a release saying AZT had *not* been approved, the FDA had panicked and gone to Parkman. Who knew? "I think that behind the scenes something definitely happened," says Brook.

Dr. Parkman was an old colleague of David Barry's. "I knew Paul Parkman from years before," Barry recalls. "I worked with him for a time at the FDA." He had even published with him in 1975.

Barry concedes that Parkman's comments helped in the meeting. "The main worry of the committee was that we would sell this drug willy-nilly to everyone, including asymptomatic patients. The background of academic and regulatory people is that industry are [*sic*] robber barons who would sell anything to anyone for money."

For most of the afternoon the committee had felt that there was no regulatory way, once a drug was approved, for the FDA to control the widespread sale of AZT. The eleven voting scientists were ready to recommend only the continuation of the Treatment IND, if that. Barry insisted Wellcome would regulate the sale of the drug so that only very sick AIDS patients received AZT. But there was much skepticism. Then the FDA's Parkman stood up and did his thing. "What Paul Parkman meant, when he got up, was, 'Look, although we can't enforce it, *I know these people* and if they say they can do it, they're gonna do it,'" says Barry.

Of course, no one on the FDA's advisory committee knew just how well Parkman knew Barry. Given the song and dance at the beginning of the day about revealing the relationships scientists had with Wellcome, it was a curious omission.

It was late and the people around the room were getting restless. Parkman's statement made it clear which way the FDA wanted the vote to go. Chairman Brook then began a series of questions to be voted upon. "Does the committee agree that the data from the controlled trial of AZT adequately demonstrate a significant clinical effect?" This question focused on the original experimental data that showed that only one AZT patient compared to nineteen placebo patients had died during the trial. A show of eleven hands said yes.

The next question: "Do the additional data accumulated since the end of the trial support or modify this conclusion?" This revolved around the new, confusing mortality figures, which actually showed a growing number of people on AZT dying. Stephen Straus answered: "I think the data since the end of the study temper my enthusiasm that the effect may increase with time; if anything, it may stabilize or decrease with time." Brook added that the data of the past four months since the ending of Phase II had not yet been analyzed. "The data are just too premature and the statistics are not really well done." Lemon reiterated that "after sixteen to twenty-four weeks—twelve to sixteen weeks, I guess—the effect seems to be declining with regard to a number of different parameters." This was absolutely critical. Lemon was saying that AZT appeared to buy just a few months of possible improvement for people with AIDS. Three to four months to be exact. Was that all? After all the hoopla, the shouting, the self-congratulations, was that it?

Brook then said: "I agree with you that it is really an unknown for us. There are so many unknowns that it is hard to exactly know the truth. We do not really know what will happen a year from the beginning. The drug may actually be detrimental. We do not know."

Brook asked: "Who is in favor of supporting the contention that additional data since the end of the trial support the conclusion?" No one was willing to say yes. "They modify it," said Frederick Ruben. "They temper our enthusiasm for the original study." Okay, said Brook, we will phrase it that way. It was a vote of no confidence in AZT, but a minor one.

Then came a very important question: "What patient population has been shown to benefit from this drug?" The committee split on it. Most wanted to define the population extremely narrowly—those very sick AIDS patients with T-4 cell counts below 220, who had just had pneumonia. A few others wanted a wider definition. This was a high-stakes game. The wider the definition, of course, the bigger the potential market for AZT. Wellcome's eventual goal was to sell AZT to all the 1.5 million people infected with the AIDS virus, especially the vast majority of seropositive people who were asymptomatic and still clinically healthy. This was *the* critical question for Wellcome. Brook asked for a vote: "Anybody in favor of voting for answering yes, the patient population that has been shown to benefit from the study is those who met the criteria for inclusion in the study, including depressed T-4 and the PCP and ARC patients, as they were defined by the study criteria, raise your hand." Ten in favor, one against. It was a vote against Wellcome, a vote to restrict the market for AZT.

But Wellcome knew the vote was moot. The company had voluntarily given AZT to four thousand people with AIDS on the Treatment IND. Only a fraction of them fit into the tiny market niche just approved by the committee.

So it went. There were votes on concerns about dosage (yes), concerns that resistance to AZT might develop (yes), concerns about safety (yes), concerns about postmarketing studies of safety or efficacy (yes), concerns that the risk of AZT might outweigh the benefits (yes). Then finally Brook asked the question: "Based on all the information presented, does the committee feel that AZT should be approved for marketing at the present time?" He wondered whether, "by approving it now, we may release a genie out of the bottle and it may be something that we may regret." They voted: ten to one in favor. Only Brook voted against. He was stunned. At 4:05 the meeting was adjourned. People had planes to catch.

It was the most expensive drug of its kind ever: $10,000 per person per year forever for the only U.S.-government-approved drug against AIDS—AZT.

The announcement on February 13, 1987, came out of Burroughs Wellcome's parent headquarters in London, not the U.S. subsidiary in North Carolina. The short press release, issued by "Wellcome, plc," said, "Wellcome is considering a provisional price for its anti-AIDS drug, Retrovir (AZT), in the event of its approval by the USA Food and Drug Administration. It is anticipated that the price per bottle (100 × 100-mg capsules) will be around $188 into respective distribution channels throughout the world. As a result of variations in dosage regimes and local marketing conditions, the cost to the patient will vary."

The next paragraph read: "In establishing its price, Wellcome has taken into account a number of social and economic factors." Which social and economic factors, the company didn't mention.

Nor did it do its math publicly. The press release did not do the calculations for what it would actually cost the average person with AIDS. Other people did and the price for AZT came out to around $10,000. The price was so high, it simply amazed people into silence. No one had anticipated this high a price, no one outside Wellcome, at least.

In the United States, company spokesperson Kathy Bartlett told reporters that the people then receiving AZT for free from Wellcome would have to begin paying for the drug within a month. The forty-five hundred people would have to find $45 million over the next twelve months to pay for their treatment.

It wasn't as if no one had been warned. David Barry deliberately mentioned the figure of $80 million as the cost of developing AZT during the FDA review. Barry didn't break out those costs, however. Neither did the press release. In fact, Burroughs Wellcome would *never* explain what AZT really cost to develop, not even under congressional pressure. The world just had to take its word for it: $80 million.

Dr. Jerome Horwitz was also surprised at the $80 million Burroughs Wellcome said it spent to develop AZT. Horwitz was the man who had invented AZT—a quarter century ago. While Sam Broder was being lauded in the press as Mr. AZT, and David Barry was setting the stage for making AZT a billion-dollar drug, Horwitz sat quietly in Detroit fuming.

Back in 1963, Horwitz, then forty-four, was still a contender for the big time in cancer research. The Detroit Cancer Foundation, where Horwitz worked, was in the minor leagues of American science. It certainly wasn't one of the National Institutes of Health, where brilliant stars in their expensive labs competed to be the next Jonas Salk. But Horwitz was doing okay. He'd often observe that he'd done pretty good for a Detroit street kid, educated in the public schools when they still taught you something. The same schools that Sam Broder would attend a generation later.

Horwitz received his Ph.D. in organic chemistry from the University of Michigan in Ann Arbor back in 1950. He now had his own lab, a bunch of assistants to run tests, and a grant from the National Cancer Institute.

But the work wasn't going right. For two years he had been searching for the one compound that would selectively kill cancer cells without mass-murdering the rest of the body's cells. Horwitz's research technique, randomly searching for chemical compounds, was leading nowhere. It may have been standard operating procedure in science, especially cancer research, but the random screening was proving to be a dead end. It was boring, tedious, monotonous work.

There had to be a better way. After all, cancer was really just a wild, frenetic explosion of normal body cells, growing beyond all restraint. Block the reproduction of these cells, Horwitz reasoned, and the cancer stops. That might be accomplished by introducing a "fake" compound right into the DNA of the cell. Stop the DNA from reproducing and the cancer would be stabilized. That would, at least, arrest the disease. Horwitz decided to design his own killer compounds.

So on a cold Michigan morning, Horwitz created the chemical compound AZT, azidothymidine. His research was "elegant": simple, clear, and focused. For one key chemical in the genetic chain that was critical to the reproduction of cancer, Horwitz substituted a phony.

On paper, the logic was impeccable. In reality, it simply didn't work.

Absolutely nothing happened to the mice tumors when AZT was injected. Tests showed that AZT was biologically inactive, a dud.

That moment of failure in his lab was frozen in time for Horwitz. "It was a terrible disappointment," he said quietly decades later. "We found no use for it in cancer research."

When the experiment ended in failure, so, in a way, had the first half of Horwitz's life. Disgusted, he turned on AZT. "We dumped it on the junk pile. I didn't keep the notebooks."

So worthless was AZT to Horwitz that he didn't even think it was worth patenting. It didn't do anything, certainly not anything anyone cared about. It was this decision that transformed a defeat into a tragedy that would haunt him for the rest of his life. For in the end, AZT might have made Horwitz a contender after all.

Twenty-four years later, when politicians, public health officials, and scientists gathered to congratulate themselves on the discovery of a breakthrough drug that promised to combat AIDS, Horwitz would not be on the stage with them basking in the glow of TV klieg lights. By then Horwitz had disappeared into a sea of obscurity.

In his seventies, Horwitz is now retired from the Detroit Cancer Foundation and spends most of his time with his wife. From time to time she asks him, "Jerry, why didn't you just patent it?"

Sam Broder, to his credit, felt betrayed by Wellcome's behavior. "I felt very, very deeply sad," he now says. At the time, scientists working on AZT at the NIH and the FDA didn't think much about how Wellcome would price the drug. "We didn't pick up fast enough on the cost issue," he says. "The Burroughs Wellcome price was not something anyone could have anticipated."

But Broder, back in 1987, still went on to defend Wellcome. "A deal is a deal," he said. "It was right to have a drug company sponsor. But we didn't pull strings at the beginning and we couldn't do it at the end." Broder knew that there was something fundamentally wrong about charging $10,-000 a year for a drug, any drug, but he couldn't, at that time, bring himself to conclude that his own participation in the development of AZT had contributed in any way to the astonishing price of the only drug legally available to treat AIDS. Broder couldn't see that his decision in 1984 to support only those few drugs with big drug company sponsors would inevitably lead to the development of the most expensive drug in the world. It took three more years, until 1990, for Broder to realize how royally he'd been had.

Burroughs Wellcome aggressively defended its $10,000 price, constantly repeating the $80 million figure. "We spent as much money to develop this drug as we have spent on any other," said Barry. "We did two years' worth of work in a few months. We had a hundred people working on it before the FDA approved it for sale. Now we have seven hundred people, minimum, working on it."

The company emphasized that the market for AZT was uncertain. New drugs could appear at any time. Wellcome president and CEO T. E. Haigler, Jr., went on record saying that "the full usefulness of Retrovir (AZT) is unknown. Efficacy and speed of introduction of other therapies are unknown. Our financial returns are uncertain."

Burroughs Wellcome even asserted that AZT would actually save money by cutting the medical cost of treating AIDS patients. It said that nearly $400 million could be saved by individuals, government health plans, and private insurance companies if twenty thousand people with AIDS took AZT. This was just in the first year. No one bought the argument, but there were a few grudging smiles in the drug industry for Wellcome's gall in trying.

Thomas Kennedy, Wellcome's vice president for corporate affairs, its chief public relations person, said at that time that "a drug usually takes six or seven years to develop from beginning to end. We have made all these commitments on patient data of one year. We hope that the ongoing clinical work will show the drug to be of considerable help, but we can't be sure." Ergo, the high price designed to recoup costs as quickly as possible.

But Kennedy also threw a bit of light on the mysterious $80 million figure. He admitted that only a portion of it, maybe $30 million, had actually been spent. The other $50 million was what the company *expected* to spend in the first year of production. This was very different from what Wellcome had said in January at the FDA advisory meeting. At that time, David Barry said that the $80 million was for "direct costs" of AZT, including R&D and the trials.

Henry Waxman's congressional office was swamped with phone calls complaining about the $10,000 price of AZT. Hundreds of his constituents were begging him to do something. They were getting the drug free now. How were they ever going to find $10,000 year after year to keep themselves alive? Please help, they asked. Do something, they pleaded.

Waxman called a hearing of his Subcommittee on Health and the Environment less than a month after Burroughs Wellcome announced its price. He asked Wellcome CEO T. E. Haigler, Jr., and David Barry to come to Washington and explain why AZT cost so much.

On March 10, 1987, in room 2322 of the Rayburn House Office Building, Waxman began by asking if $10,000 is "a fair price? Who will pay for the people who are now being treated for free?" he added. "Who will pay for the people who will become ill after the drug is approved? Who is responsible for people who cannot pay?"

Waxman proceeded to grill Haigler on the cost of AZT. Where did the $10,000 price come from? He began by reminding Haigler that Wellcome had received orphan drug status for AZT, "which should contribute as much as a 72 percent tax subsidy to your clinical costs." (In 1983, Waxman had sponsored the Orphan Drug Law, which subsidized pharmaceutical companies if they did research on drugs to treat rare diseases, "rare" being defined as affecting up to 200,000 Americans.) In addition, Waxman pointed out that the company would get a 25 percent tax credit for increased R&D. So, Waxman asked, "After taxes, how much do you estimate that it cost to get AZT to the point of manufacture?"

Haigler's entire testimony was an effort not to answer that simple question. It was verbal fencing all the way, with Waxman returning again and again to the cost issue and Haigler answering again and again, "I'm sorry. I can't respond to that," or "I do not know the answer to that."

Waxman quoted *Barron's,* the financial weekly, as predicting that Wellcome would make $200 million in profits from AZT in the *first year.* When Waxman asked Haigler if he agreed with the *Barron's* estimate, Haigler responded with, "I'm sorry, who?"

It was strange watching this exchange. Haigler apparently hadn't read an article mentioning his own company in one of the most influential financial publications in the country.

Representative Ron Wyden from Oregon then caustically asked Haigler why he didn't just set the price at $100,000. Haigler said, "Well, I think that—you know. How can I answer that question?" Wyden followed with, "I must tell you, I'm still unclear about how you arrived at $10,000, rather than $30,000 or $24,000. I appreciate your feeling that $100,000 is unfair. But I must tell you that I think the pricing system is close to a random system."

The stock market didn't give a damn *how* Wellcome calculated AZT's price. It just loved the cash flow. In London, Wellcome's stock rose 12 percent the day of the $10,000 price announcement. It jumped 77 cents to $7.97. In New York, Jonathan Gelles, a pharmaceutical company analyst for Wertheim & Company on Wall Street, said, "We expect Retrovir to be selling at a rate that would make it the company's largest contributor to revenue and earnings by December and that the profit margin will be three times the company's 13 percent average." That meant a profit margin of about 40 percent. He estimated sales in 1988 at $130 million. If the company produced enough AZT for 30,000 AIDS patients, sales would climb to $200 million. If the number of people getting AIDS doubled by 1990, as expected, Wellcome would be generating about $300 million a year, every year, until another antiviral drug was approved by the FDA. By the fall of 1990, a competitor had yet to be found. The number of people with AIDS exceeded predictions and pushed quickly past the 100,000 level. By Christmas 1991, the number of PWAs was expected to double to 200,000. By then Burroughs Wellcome would be taking in upwards of $500 million a year, each year, for AZT. Jerome Horwitz's baby was heading for the Drug Hall of Fame, heretofore restricted to Valium, Tagamet, and a few other billion-dollar drugs.

Marketing glitz. That's what Burroughs Wellcome used in peddling AZT around the country. Not content to passively depend on the natural market for the drug—the tens of thousands of people with AIDS—Wellcome launched a huge advertising campaign.

But a respected pharmaceutical company can't simply use Michael Jackson to sing its praises. It has to promote its message in scientific forums and "educational" programs.

The *Ray of Hope: Retrovir* video was one such educational effort. Sponsored as an educational service, the video was sent free to specialists in hematology, oncology, and infectious diseases, as well as to certain physicians in the twelve American cities where AIDS was most prevalent. It was the third such mailing on AZT done by Wellcome, at considerable cost.

Donna Mildvan was the host of the video show. After an opening of brave music and a shaft of light signifying the "ray of hope," she appears sitting in a chair, a vase full of flowers carefully placed in the background to frame her face. Mildvan is identified on screen simply as a doctor from Beth Israel Medical Center, New York. She begins by saying that "the AIDS epidemic threatens to be one of the most devastating in the history

181

of mankind." Quietly and slowly she explains the progress of AIDS research and says researchers have now "developed Retrovir, the first effective antiviral therapy for the treatment of AIDS and AIDS Related Complex."

Through her entire discussion, Mildvan refers to AZT as Retrovir, Wellcome's brand name for AZT. She never once uses its generic name, zidovudine, or its chemical name, azidothymidine.

Sam Broder does the same. He is shown seated with a white lab coat on, hands clasped, head tilted, talking very slowly about the Phase I safety trial.

Then the video jumps coasts to Dr. Paul Volberding in San Francisco, who talks about the Phase II trial. Volberding is in shirtsleeves.

As the video drones on in somber tones, Douglas Richman appears in San Diego. He is the only talking head who refused to use the name Retrovir. Instead he calls it zidovudine.

David Barry then appears, talking about Retrovir again.

Then it's back to Donna Mildvan, still sitting in her chair, lemon suit on, speaking slowly and distinctly. She ends her hosting job with, "Retrovir is our first weapon against AIDS. It is a ray of hope for us all."

Nowhere in the video does it say that Mildvan, Volberding, or Richman were PIs compensated to run AZT in the Phase II trial. Nowhere does it say that their respective universities and teaching hospitals received substantial "overhead" funds for the effort. Nowhere does it say whether these doctors received honorariums for this educational video on behalf of AZT.

# Acting Up

Nora Ephron couldn't make it, so Larry Kramer filled in. He had a lot to say, and the converted school auditorium at the Lesbian and Gay Community Center on Thirteenth Street in the Village was a good place to say it.

Kramer was just back from Houston, where his big new play, *The Normal Heart*, had been staged. As he watched from the audience, Kramer had seen himself do screaming battle with his old friends at the Gay Men's Health Crisis. His years of pleading for more radical political action, his sense of betrayal at their rejection of him, his anguish as friends and lovers died in front of his eyes, were all displayed for everyone to see. It was one of those rare plays that show powerful personal emotions erupting against a tableau of harsh political reality.

Kramer was invited down to Texas by Mary Lou Galantino, a fan who was also physical therapy coordinator at the Institute for Immunological Disorders, the first AIDS hospital in the country. It was run by Dr. Peter Mansell, whom Kramer knew to be a fighter. Mansell told him a story that Kramer would never forget.

The AIDS hospital, just outside Houston, was state-of-the-art. It was for-profit, owned by AMF, a Beverly Hills company that had a chain of hospitals. The institute had beds for 180 people with AIDS, but only 6 were currently residing.

Texas was a state with a large gay population and a large number of people with AIDS. It was perfectly logical for AMF to set up an AIDS hospital there. Unfortunately for AMF, Texas was also one of the only states that didn't reimburse AIDS patients for their hospital medical care. Without private insurance, a person with AIDS was out of luck. Most of the PWAs in Houston didn't have insurance. Mansell was treating 150 patients every week as outpatients for free. His hospital was quickly going bust.

Mansell was deeply depressed over the wasted medical facilities. But he was furious at something else—the FDA. He told Kramer that there were at least five drugs just as promising as AZT, with far fewer side effects. Yet the FDA wouldn't let him use them. These drugs, AL 721, Ampligen, HPA-23, DHPG, MTP-PE for Karposi's sarcoma, had each passed Phase I testing for safety but were not being given to patients. It was another example of wasted medical care. Safe drugs couldn't be given to terminal patients, people with AIDS.

When he got back to New York, Kramer hit the phones. He called everybody he knew. If he was going to give a talk, then it was going to be a hellfire-and-damnation speech.

That night, Kramer warmed up his audience by describing what had happened in Houston. "There are drugs out there, *safe* drugs, and we can't get them," he said. "Our people are dying and we can't get safe drugs."

Kramer laid it all on a heavily bureaucratic FDA. He told the audience that Mansell had showed him a protocol application, for example, that was rejected by the FDA because four words, literally four words, did not meet the approval of the government bureaucrats. Each time Mansell had to redo the entire protocol and resubmit it. It took eight more months before he received a reply. This happened again and again, and each time he had to submit eighteen copies of each protocol. It was an unbelievable mess in Washington, Kramer shouted. The bureaucracy was running wild while people with AIDS were dying.

Kramer told the audience that in 1980, the head of the FDA had said publicly: "Ribavirin is probably the most important product discovered during the intensive search for antiviral agents." Then Kramer screamed, "It's 1987 and we still can't get it." He quoted a *Village Voice* article written the week before that said, "It's astonishing that ribavirin wasn't chosen before AZT." Kramer continued with, "Leading researchers I have talked to explain this one way: The FDA doesn't like the difficult, obstreperous head of ICN Pharmaceuticals, which manufactures ribavirin, while Burroughs Wellcome, which makes AZT, is smooth, politically savvy, with strong PR people."

Kramer moved on to AL 721. "AL 721 isn't even a drug—it's a food! How dare the FDA refuse to get it into fast circulation when it has proved promising in Israel at their famous Weizmann Institute? Indeed, Praxis

Pharmaceuticals, which holds the American rights to it, could put it out as a food, but they apparently are gambling for big bucks by waiting for FDA approval to put it out as a drug, which is going to take forever because Praxis doesn't appear to have much experience in putting out drugs at all."

Kramer told the audience that they were being misled. "Almost one billion dollars is being thrown at AIDS, and it's not buying anything that will save two-thirds of the people in this room," he told them. We want, we demand, all the drugs that are safe and available. "Give us the fucking drugs!" he yelled.

Then the furies began to really leap out of Kramer. Raising his voice to shouting pitch, stabbing the air with his hands, he said they had to *do* something about this. They had to do something right now.

But, he said, lowering his voice, putting his head down as if in shame, "we have always been a particularly divisive community. We fight with each other too much, we're disorganized, we simply cannot get together. We've insulted each other. I'm as much at fault in this as anyone," he confessed.

Kramer then turned to the enemy within the community, his own enemy, the GMHC. With scorn and anger pouring forth again, he told the audience that while the GMHC was the biggest and most powerful AIDS service organization in the country, it remained basically a very conservative, very frightened organization, afraid to offend the powers that be. "But we desperately need leadership in this crisis. We desperately need a central voice and a central organization. But in this area of centralized leadership, of vision, of seeing the larger picture and acting upon it, GMHC is tragically weak," he said sadly. "It seems to have lost the sense of mission and urgency upon which it was founded"—upon which Kramer had founded it.

What was needed? Kramer demanded. He'd tell them. Look at the front page of the *New York Times* that day, he told the audience. Two thousand Catholics in the halls of the governor's mansion in Albany, "with their six bishops. Two thousand Catholics and their bishops marching through the halls of government. That's advocacy," he shouted. "Why are we so invisible, constantly and forever?"

Kramer said that *they* now had to protest. *They* had to picket and risk arrest. Then he said that in the audience was a man who could show the way. This man wasn't ashamed to get arrested. "He uses his name and his fame to help make this world a better place. Martin Sheen. Stand up, Martin. The best man at Martin's wedding, his oldest friend, died today, from AIDS."

It was a bravura performance. It was Moses down from the mountain casting scorn on the idol worshipers, demanding that they do the right thing. Kramer went from outrage to sadness to outrage again. Every few moments, as if he himself were not even in control, the furies would shoot out and his anger would boil over.

It was clear what Kramer wanted to do. He ended his sermon with a quote from Surgeon General C. Everett Koop: "We have to embarrass the administration into bringing the resources that are necessary to deal with this epidemic forcefully." We have to embarrass them. To do that, Kramer wanted a new group that would embrace his own tormented soul, his own furies. He wanted an organization that would break the rules and *fight* for what was right. He wanted anger. He wanted outrage. His dead and dying friends—*their* dead and dying friends—deserved no less.

If there were 200 people on that Tuesday night in March 1987, there were 350 on Thursday. Kramer held center stage, but it seemed that all 350 people had something to say that night and actually managed to say it. It was a foretaste of the kind of organization that would soon be created.

Kramer looked out and recognized a lot of old friends from the now-defunct AIDS Network. But there were others as well, younger gay kids in their early twenties, very hip, very vocal, and very angry. To Kramer's amazement, they were as angry as he was! In time, most older gay men, people in their late thirties and early forties, would drop out and this younger generation of activists would take over the fight. He didn't know why his own generation gave up. Maybe they were just sick and weary and burned out after years of beating their heads against the political wall.

But tonight was the beginning. The crowd, the young ones especially, wanted something newborn, in their own angry image. A community protest group, that's what they wanted. It would be outside both the government establishment and the gay establishment. The crowd wanted to break with both the external "enemy," the biomedical establishment, and their elders, the gay establishment. And they didn't feel they had to be polite about it.

After endless hours of talk and debate, the crowd somehow focused on a single mission for the new group—to fight for the early release of all experimental drugs that could treat AIDS. Only treatment could save their lives. Only access to that treatment could save their community. The NIH, the FDA, maybe even the drug companies were stalling, said Kramer. They would shake them out of their standard operating procedures.

But what to name themselves? Everyone was talking at the same time. Names kept flying through the air. Then out came ACT UP! Yeah, that felt right to the crowd. That's what they were going to do. Make waves, make trouble until people listened. ACT UP. The AIDS Coalition to Unleash Power. Its motto would be "united in anger and committed to direct action to end the AIDS crisis."

For the first time in its fight against AIDS, the gay community was deliberately turning to civil disobedience. In the process, it would help launch a broad social movement that would begin to change medicine as the United States had always known it. For the first time, a politically savvy group of sick people and their friends were about to fight for their own medical agenda. They were going to fight for their own lives, rather than wait for somebody in a faraway laboratory to help them. Those PWAs who fought the hardest would tend to live the longest. They would also tend to use AZT the least.

Several weeks after Burroughs Wellcome announced that AZT would cost $10,000 a year, 250 members of ACT UP stormed into Wall Street blocking traffic for hours. An effigy of FDA Commissioner Frank Young, made in Joe Papp's Public Theater workshop, was hung in front of Trinity Church, in the heart of the financial district. The demonstrators passed out thousands of fact sheets condemning Burroughs Wellcome for pricing the only available anti-AIDS treatment at such an outrageous level. Then ACT UP did something that young white people hadn't done in America for most of the eighties. They sat down in traffic during rush hour for a social cause and got arrested for it.

How was this possible? This was Reagan's America, where polls told everyone that young people were the most conservative segment of the population and where political protest was something parents did a long time ago. Wall Street was where greed was godly if not god and where twenty-five-year-olds were hoping to make a million dollars a year. It wasn't where you sat down in front of traffic to protest a social policy and get a police record.

The ACT UP demo made national news, but not at first. The *New York Times* and the tabloids didn't write it up. Only the AP wire service ran a piece and even then the AP got it wrong when it attributed the action to the old AIDS Network. Dan Rather did get it right later when he gave credit to ACT UP for forcing FDA Commissioner Young to promise to speed up drug testing.

It was a lesson well learned. After seven years, people were discovering how to get the issue of AIDS on TV. Indeed, getting on TV and into the newspapers quickly became a central goal for the new organization. It was its key tactic in forcing change through protest.

This first major act of civil disobedience in the long fight against AIDS struck a deep chord within the gay community, which was already prepared to shift to more militant tactics in its drive to get the government to deliver treatments for the deadly disease. A strong sense of frustration was evident even among the more moderate, long-established gay lobbying and advocacy groups. They had made big contributions to liberal politicians who obliged them by increasing funds for AIDS research. But what good was that if drugs weren't being made available? It only meant subsidizing scientists and government bureaucrats who had their own agendas. The political process wasn't working for the gay community. It wasn't delivering the goods.

It even worked against them at times. In October 1987, California activists witnessed their liberal Senator Alan Cranston, whom they'd supported for years, vote for a Jesse Helms measure that prohibited federal AIDS education money from going to any group that might "promote or encourage" homosexuality. It passed the Senate 94 to 2. Of all the things that were desperately needed to fight AIDS, education was the single most important one. Not only was the vote a slap at who gays were, it was idiotic in terms of national health policy. They expected better from Senator Cranston.

The ACT UP action on Wall Street was applauded in California and elsewhere around the country. Civil disobedience quickly spread to Washington, D.C., where sixty-three gay leaders were arrested in June for protesting Ronald Reagan's record on AIDS. The police, in what seemed to the activists a slap in the face, wore yellow rubber gloves, as if to avoid contamination. In San Francisco, a two-year-old AIDS Vigil in front of the Federal Reserve Building at U.N. Plaza suddenly turned more confrontational. People began deliberately flaunting the law in civil protest and were arrested.

Within months of the Wall Street action, ACT UP chapters appeared in Los Angeles, Boston, and Philadelphia. By the end of the year, ACT UP had as many as four thousand members around the country and was growing fast. It would have forty chapters by the beginning of 1990 and ACT UPs would appear in Toronto and London. For anyone who had lived through the sixties, the vibes were unmistakable. Social protest was in the air again. The "AIDSies" had given birth to a genuine social movement, the most important of the decade.

Right before the 1987 Christmas holidays, Kathy Bartlett, Burroughs Wellcome's main PR person, sent out a news release. "Burroughs Wellcome Co. today announced a 20 percent reduction in the price of its anti-AIDS drug RETROVIR brand zidovudine, also known as AZT. This reduces the price for the drug to the wholesale distributor from $187.80 to $150.24 for a bottle of 100, 100-mg capsules."

The release went on to say that the reason for the cut was the savings Wellcome was now making due to a drop in production costs. The company had made "substantial strides" in expanding its manufacturing facilities for AZT both in its own plant in Greenville, North Carolina, and at its Dartford, England, facility.

It quoted president and chief executive officer T. E. Haigler, Jr., as saying, "We are delighted that the efforts of our production people and our suppliers have brought us to this point long before we thought it would be possible."

What Haigler didn't mention was the embarrassment Wellcome felt from the March 10 hearings on AZT's price held by Congressman Henry Waxman. Waxman had grilled Haigler like a fat steak at that hearing, pushing him again and again to reveal the cost structure of the drug. Again and again, Haigler had refused—in front of dozens of newspaper and TV reporters.

Haigler also didn't mention in the press release the ACT UP demo on Wall Street on March 24, the first demonstration by a patient group against the cost of a drug specifically designed for them. Wellcome had produced dozens of drugs over the years, but no group of patients had ever taken it to task for the price it charged them. This was somehow very different. But it didn't make it into the press release that day.

Dr. Iris Long was an unlikely heroine. She was a fifty-three-year-old married woman who rarely finished her sentences. What she did say sounded as though she were speaking through cotton. Long may have been the straightest member of ACT UP. She was also perhaps the most important.

Long has been behind the most significant changes the United States has seen in its biomedical research system in decades. She gave ACT UP the scientific knowledge and, hence, the power to launch a series of critical actions that have altered how research is performed and how drugs are developed. Her goals were to speed up drug development and expand access to treatment for people with AIDS. The result has been to dramatize the need for drastic transformations of the FDA, the NIH, and the nation's most important medical schools and teaching hospitals. The pharmaceutical industry has also gotten a kick along the way. But in the strangest of ironies, the industry stands to benefit almost as much as the public from what ACT UP has done.

Long was a pharmaceutical chemist for twenty years before she decided she needed to do something completely different, something that involved people, not lab rats. For many years she had worked on nucleosides and even knew Jerome Horwitz, the man who created AZT, ddI, ddC, and other similar compounds. "We were all nucleoside chemists," she says. "We put various groups on the nucleoside, such as sugars, to build new compounds. It was easy to get a lot of new products." Long was at Sloan-Kettering when Mathilde Krim was there, although they never met and worked in different departments.

Long's decision to now do something that would benefit people is the kind that often comes to people in their forties or fifties, when compassion and generosity displace the need to prove oneself, to make one's mark. Long's midlife crisis was ACT UP's gain.

Long first started volunteering at the new Community Research Initiative, the first PWA-doctor organization to do actual drug research on treatments for AIDS and its opportunistic infections. She worked at setting up the IRB, the Institutional Review Board, that watched over the safety of human subjects in trials. At the same time, she helped out at the PWA Health Group, the first major buyers club in the country. She helped get out the first big buyers club drug, AL 721.

At both places, Long discovered what people with AIDS wanted— access to treatment, access to drugs. They were desperate. In the AIDS community, access to drug trials *meant* access to treatment. There were no other alternatives. But no one knew where the trials were because the NIH, the FDA, and the drug companies never publicized the sites or the criteria for entry. That was the province of the local PI, who guarded that power closely. Control over patients was the key to PI power. It forced the drug companies and the government institutes to come to the PIs to test out their drugs. Opening access widely to drug trials would seriously erode that power. The PIs opposed it.

In June of 1987, Long went to one of the first ACT UP meetings. "It was rather exciting," she says. Just a few weeks before, ACT UP had had its first demonstration at Wall Street, protesting the price of AZT. At that first meeting, Long watched Larry Kramer give vent to his most vituperative self. "Where are the drugs the government promised?" he asked. "After we got them millions of dollars for their experiments, what do we get? A ten-thousand-dollar drug! What about all the other drugs out there?" Long, who lived in a quiet section of Queens, was totally taken with the scene of several hundred people packed into the Lesbian and Gay Community Center, all talking and shouting at the same time. The energy level was enormous. She loved it and stayed.

But what could she do to help? She could scout every territory. Long could find out where the drug trials were being held and tell people how to get into them. Long knew the drug development system because she had worked within it for decades. She was an expert, the first expert ACT UP had on "the system." She could form what John James had been calling for in his newsletter on the West Coast—the AIDS community's own group of research experts independent of the drug companies and the NIH. Long didn't disappoint. She had found her calling. She knew what she wanted to do for the second half of her life.

So where were the drugs? In June of '87, they were mostly in the trials being run by Tony Fauci's NIAID. They were in Dan Hoth's ACTG system. Long did what no other AIDS activist had done before. She called up and asked for a list of the trials.

Her first list from NIAID was the July '87 one. It contained all current trials, the targets for enrollment, the number of people actually enrolled, and the places where they were being held.

They were also total bullshit. Long was flabbergasted as she read down the list. There were so few patients enrolled! Hardly anyone was in them. Only 844 people were in the entire government effort. That meant only a tiny fraction of all PWAs were getting any treatment. It was astonishing. Worse, 86 percent of all these people were on AZT. Long couldn't figure out where all the other drugs were. Everyone had assumed that they were being tested out also. What had happened to AL 721, to GM-CSF, to HPA-23, to dextran sulfate, to ribavirin? Why weren't they doing other antivirals or immune modulators or drugs to fight the opportunistic infections that did the actual killing of PWAs?

There were other questions that came to Long's mind. What were the investigators doing with the government's money if their trials were so underenrolled? Where did the NIAID grant money go if only 5 or 10 percent of the slots were actually filled? Did NIAID keep the money? Did the hospital? Did the university? Did the principal investigator? Long didn't know the answers. No one else had asked them.

A Treatment and Data subcommittee of ACT UP's Issues Committee existed at that time, headed by Herb Spires. Long began going to these meetings. So did Jim Eigo and Mark Harrington, who were soon to become her two disciples. Harrington would later say that their mission was to translate Iris Long to the world. In that they would succeed.

Eigo first showed up at an ACT UP meeting in October of '87. He didn't know what to do exactly and kept quiet for several meetings. In his mid-thirties, Eigo was older than most of the men and women in ACT UP, who were closer to twenty-three than thirty-three.

Eigo heard Iris Long talk about a meeting she had just attended of an FDA advisory committee. She told the ACT UP audience that she was very upset because the FDA committee had failed to recommend approval of DHPG, a drug which, she said, community doctors all over the country already knew to be effective against CMV-induced blindness. A few brave frontline doctors were already giving DHPG to their patients. Long was furious and said at the end of her talk that she had a study group that met before the regular Monday night ACT UP meetings. Please come and help, she said.

Eigo went the next Monday night. "I was kind of searching for my niche in the group," he recalls, "and I said I was a writer." He told Long that she had great ideas and he could help by getting them in shape and putting them out in a series of papers.

Long said great. Then she showed Eigo the July trial enrollment list she had received from NIAID. She told Eigo that NIAID wasn't telling any people with AIDS anything about its own trials. It was all a secret. Thousands of PWAs were trying to get into the only treatment they knew of, the testing going on in the ACTG trials, and NIAID wasn't telling them how to do it. There was no communication between NIAID and the PWAs or their doctors. It was a story as old as the AIDS epidemic itself.

Trial enrollment was left entirely in the hands of the principal investigators, who were expected to supply their own patients. How they found their patients and what criteria they used for choosing them was left up to the PI. Yet it was clear to Long from the accrual numbers in the July NIAID report that the PIs were doing a miserable job of getting those patients. Long wondered if this was just some anomaly or if this was true for all research in the country. Were PIs who were testing drugs in cancer, for example, slow in enrolling patients in their trials? She wondered why people with life-threatening diseases weren't being told about trials for possibly effective drugs. Why was access always controlled by the PI and his institution?

Eigo couldn't believe it either. Then Long gave Eigo his first ACT UP mission: write a one-page plan for creating a registry of all AIDS-related clinical trials in the New York area. Eigo knew nothing about this stuff and told her so. Just use your head, Long answered.

Eigo did and barely found enough information to fill up the page. Long said it was fabulous. "Next week come back with three pages." Eigo really got scared. "I don't think I have anything left to say," he told Long. She smiled and said, "No, no, no. Just do it." The next week there were three pages.

The T&D subcommittee gathered lots of string on ongoing trials. Long knew that every medical institution that administers drugs to humans in clinical trials must have an IRB, an Institutional Review Board. The job of the IRB was to protect the patients. The hospital's director of pharmacy was usually the person in charge of procuring and dispensing the drugs for clinical trials and usually sat on the IRB.

Eigo and other members of the subcommittee began calling every director of pharmacy in the New York area to find out whether the institution was conducting trials on AIDS drugs. It wasn't difficult but it was tedious work, copying names and numbers out of the directory of the Greater New York Hospital Association. By the spring of '88, sixty-six hospitals had been contacted.

Then Long asked Winston Sexton, a member of T&D, for help. Like so many people in ACT UP, Sexton was superbly credentialed. He had a degree in computer science from Columbia University and worked as a software writer. Long asked him to write a special program for an AIDS

Treatment Registry (ATR) computerized database. PWAs in search of drug treatments would only have to call up the file on a computer screen to get the information.

Long wanted to include the most detailed information possible to help PWAs decide whether they wanted to get into a specific trial and how to do it. So she asked for the following to be put on-line: the drugs being tested; criteria for inclusion in the trial; drug-taking restrictions; trial sites; names of principal investigators with contact information; protocol code numbers; the total enrollment number; trial commencement and termination dates; each drug's FDA approval status; whether the trial was placebo-controlled; trial design; whether the trial was still open or closed.

She wanted to get the information out via computer and printed paper to people with AIDS, their doctors, AIDS advocacy and service organizations, the gay community, and any other communities that would be interested in it.

By February 1988, Eigo's one-page report on AIDS trials in the New York area had grown to ten pages. ACT UP then submitted it to the Presidential Commission on the Human Immunodeficiency Virus Epidemic, better known as the Watkins commission after Admiral Watkins replaced its original chairman following his resignation. Iris Long's report was a critique of the information available from the government on trial access. It said that if PWAs had such a difficult time getting information in New York City, it must be much worse in the rest of the country. What was needed was a national registry of all clinical trials for all AIDS drugs—both government and private drug company trials. The Watkins commission heard Iris Long out and soon endorsed her idea.

This decision to appear before the Watkins commission was itself a major turning point for ACT UP. A fierce debate over whether to participate in *any* government process had shaken ACT UP in the weeks preceding Iris Long's testimony. It was typical of the early months of ACT UP, before people learned to trust and accommodate one another. The organization practiced democracy-as-anarchy at its meetings, with everyone entitled to a voice and insisting on taking it, often all at once; there were no formal leaders, just "facilitators." ACT UP saw itself as working outside in the street, yelling at the powers that be, not working hand in glove with them. The March demo on Wall Street fit their self-image at that time, not talking to a bunch of President Reagan's appointees.

In the end, ACT UP voted to send Bill Bahlman, who was on the powerful Issues Committee, to monitor the president's commission. When Watkins took over and surprised everyone in Washington with his open mind on AIDS and AIDS treatments, ACT UP voted to send Long to testify.

Long next testified at an April 1988 Weiss committee hearing on "Therapeutic Drugs for AIDS: Development, Testing, and Availability." As part of her testimony, she again recommended a national registry for AIDS trials. When the final draft of the Weiss committee's report was released in June, it too came out in favor of a trial registry. Weiss, Waxman, and Senator Ted Kennedy began to push very hard for the idea.

In the fall of '88, Congress endorsed the concept of a national AIDS treatment registry and made it part of the omnibus health legislation. Congress, basically copying ACT UP's specific recommendations for publicizing AIDS drug information, ordered the NIH to set one up. In many ways, Iris Long through Jim Eigo and ACT UP wrote that legislation. In July of 1989, NIAID put out its portion of a national AIDS trial registry, which focused on its own government protocols. NIAID set up a hotline—1-800-TRIALS A—that anyone could call for information. NIAID was willing to download its computer files over the phone lines to any caller's home computer, making trial information available. But, in keeping with its history of not being in touch with the needs of the AIDS community, NIAID underestimated the demand for such information. It didn't staff its phones adequately and in the first week anyone calling usually got a busy signal. After a month, the staff was doubled and the system worked smoothly. It would have been easy for Fauci's people to simply phone ACT UP and ask about the probable response to 1-800-TRIALS A.

In August of '89, the FDA came out with its portion of the registry dealing with trials being conducted by private drug companies. The FDA National AIDS Registry was a disaster. Much of the information mandated by Congress was left out. It appeared that the FDA, knowing that drug companies felt threatened by the loss of what they considered proprietary information, deliberately misconstrued and obfuscated details necessary for PWAs to successfully use its registry. For example, the congressional legislation specifically said that the sites of all trials must be listed. The FDA interpreted this to mean the state where the trial was being held. It was not very helpful.

Fortunately, ACT UP came out with its own, easy-to-read, detailed registry, the AIDS Treatment Registry, for New York and New Jersey even before the FDA issued its useless product. Shortly after that, the ATR floated away from ACT UP as an independent not-for-profit organization headed by Iris Long. The ATR rented a loft only a block away from the building on West Twenty-sixth Street that houses the CRI, the PWA Coalition, and the PWA Health Group. It's a noisy and gritty neighborhood, the New York fur district actually, but the rents are cheap and there is a certain style about it that appeals to the hip young ACT UP members, many of whom live "downtown" in the East Village. They prefer calling the industrial area by a more chic name—Chelsea. Jim Eigo, an East Village denizen, is among several ACT UP members who are on the board of directors for the ATR. Joe Sonnabend and Michael Callen are on the ATR Advisory Committee. The only trouble Long has is finding enough money to print enough copies to keep up with demand.

Until ACT UP, no one outside the system of big science as it is practiced at the NIH and the major medical institutions around the country had ever taken a serious critical look inside the clinical trials network system. For over forty years, ever since Congress set up the NIH after World War II, investigator-initiated research had been the norm. No questions were asked by any public or private body about how PIs went about testing new drugs on humans. No one asked how efficient their system was. No one asked how ethical it was. No one suggested changes. Until ACT UP.

As Iris Long began to review the monthly lists of ACTG trials sent to her, the secrets of the PI kingdom revealed themselves. It was an unexpected horror show. Underenrollment and lack of access to drug trials were the least of the problems afflicting Tony Fauci's nominal domain.

Long, Jim Eigo, and Gary Kleinman of the T&D subcommittee decided to do a formal critique of the NIAID clinical trials program. They focused on the hospital sites doing trials in the New York area.

Dan Hoth, head of the AIDS Program at NIAID, wasn't particularly forthcoming when Long and Eigo began requesting information. In fact, when ACT UP requested minutes of key meetings, they were at first refused. When ACT UP went through the Freedom of Information office at NIAID, the minutes arrived in New York—with pages full of material whited out.

At this point, ACT UP made its first approach directly to Tony Fauci to protest the whiting out. Bill Bahlman, the ACT UP representative who was monitoring the Watkins commission, played go-between and set up a meeting between Fauci and Jim Eigo. It was the first direct contact between ACT UP and NIAID, the beginning of a dialogue.

But not a very satisfactory dialogue. Fauci said that the information requested by ACT UP on the trials was restricted to the PIs running them. Fauci did admit that it was these investigators who had pressured NIAID to white out large sections of the minutes. The PIs had complained that they would lose their privacy if outside groups could see what was being discussed in private. Outsiders wouldn't understand and would make trouble. That was the message. In short, the PIs preferred to operate in a closed, secret world of science that they completely controlled. They wanted no external interference, even from the patient population they were experimenting on and for whom, presumably, they were doing all their work.

Long and Eigo were still able to come up with enough data to show clear patterns within the trials being undertaken in the New York area. What they found was truly unbelievable. There were very few trials for drugs against the opportunistic infections that actually afflicted people with AIDS. Those that did exist had minuscule patient enrollment. Hardly anybody was in them! "Those things that were killing off people were not being studied," says Eigo. Nearly all the PIs were interested in one thing—the glamour field of retrovirology. They only wanted to run trials with AZT.

ACT UP basically discovered that the entire government clinical testing system was testing one drug—AZT. In fact, Tony Fauci's ACTG network was an all-AZT show. Nearly half of all people enrolled were in just one trial, number 019, testing AZT in people with the AIDS virus but showing no symptoms of infection. Trial 019 quickly became known as the "asymptomatics" trial. It was designed to see whether AZT slowed the onset of full-blown AIDS. Another trial, 016, was designed to see whether AZT curbed the onset of severe AIDS infections in people with mild symptoms. The vast majority of the rest of the trials included AZT either in direct comparison to another drug or in combination with other drugs. Long and Eigo discovered that by early 1988 practically 80 percent of all the four thousand slots in the ACTG network were for AZT trials.

Within science, AZT joined the AIDS virus in a medical mantra that was repeated over and over again: "There is one cause of AIDS: the AIDS virus, or Human Immunodeficiency Virus—HIV. There is one treatment for AIDS: AZT."

AZT both reflected and reinforced the basic paradigm within which almost all AIDS research was to take place. The hot fields in virology in the eighties were molecular biology and protein biochemistry. The biggest players were in those fields. Molecular biology focuses on nucleic acids, DNA and RNA, hence the focus on nucleoside compounds such as AZT.

It was simple, it was elegant. That's where the grant money flowed, that's where the articles being published in the best journals originated, that's where the awards for brilliance were.

The HIV-AZT litany became dogma. As one scientist prominent in AIDS put it: "If you don't swallow the dogma and repeat it word for word, to everybody around you, in your hospital, in your institution, you get cut off. It's very, very difficult to continue doing research unless you have private funds."

There were a few other problems with the dogma. Local doctors prescribing AZT to their AIDS patients were discovering that virtually half could not tolerate it. It was too toxic and killed off too many of their bone marrow cells, destroying their blood.

French scientists were discovering that AZT's effects were ephemeral. They lasted three to six months and then the patients' T-4 cell counts fell back to their original low level, sometimes even below it in a rebound effect. This was for the half of PWAs that could tolerate the drug.

Douglas Richman, one of the original PIs of the Wellcome Phase II AZT trial, discovered viral resistance to AZT developing after about three to six months. AZT lost its effectiveness quickly after twenty-four weeks.

Finally, AZT wasn't stopping *Pneumocystis carinii* pneumonia—the real AIDS killer. Some 80 percent of all PWAs were coming down with PCP at this time, and 65 percent of all AIDS deaths were due to it.

So why was practically all of Tony Fauci's ACTG clinical trials system clogged with AZT? The PIs wanted the glamour of antiviral research that AZT provided them. Besides, Sam Broder, Mr. AZT himself, had made it a made-in-the-NIH drug in the eyes of the public. The NIH could claim credit for it. Tony Fauci could claim credit for testing it. The message coming out of the government drug trials to the PWAs was simple: "We are writing you off. You are going to die anyway, so we're putting our resources elsewhere."

ACT UP made good use of the Freedom of Information Act to pry open NIAID's closed trials network. Through the FOIA, Long, Eigo, and Kleinman were able to get rough figures on women, minorities, and children with AIDS. What they found was again shocking. By early 1988, it was clear that AIDS was becoming a disease of blacks and Hispanics, of IV drug users and their sex partners. Nearly half of all cases were now in these categories. But only a minute percentage of the patient population enrolled in the ACTG trials in the New York area were minorities.

What was happening was SOP, standard operating procedure. Clinical trials for decades had been carried out in the same major university-linked teaching hospitals around the country. Not only was there an old-boy network of PIs, there was, of course, a corresponding network of private medical institutions. Just as a few PIs received most of the contracts to test drugs from both the government and the drug industry, so too did the medical institutions to which the PIs were connected receive the vast majority of grant and private contract money to run drugs.

These university-based private teaching hospitals were usually in middle-class neighborhoods and had white middle-class patients in their beds, with a sprinkling of working-class people. This was their traditional source of patients for all drug trials. It had worked for decades and it would work now, they believed.

At New York University Medical Center, for example, one of the four ACTG sites in New York, 3.6 percent of the patients enrolled in eleven AIDS drug trials were black or Hispanic. NYU Medical Center, a private hospital, is physically right next door to Bellevue, the flagship of New York City's public hospital system. NYU is supposed to have a special relationship with Bellevue, a kind of "sister city" relationship. Bellevue has the best facilities and best staff of all the municipal hospitals. It also has the greatest number of AIDS patients. Most of those patients were black and Hispanic IV drug users. NYU, however, rarely took any AIDS patients from Bellevue. The result? NYU's clinical trials were all tremendously underenrolled because Bellevue's minority patients were excluded.

This situation was the same for women. Iris Long was able to discover that only ten out of thirty-nine ACTG trials had any women in them. Of the 2,681 PWAs enrolled in the New York region, only 5 percent were female. NIAID's logic was that AIDS was a disease of gay men, so why worry about women?

That made sense for the first six years of the AIDS epidemic, but by the time the government finally got around to building a clinical trials system, the course of the epidemic had changed dramatically. The incidence of AIDS in gay men was leveling out in San Francisco and New York while it was rising dramatically in black and Hispanic IV users and the people who slept with them. The AIDS population was sharply changing to include many more women and children.

The PIs were totally out of touch with reality. NIAID's Tony Fauci and Dan Hoth were out of touch. So was the FDA's Ellen Cooper. They didn't know what was happening to the direction of AIDS on the streets of New York or any other big city in the country.

So the trials were poorly designed. They were chronically underenrolled. They missed the big shift in patient population. They were sexist and racist in the sense that the humans in the trials were not representative of those who were coming down with AIDS. And the investigators were so locked into doing things *their* way, the standard way, the way that had workèd for so long, they couldn't see it.

They refused to see it. Long, Eigo, Kleinman, and the Treatment and Data subcommittee finished their report in late March of 1988. They sent it in early April to Tony Fauci and all thirty of the principal investigators in the ACTG system.

In an accompanying letter that Eigo drafted, he called for a new system of "parallel" trials that would take place alongside the usual Phase I and II clinical trials. The parallel trials would be for populations excluded from the regular clinical trials for AIDS drugs. These people would include black and Hispanic minorities, IV drug users and their sex partners, and urban and rural people living far from teaching hospitals. It would also include the AZT intolerant, the 50 percent of PWAs who couldn't stand to take AZT and therefore couldn't enroll in practically any of the ACTG trials. The proposed parallel track of clinical trials would also include the growing numbers of people who could, at the beginning, take AZT but were now becoming AZT-resistant. All these people would go into a different set of trials so that they too could access treatment. This was the first time that a parallel track proposal was mentioned on paper, although Martin Delaney of Project Inform had also been talking about a similar concept in the months preceding.

ACT UP didn't receive a single reply to either its report or Eigo's parallel track idea. Nothing. "We didn't even get a response from the local investigators even though [in preparing the report] we had met with Fred Valentine and lots of his assistants at NYU," says Eigo.

Despite the silence, the Treatment and Data subcommittee (it became a full committee in ACT UP later in 1989) continued to expand its analysis of the government clinical trials system. A report was done on the use of placebos in trials on children with AIDS. These experiments always required that the end point, the proof, be death. In this case, dead babies. It was grotesque, especially so since AZT was already accepted as standard treatment. Ellen Cooper at the FDA insisted on separate trials for testing

AZT in children, and insisted on double-blind, placebo-controlled trials at that. All the trials with children included placebos.

ACT UP also discovered that Margaret Fischl, who had coordinated the placebo-controlled Phase II trials for Burroughs Wellcome, was also a PI for an ACTG trial on Bactrim. Despite the proven effectiveness of Bactrim and Septra against *Pneumocystis carinii* pneumonia over the years, Fischl insisted on a placebo. Joe Sonnabend had been prophylaxing with Bactrim since 1982. Dozens of other community doctors were also using Bactrim, as well as aerosol pentamidine. Cancer specialists had been using Bactrim and Septra to fight PCP since the seventies. Yet Fischl insisted. Twenty-eight people who received placebo died in her experiment to prove what virtually everyone already knew. It was senseless science. It was irresponsible, unethical science. It should never have been permitted by the Institutional Review Board that presumably approved of the trial design.

The critique of Tony Fauci's clinical trials system and the compilation of the AIDS Treatment Registry were used in the next year and a half by ACT UP to hack away at the biomedical research establishment. Together these documents composed a single, powerful message to those in charge of the clinical trials network, the people at the NIH and the FDA, the PIs, and the drug companies. In essence ACT UP said that it was no longer sufficient for scientists and bureaucrats to design the programs that were supposed to get PWAs drugs and treatments for AIDS. They had failed in the past and they would fail in the future because the scientists and bureaucrats didn't know what was happening in the real world. ACT UP demanded the right of participation in trial design by people with AIDS. For the first time ever, people with a disease were demanding the right to help structure the scientific experiments designed to help them. This was the kind of empowerment envisioned by Michael Callen in its most elemental form.

There really was no choice. As more and more people with AIDS learned about the various NIAID trials through ACT UP's AIDS Treatment Registry, fewer and fewer enrolled. PWAs didn't want to take a chance on getting placebos and dying. They wanted treatment in order to live, not to play science roulette and chance dying. Both government and drug company trials became chronically underenrolled. The PIs began to lose control.

Alternatives became available—underground alternatives. By 1988, there were over sixty drugs being discussed in the drug underground as possible treatments against AIDS. Many were already available through buyers clubs. PWAs increasingly didn't have just one choice of treatment.

They had several. They didn't have to enroll in government or drug company trials. So many stayed away or dropped out or cheated by taking other drugs that the ACTG system began to spin out of control.

Trial 019 suffered most. It was the largest clinical trial of AZT in the United States, the most important in NIAID's entire ACTG system. It was supposed to have had 1,562 patients enrolled in nineteen medical institutions by year-end 1987. Instead it had 755. In New York and San Francisco, the accrual rate was as low as 10 percent.

Trial 019's problems began back in September 1986, when the code was first broken on the AZT Phase II trial. Scientists from both Burroughs Wellcome and the NIH agreed that the next step should be testing the drug to see whether people with the AIDS virus but showing no symptoms could be helped. AZT might slow the progression of the disease. At that time, the Centers for Disease Control offered to do a trial. It wrote up a protocol and wanted to start enrolling by March 1987.

But the CDC had no experience in conducting clinical trials and no money to finance the effort. Then Tony Fauci wrested away control over all clinical trials for AIDS drugs for his institute, NIAID, even though it, like the CDC, had no prior experience in conducting big clinical trials.

In February 1987, the asymptomatic trial was shifted to NIAID. A new protocol was then written by Dr. Paul Volberding at San Francisco General Hospital. Volberding became the principal investigator of what became NIAID trial 019. It took four months, until May, for that protocol to circulate among other AIDS experts, administrators, etc., for comment.

Then Burroughs Wellcome refused to provide AZT for this purpose. The supply of the drug was still scarce and Wellcome said that the available drug should first go to the very ill. In March, the company sold NIAID some AZT but left it up to the government to package and label it.

Then problems at the various hospitals delayed enrollment. At Volberding's own school, the University of California at San Francisco, it took three months for the protocol to pass the Institutional Review Board. At Sloan-Kettering in New York, a shortage of nurses led to a two-month delay in enrollment. At Mount Sinai in New York many doctors and nurses simply refused to work with AIDS.

When Volberding and his trial 019 were finally set to go, people with AIDS didn't rush to enlist. Many who were asymptomatic saw no urgency in taking a toxic drug that would kill their bone marrow cells, make them anemic, and generally suppress their immune systems.

Those who did want AZT were put off by 019's placebos—half of those enrolled would be given sugar pills as a control to test the AZT. If the PWAs wanted AZT, they wanted AZT, not a placebo. They wanted treatment, not martyrdom, and they had a 50 percent chance of receiving a placebo and becoming martyrs in Volberding's trial 019.

By this time, Burroughs Wellcome was producing enough AZT to sell it all over the country. Doctors began prescribing it for their patients. The initial response was appalling. AZT's toxicity was tremendous. At the FDA-recommended full dose of 1200 milligrams per day, half their AIDS patients became deadly sick and had to be taken off the drug immediately. The other half required blood transfusions several times a week.

In San Francisco and New York, about fifty community doctors with large gay and AIDS practices began lowering the dose. Instead of the full 1200 milligrams a day, they first cut it in half to 600 milligrams, then in half again to 300. While trial 019 was using 1200 milligrams of AZT, they were prescribing a fraction of that. It was all done by trial and error.

All of these doctors believed in early and aggressive treatment of AIDS and prescribed several different drugs in combination. AZT was added to a "cocktail" that often included an anti-PCP drug such as Bactrim or Septra, an antiherpes drug, usually acyclovir for CMV retinitis, and another antiviral drug, such as AL 721 or dextran sulfate. In 1986 and '87 especially, an AL 721 knockoff was almost always included in the cocktail.

Peter Staley was twenty-six and trading bonds on Wall Street in 1987 when he began taking AZT full dose right after the FDA approved it. In two weeks, however, he saw his red blood count fall by half. Scared, he persisted. Then, like so many other people with AIDS taking 1200 milligrams of AZT daily, he became severely anemic. He was very tired all the time. He even started sleeping at his trading desk. So Staley, who grew up on Philadelphia's Main Line, stopped taking AZT. It was threatening his livelihood, if not his life.

But Staley's health continued to get worse as his AIDS progressed. In 1988, after about a year off AZT, his T-4 cell count fell to 105. By this time, however, after seeing AIDS activists in action at the Wall Street demo protesting Burroughs Wellcome, Staley had quit Wall Street and joined ACT UP.

This move plugged Staley into the medical underground, where he heard that some doctors were prescribing much lower doses of AZT. He tried it again. After a testing period, Staley and his doctor found that he could tolerate only 300 milligrams a day, a quarter of the recommended dose. Any more than that and Staley's anemia and drowsiness returned.

But AZT still appeared to help at that low dosage. Staley couldn't be sure. He was taking a cocktail of several drugs, including one to ward off PCP and one to fight CMV. But his health did stabilize. His T-4 cell count rose to 700 and he greeted 1989 well enough and feisty enough to lead many of ACT UP's largest demos.

Ironically, community doctors salvaged what was becoming a very negative opinion of AZT for Burroughs Wellcome and the government. By experimenting with their own AIDS patients, the doctors were able to bring down the dosage to more tolerable levels. Although half their patients couldn't tolerate any AZT, the other 50 percent found they could take it without being forced to undergo blood transfusions all the time. This increased the demand and market for AZT throughout the country, sending tens of millions of dollars in profits into Wellcome's coffers. The reputations of Sam Broder and Tony Fauci were enhanced, if not salvaged, along the way.

Iris Long, Jim Eigo, and the Treatment and Data subcommittee of the Issues Committee of ACT UP called its first "action"—a massive demonstration against the FDA in Washington. Shut it down.

ACT UP coordinated the demo with a coalition of other AIDS activist groups. The Media Committee of ACT UP, headed by gossip columnist Michelangelo Signorile, printed up 550 glossy press kits. Signorile, who joined the group in January, booked ACT UP people on local television talk shows across the country. Getting media attention for the demo was as important as the demo itself. More important.

On September 2, 1988, the FDA got wind of the impending demonstration and sent two people from its Consumer Affairs department to meet with ACT UP. This was the first official meeting between ACT UP and the FDA. "These Consumer Affairs people," says Jim Eigo, "tried to facilitate things but they didn't know near as much as we did." He sent back word that ACT UP would prefer to talk with people who really knew what they were talking about.

A week before the demo, on October 5, the FDA invited ACT UP to a talk in Rockville, Maryland. Commissioner Frank Young and eleven of his staff members, including Ellen Cooper, were there. Six ACT UP people from New York and five others from ACT UP/LA and the GMHC flew to Washington.

This was the first time for any of the ACT UP people to actually be in the building housing the FDA headquarters. They were amazed! It looked worse than the New York City subways. It was shabby, run-down, with miserable, crowded meeting rooms. It surprised the hell out of them.

Commissioner Young listened closely to the critique and agreed with everything presented to him. Young appeared to be ACT UP's friend in much the way that a used-car salesman appears to be a friend. He said yes 100 percent of the time. He also didn't have any great knowledge of the issues Eigo and Harrington were discussing. In fact, both came away from the meeting believing that Frank Young was *not* where the power was in the FDA. "Certainly you want his okay for any changes you propose, but the real power for most AIDS drugs was in Ellen Cooper," says Eigo. "Certainly for all antiretroviral drugs and for all the drugs to fight opportunistic infections associated with AIDS, Cooper was the one."

Cooper wasn't shy about disagreeing with the ACT UP contingent at the meeting. She blasted them time and again for not knowing details or for not knowing that the FDA didn't even have jurisdiction in certain areas. Eigo liked Cooper. "One of the things I admired about Cooper was that I felt she was honest, or at least not afraid to critique those of us in the room to our faces when she disagreed with us. That was a refreshing contrast to Frank Young, who would say nothing against us to our faces."

Cooper thought Eigo and Harrington were way off base. They didn't know the system and she told them so to their faces. They resented the FDA's authority yet wanted it to do more for them. "My reaction was, ya know, which way do you guys want it?"

The meeting left both sides unsatisfied. The FDA hoped it would stop the ACT UP demonstration. It was wrong. On October 11, one thousand demonstrators showed up on Fishers Lane, Rockville, Maryland, and the FDA was shut down. Always with an eye to the camera, several smaller demos were carried out over a period of nine hours. At one protesting the FDA's failure to release sixty experimental drugs to people with AIDS, ACT UP members held a "die-in"; they lay down in the street and held paper tombstones over their heads that read: DEAD FROM LACK OF AL 721; I DIED FOR THE SINS OF THE FDA; DEAD—I NEEDED AEROSOL PENTAMIDINE; DEAD—AZT WASN'T ENOUGH; DEAD—AS A PERSON OF COLOR I WAS EXEMPT FROM DRUG TRIALS; I GOT THE PLACEBO—RIP.

They chanted, "Arrest Frank Young"; "Shame! Shame!"; "No more deaths." About 360 Montgomery County and federal police officers were on the scene, many of them wearing yellow rubber gloves to "ward off" AIDS infection. Many had riot gear on, with batons and shields. They formed lines in front of the FDA building and the demonstrators crashed through them. In all, 176 people were arrested, mostly on loitering charges. They were quickly processed and released at a Metro subway station. As far as choreography goes, both the police and the demonstrators played their proper roles and no one was seriously hurt. Ronald Reagan's effigy was burned and a glass door was broken. Six demonstrators snuck into the building briefly as the cameras rolled. A quarter of the FDA employees didn't show up that day and many of the rest spent hours looking out windows at the angry ACT UP demonstrators below. It was *not* business as usual. ACT UP had made its point.

An eighties media savvy permeated ACT UP so strongly that Ronald Reagan's handlers might have been jealous. It was a logical outcome of the group's membership—mostly young, white gay men in their twenties working in advertising, television, magazines, newspapers, and Broadway, ACT UP members *were* the media in many cases.

Powerful visual images became part of ACT UP's repertoire from the very beginning. It created the SILENCE = DEATH graphic with a pink triangle floating on a black background; the triangle was the symbol used by the Nazis to identify homosexuals in the camps. The logo was put on T-shirts, buttons, posters, and stickers that were plastered all over the country. By inventing a stark visual symbol for their AIDS protest, ACT UP successfully forced people to confront their own inaction toward the disease and their own feelings toward gays.

ACT UP was remarkably creative in its protest activities, raising them almost to an art form, performance art. At the FDA demo in October 1987, in addition to inventing the die-in, they also traced chalk outlines of members lying on the street, the way police do with bodies. Inside the chalk outline ACT UP people wrote the name of one person who'd died from AIDS. It was theater with powerful imagery.

When Northwest Orient Airlines announced it would not allow people with AIDS to fly on its airplanes, ACT UP invented the phone zap, a telephone campaign that flooded the airline's switchboard with calls protesting the new policy. Dozens of people called twenty-four hours a day. False reservations were also made, wreaking havoc inside Northwest.

Finally ACT UP took to the streets of New York to demonstrate in front of Northwest's office. Chanting, "If you get sick in the air/Don't expect Northwest to care," the demonstrators made sure TV cameras were rolling and newspaper reporters were on hand before the action started.

Northwest began losing riders from the phone zap and the bad publicity. Meanwhile, its competitors called up ACT UP one by one to quietly reassure the group that they continued to fly anyone, including people with HIV. Northwest caved and reversed its policy.

There was also a childish, adolescent side to ACT UP that sometimes proved counterproductive. The name itself suggests self-indulgence, and weekly meetings were an exercise in both social activism and personal narcissism. Each of the three hundred to four hundred people packed into the converted school auditorium in the Village insisted on having his say. Meetings went on for hours without producing any consensus.

Worse, personal insults became a major tactic of ACT UP. Ronald Reagan was a "murderer." Ed Koch, mayor of New York, was a "killer." While Mathilde Krim was talking with Ted Koppel on *Nightline,* ACT UP members were screaming, "Stop the Inquisition," and more pointed obscenities at Cardinal O'Connor of St. Patrick's Cathedral in Manhattan, one of ACT UP's favorite targets because of his stand against homosexuality.

Perhaps it was the presence of middle-aged Iris Long, but the Treatment and Data group suffered less from the paranoid petulance of ACT UP. Jim Eigo, too, was older by a good ten to fifteen years than the average member of ACT UP. "Negotiation" was not an obscenity to him, or to Mark Harrington and others in T&D.

Eigo, Harrington, and Larry Kramer took the lead in actually arranging for powerful figures in the biomedical research establishment to meet ACT UP members and learn what was *really* happening in the world of AIDS outside their ivory towers.

Dr. Burton Lee was an old friend of George Bush. Before he was appointed personal physician and AIDS adviser to the president he served on Ronald Reagan's Watkins commission on AIDS. At that time Lee was a renowned researcher at the Sloan-Kettering Institute for Cancer Research. The walls of his office were full of Bush photos and Bush–Lee photos.

So a week after Lee joined the Watkins commission, ACT UP decided to invite him up to New York to educate him on what was happening in the streets. To their surprise, Lee quickly accepted. Straitlaced Dr. Burton Lee soon found himself walking down garbage-strewn East Ninth Street in the East Village. Needless to say, it was the first time Lee had been in this neighborhood in his life. Just a few blocks away, Tompkins Square Park stood as testimony to New York City's Dickensian decline during the Reagan years under the stewardship of Mayor Edward Koch. Nearly a hundred homeless people actually lived under the trees in the park. Tents of cardboard and plastic were everywhere, making the area look like a Manila slum. "Ment-chems" were everywhere, the city's underclass of mentally ill and chemically addicted lost souls, the true homeless of New York.

Across the street on Avenue B, the Christadora House, once a neighborhood community center for waves of immigrant children, stood transformed into a pricey condominium where apartments went for hundreds of thousands of dollars. Gentrification was sweeping through the area, driving the working poor out to more remote sections of the city and the ment-chems into the park. The abandoned buildings they had been occupying were suddenly valuable real estate. A coat of new paint, a little plastering, and a bit of exposed red brick attracted the young, the hip, the cool, the artistic, and the kid millionaires from Wall Street. A number of them belonged to ACT UP.

Just around the block from the Christadora House, Lee walked up a flight of stairs and found himself facing about fifteen members of the gay community. There were people from ACT UP, from GMHC, and from various gay minority groups. Lee came in very full of himself. He was the scientist from Sloan-Kettering deigning to travel to the provinces to talk to peasants, or so his attitude was perceived by many of those present.

Yet as the evening wore on, Lee's persona would change dramatically. People sitting around him told story after story of the intransigence of the system, of FDA incompetence in writing protocols and enrolling people in their clinical trials, of NIAID refusing time and again to listen to their suggestions on drugs and treatments used widely throughout the gay community. Lee was told that people with AIDS and their own doctors, the people who knew the most about the disease, were basically shut out of the government process of treating the disease.

By the end of the evening, Lee was visibly moved. The bureaucratic horror stories moved him. Lee would later tell Mathilde Krim that he wouldn't mind if the whole U.S. health system was changed. He thought it stank. When he became part of the Bush administration as the president's doctor, Lee joined a large number of officials who believed that the best way to improve health care in America was to deregulate it. The idea not only fit their conservative ideology, the need for it was apparent from the reality around them. They would especially point to the FDA drug approval process, which was so cumbersome. Lee believed that the changes taking place in the treatment of AIDS should also occur in cancer, Alzheimer's, and other diseases.

This openness to a relaxation in the regulation of drug approval was supported, of course, by ACT UP and other activist gay groups. It was also supported, not surprisingly, by the drug industry, which had long complained of the time and money lost waiting for the FDA to get its act together. A funny coalition began to emerge in 1988 driven by radical forces in the gay community. It was, a year later, to come together to generate the most intense change in biomedical research in the United States in a generation.

When Burton Lee left the apartment on East Ninth Street he said he wanted to continue meeting with the people in the room. They had impressed him with their detailed scientific knowledge. Thereafter, Lee did make himself available to the gay community and its leadership. For the first time, there was some personal access to the powers in Washington that were, in no small degree, determining their actual lives. It was heady stuff for the ACT UP members that night. They were getting to sit at the table of power, after years of frustration and defeat.

Burton Lee was just the beginning. The real turning point in ACT UP's quest to be heard in Washington came with Dr. Louis Lasagna. Before the Lasagna committee hearings, ACT UP was perceived inside the Beltway as just a crazy bunch of gays blocking traffic and clogging phone lines with demands for changes in a medical system they didn't understand. After the testimony of Jim Eigo, Iris Long, and Mark Harrington, ACT UP was taken very seriously. Their critique of the FDA and the NIAID clinical trials network was precise, in depth, and in a language scientists and scientific bureaucrats understood. After Lasagna, ACT UP became a major player in the biomedical research game in D.C., effecting change in a system frozen in time.

It began with Vice President Bush. Through all of the eighties, the

Republicans had pushed for deregulation of the drug industry along with everything else. The industry's beef was with the FDA. In the distant past, the FDA's job had been to make sure that all drugs sold in the country were safe. That was okay with the pharmaceutical companies. The forties and fifties were a golden time for them, as dozens of new drugs came out of their labs, making them millions.

Then came thalidomide and the Kefauver amendments in 1962. The Kefauver amendments, named after Senator Estes Kefauver (D.-Tenn.), ordered the FDA to make sure drugs were effective in addition to safe. That meant much more testing. It practically tripled the time it took to get a new drug from the lab to the consumer and raised costs exponentially. By the mid-eighties, it could cost as much as $100 million to bring a new drug to market. Drug development inside the United States took a nosedive, as companies went to Europe to do most of their research.

Bush turned to Armand Hammer, the head of Occidental Petroleum, for help. Hammer knew a doctor who had written extensively on problems with the FDA bureaucracy, Dr. Louis Lasagna, the dean of the Sackler School of Graduate Biomedical Sciences at Tufts University.

Lasagna set up shop at the NIH, and quickly found allies against the FDA within the NCI. Sam Broder was bristling against the FDA for taking too much power unto themselves. The National Committee to Review Current Procedures for Approval of New Drugs for Cancer and AIDS, known as the Lasagna committee, was set up under the auspices of the National Cancer Institute. It had several representatives from the drug industry, including people from Burroughs Wellcome and Upjohn, several from academia, including Thomas Merigan from Stanford, and a couple of regulatory lawyers.

The Lasagna committee opened on January 4, 1989, in conference room 10, Building 31C, on the NIH campus. It took less than ten minutes for Sam Broder to start blasting the FDA as obstructionist. He charged that the FDA was usurping powers from local physicians by deciding on all the uses of a drug. Broder said that the FDA thought it should approve virtually every single possible use of a drug before it allowed it to be sold on the market. That was how the FDA was defining its role in proving effectiveness. Broder said it was ridiculous. He said that 99 percent of what a drug is used for is discovered in actual practice by doctors in the community. The problem, according to Broder, was that since the 1962 Kefauver amendments, the FDA had defined its role much too broadly.

Tony Fauci also spoke at the hearing, but he pulled all his punches. His responses were pure bureaucratese. Yes, there are many serious problems, he said, but they've been addressed and we should see the improved results very shortly. How many times has that sentence been spoken by one bureaucrat to another bureaucrat? It had probably been spoken by most of the people in that room. Lasagna didn't like the hackneyed response. Neither did Broder. Unfortunately, Fauci ran the institute at the NIH that did practically all the government AIDS research in the country.

The second meeting of the Lasagna committee, on February 1, was Ellen Cooper's chance to defend herself. She didn't get much of a chance. Instead, Cooper found a roomful of angry ACT UP people holding signs that read, FDA, SEE THE LIGHT: DHPG WORKS. The room was blanketed with flyers about the drug DHPG, condemning the FDA for five years of inaction on it, even longer than AL 721. Community doctors had found DHPG to work very well against the AIDS infection CMV retinitis, which invariably leads to blindness.

In a dramatic confrontation with Cooper in front of the entire committee and the press, ACT UP demanded that PWAs be given a voice in all drug approvals relating to AIDS. Throughout Cooper's testimony, ACT UP interrupted with demands that PWAs be given the choice of using what the community considered an effective drug, not just what the FDA or the NIH selected. Voices shouted out, "Why does the FDA continue to refuse to approve a drug that stops blindness 80 percent of the time?"

Cooper was sitting right in front of Louis Lasagna, trying to answer the harsh salvos from Broder, but all around her people were screaming in her face.

As she sat there trying to concentrate, it was easy to remember how this monster of a problem had started out so sweetly. Back in 1984, a company called the Syntex Corp. of Palo Alto, California, started developing a drug called ganciclovir, or DHPG. It appeared safe and showed some effectiveness against cytomegalovirus retinitis. There were still only a few thousand cases of AIDS at that time. The FDA granted Syntex a Compassionate Use approval to offer DHPG to people with AIDS who had CMV retinitis. Others began taking it for CMV colitis and CMV encephalitis. Under the Compassionate Use restrictions Syntex gave it out free. It did not do FDA-approved clinical trials of the drug, although Syntex did try to collect data from PWAs.

It soon became clear that up to 40 percent of all people with AIDS

211

come down with some form of CMV. By 1988, six thousand people were taking DHPG to curb their CMV. That's when it "got out of hand," according to Cooper. "Just more and more patients were added on without systematically studying the drug. The word got out; people were losing their eyesight and wanted to try it. But we didn't have the data to say that it worked."

It was an ironic situation. Thousands of PWAs were saying that DHPG worked against CMV, but the FDA didn't have the *right kind of data* to prove it.

Syntex found itself in a bizarre situation. In order to provide the FDA with the standard kind of data the regulating body usually required to approve a drug for commercial sale, Syntex would have had to perform a double-blind, placebo-controlled experiment. That would mean, however, allowing those people getting the placebo to actually go blind. With the overwhelming evidence involving thousands of people with AIDS showing DHPG to be effective, it would be completely unethical to do a placebo trial. Catch-22. Besides, who would enroll in it?

In October 1987, the same FDA advisory committee that had recommended approval for Burroughs Wellcome to sell AZT turned down Syntex on DHPG. Dr. Itzhak Brook was the chairman again. The committee looked at the data presented by Syntex; it showed that while 90 percent of untreated AIDS patients progressed to blindness, 80 percent of those treated with DHPG improved or stabilized. But the data wasn't systematic. It wasn't from a controlled study.

Only two members of the committee voted for approval of DHPG. Both were ophthalmologists. No one on the FDA committee seriously questioned that the drug worked. Yet in the end, they voted no.

The FDA can override an advisory committee recommendation. It chose not to. "We can't get into the business of approving drugs on the basis of testimonials," Cooper later explained. Then Cooper added, "But if I was out there treating patients, I would use it. It's a different role. You need different data."

The decision infuriated PWAs. It angered their doctors and their ophthalmologists. Tremendous pressure was put on the FDA to do something. The no vote also sent a signal to drug companies to be wary of Compassionate Use. Getting drugs approved by the FDA on this basis could clearly be a serious problem.

Over the next year, Syntex and the FDA worked out three new DHPG trials that would be undertaken to generate the "proper" data. In the fall of 1988, thirteen months after the FDA advisory committee turned down Syntex, protocols were announced. Members of ACT UP read them and quickly discovered that many people who had been receiving DHPG free for years were now going to be denied access to the drug. Even Ellen Cooper concedes the point. "It was perceived in the community, and certainly in some respects, ya know, rightly so, that there were patients who weren't eligible. Ya know, two months ago they could have gotten the drug under Compassionate Use and now they can't get it. Okay?"

ACT UP obtained copies of the Health and Human Services press release on the DHPG protocols before the official release date of November 30, 1988. The activists wrote a seven-page critique, pointing out that the protocols were coercive, unnecessary, a waste of time and money, and unsafe.

Then came February 2 and the Lasagna hearings, when ACT UP zapped Cooper. "We were between a rock and a hard place then," remembers Cooper. "At Lasagna, there was a pretty significant demonstration inside about the drug. Ya know, signs about DHPG and going blind. It became most active when I was speaking."

Cooper almost quit the FDA after the zap. She told FDA Commissioner Young shortly after the hearing that she was getting nothing but grief from AIDS activists. They were making her life miserable, she said, and didn't appreciate the seventy-hour weeks she had put in year after year. Cooper was so down when she talked with Young that he thought she was going to quit within six months. She didn't.

After the demonstration at the Lasagna committee, Cooper had a meeting with Martin Delaney and several community doctors from New York to discuss DHPG. "We were certainly aware of the frustrations in the community," says Cooper. "We weren't as aware [that] the way some of the protocols were written that particular types of patients were falling through the cracks."

This rather amazing statement meant, in essence, that the DHPG trials had been drawn up without any input from the people it was supposed to help, or from their doctors. This was 1989, nine years into the AIDS epidemic. "The docs were tellin' us that there really were people they couldn't fit into any of these studies," says Cooper. "That was a very productive meeting. This was the first serious meeting to take place on ganciclovir with these doctors."

Cooper then returned to Syntex and said, "Look, can we get data from anywhere to see if it can give us enough?" Looking back later she would explain, "We needed data, on which to hang our hat as far as efficacy was concerned."

Then, according to Cooper, somebody said that Douglas Jabs at Johns Hopkins had just published new data on the drug. He didn't use controls, but his data was well documented. That was the solution. The FDA had finally found just enough new data it could describe as "sufficient" to get the DHPG approved. It wasn't exactly the scientific method at its best, but . . . "Jabs had enough patients who were treated and enough patients who were untreated and had seen them often enough that our analysis of that was adequate to say the drug worked," says Cooper.

On May 1, the FDA convened its advisory committee again. Syntex still had no clinical trial data. The general profile of DHPG was the same as it had been for years. What was new was this single study of one doctor's use of the drug in his practice. It was enough of a fig leaf for the FDA. The advisory committee then voted to approve DHPG for sale to PWAs who had CMV retinitis.

This was the second time that the FDA had bent its rules of drug approval. With AZT, Ellen Cooper reached an accord with David Barry of Burroughs Wellcome, permitting a lower level of data to be submitted to the FDA's advisory committee meeting. With DHPG, Cooper made her deal with the AIDS activist community rather than the corporate manufacturer of the drug. Political pressure pushed her in both cases to negotiate. The rock-solid rules of the scientific method proved to be quite plastic, protestations notwithstanding.

It was a clear victory for ACT UP. One of its first.

The third and final hearing of the Lasagna committee was set aside to hear testimony from AIDS activist groups. Martin Delaney from Project Inform was there. Jeffrey Levi, the executive director of the National Gay and Lesbian Task Force, had a speech ready. Mervyn Silverman was standing in for Mathilde Krim. ACT UP fielded three speakers, all from Treatment and Data: Jim Eigo, Iris Long, and Mark Harrington. After their testimony, ACT UP would be legitimized. It would increasingly be perceived by the players in the biomedical game as an interest group to be dealt with.

Its analysis of the system, the FDA and the NIAID clinical trials network, would show that ACT UP had learned the "inside" rules of the drug development game. To the scientists and bureaucrats at the Lasagna committee hearing, that meant that ACT UP could be brought *into* their world and issues and policies could be discussed and debated, even changed, in language they understood. It was a significant breakthrough, coming nine years into the AIDS epidemic. ACT UP was on the verge of bringing people with AIDS inside.

Jim Eigo led off by providing a deep analysis of what was wrong with the FDA, especially its supervision of clinical trial protocols. It was music to the ears of an audience ready to criticize the FDA. They were impressed. Eigo began by saying that ACT UP was not against all regulation: "We don't want ourselves and our friends to die from taking unsafe drugs and we disagree with the radical deregulators of the right who would abolish all efficacy requirements." ACT UP was against ineffective regulation, Eigo said. It was against an FDA that denies approval of a drug even when it is widely recognized as useful (as in DHPG). The FDA had to realize that for a major segment of the U.S. population clinical trials had become health care. Access to those trials often meant the only available treatment to thousands of people.

Eigo then went on to say that the FDA didn't make available enough information on drug trials to give PWAs the choice of entering those trials for treatment. The FDA also didn't tell drug companies the kind of data it wanted in order to grant drug approval. "An FDA official told us recently that FDA's antiviral people aren't themselves sure what an efficacy trial is," Eigo said. Drug company executives were terrified, he said, of repeating the Syntex experience.

Eigo moved on to the issue of placebos. He said that the FDA traditionally favored placebos. With AIDS and other life-threatening diseases, this meant certain death for many people. It was unethical and unnecessary, Eigo said. Drugs could be compared with other drugs, different doses of the same drug could be compared, and even the historical progression of the disease could be used to measure efficacy.

The rationale offered by scientists—that placebo trials provided the fastest and cleanest data possible—was wrong when it came to AIDS. Three major drug trials, including 019, were jeopardized, according to Eigo, because of placebos. Patients were not enrolling for fear of getting the placebo. The results were far from quick, clean data.

Eigo then tackled the FDA's propensity to force people off the drugs they were taking in order to enroll in trials. This was especially so for anti-PCP drugs such as Bactrim or aerosol pentamidine. This meant that people with AIDS were coming down with *Pneumocystis* all the time in trials, whereas before they were free of that killing infection.

Then Eigo went into a critique of the two most important FDA programs designed to get drugs to people who have no treatment alternatives. In many ways, this issue proved to be the biggest attention getter, with both Broder and Fauci criticizing the FDA for these failures.

Eigo described the FDA's Treatment IND program as simply not working. In two years, only three drugs had been released under Treatment IND and they were available only to a small number of people. "Even Commissioner Young has estimated that, at its optimum, Treatment IND would get drugs to those who need them only 20 to 30 percent faster than normal approval," said Eigo. The FDA had to loosen its definition so that only safety and *promised* efficacy were needed for a drug to receive a Treatment IND.

The FDA also had to start informing doctors around the country that while drugs under Treatment IND are "experimental," they should be used when there is no alternative. Right now most physicians were woefully ignorant, said Eigo.

Finally, Eigo said, the FDA would have to clarify just what Treatment IND was supposed to accomplish. Right now it is very foggy. Two years ago, after AZT, the program promised so much. But since October 1988, the FDA appeared to be saying that it is simply a bridge between the final phase of human trials and approval for commercial sale. That would be "a tragic narrowing of this program," said Eigo.

Turning to the Compassionate Use program, Eigo said that it too was supposed to supply seriously ill people with experimental drugs if they had no alternatives. "FDA has made no secret of the fact that it doesn't like the program," said Eigo. "Treatment IND was a partial attempt to do away with Compassionate Use."

Eigo said that the FDA often quietly collaborated with drug companies to narrow the Compassionate Use protocol to extremely sick people near death. The goal was to force everyone else into the standard clinical trials so that standard data could be gathered on the drug. This is what the FDA was doing with Schering-Plough and its drug EPO, he said. This had to stop.

Eigo completed his testimony by saying that "the same FDA that has botched its job has at times worked to deter local groups from keeping community members alive." The FDA had "made it difficult, despite the FDA commissioner's repeated proclamations of noninterference, for individuals to obtain foreign drugs."

Finally, Eigo said, the FDA should put people with AIDS into decision-making positions to draw on their experience. Eigo closed his testimony with the following: "Therefore ACT UP urges the FDA to expand all its relevant committees to include people with AIDS infection, including its extramural drug advisory panels that have in the past demonstrated their absence of compassion and knowledge of the real world of HIV infection and of special programs like Treatment IND."

The testimony was boring, deliberately so. Eigo wrote his detailed critique in the language of the people he was addressing. He was providing ammunition to powerful forces within the NIH and the administration who could pressure the FDA into changing policies that were hurting PWAs and all people with serious, life-threatening diseases. Eigo's goal was to have the Faucis, the Broders, and even the George Bushs pick up his criticisms and use them against the FDA to force it to increase access to experimental drug treatment. In that, Eigo would prove immensely successful.

Iris Long then took center stage. She told those present what was actually happening inside the trials of the NIAID clinical network.

Long began by promising that "I will give you evidence that the testing of AIDS drugs is not proceeding at a sufficient pace because of critical problems in enrolling patients in trials."

Long went on to say that she'd analyzed both the ACTG trials and private drug company trials taking place in New York State. There were three ACTG sites in New York City, the New York University Medical Center, Mt. Sinai, and Albert Einstein. Four city hospitals were satellites of these three sites.

Within the ACTG system, only 844 patients were in active trials in a state with hundreds of thousands of people infected with AIDS. Of those enrolled, 73 percent were in five trials testing AZT. That left 230 patients in the whole state for the thirty-two other open trials. New York wasn't alone. In New Jersey, 59 percent of the 93 patients enrolled in ACTG trials were enrolled in just one trial, 019, testing AZT.

Mark Harrington then offered "twelve prerequisites for a faster, more humane drug-testing system for AIDS." It was a series of final hammer blows to the NIAID clinical trials program testing AIDS drugs.

Harrington began by warning that "never before in history has the medical establishment confronted such a mobilization of angry, impatient, and well-informed citizens from communities affected by a disease. No longer will we sit and wait for scientists and bureaucrats to proceed in a research enterprise which all too often undermines the health of those in trials. No longer will trial subjects allow themselves to be used as grist for researchers' data mills."

Then Harrington moved on to his twelve demands:

1. *"Full participation of the AIDS community."*

   All too often the trial design was deleterious to the health of the participants because of the use of placebos or restrictions on the use of other drugs and because of narrowly defined patient populations.

   The motives of both government and the private drug sponsors were suspect because after nine years of drug development, the major emphasis was still on expensive, toxic antivirals rather than cheaper, more practical anti-infectives that would prevent and treat the infections actually killing people.

   Therefore, "people with AIDS and their advocates must participate in designing and executing drug trials," said Harrington.

2. *"A comprehensive, coordinated, compassionate drug development strategy."*

   NIAID's clinical trials program, after three years and hundreds of millions of dollars, had not produced a single new approved drug, according to Harrington. On the other hand, privately sponsored drugs such as alpha interferon and community-sponsored drugs such as aerosol pentamidine had successfully been developed and were widely available.

   The only solution was to form a new partnership between the AIDS community and researchers and corporate sponsors. "People with AIDS and their advocates must be full voting members of every decision-making body related to AIDS clinical trials," said Harrington. These included NIAID's ACTG Executive Committee; NIAID's AIDS Clinical Drug Development Committee (ACDDC); the FDA's Anti-Infective Drugs, Antiviral Drugs, and Vaccines and Related Biological Products Advisory Committees; and the Institutional Review Boards (IRBs) at all sites conducting AIDS and HIV-related clinical trials.

**3.** *"Equal resources given to research in anti-infectives and antivirals."*

Most of the government funds had gone into antiviral drug research. "This is fine for researchers seeking clues to the inner workings of the immune system and pursuing leads that may yield a Nobel Prize," said Harrington. It didn't help people dying of opportunistic infections.

No current trials even existed for most of the OIs.

**4.** *"An end to the quarantine of women, poor people, people in rural areas, people of color, IV drug users, prisoners, hemophiliacs, and children with AIDS from experimental treatments."*

Less than 1 percent of all the people infected with AIDS were enrolled in any AIDS drug trial, said Harrington.

**5.** *"An end to the quarantine of the AZT-intolerant."*

Half of all people with AIDS cannot tolerate AZT and they were effectively restricted from practically all drug trials because most trials included AZT.

**6.** *"Trial design must be flexible enough to allow for changing understanding of AIDS virus infection and allow subjects to receive the full standard of care for other conditions as such standards evolve."*

As treatments evolved, trials should be open enough to change to include new drugs. The patients were going to take them anyway, skewing the trials results, according to Harrington.

**7.** *"Trials must be designed for the real world: prophylaxis permitted, placebos banned, efficacy criteria flexible, and end points humane."*

Harrington went on to say that placebo trials produced bad results because no well-informed PWA would join one. In fact, entire trials, such as 005, had been scuttled for just that reason.

**8.** *"Clinical costs associated with trials and not paid for by sponsors must be paid by the government and insurance companies, guaranteeing equal access to trials for the uninsured and the underinsured."*

Insurance companies were refusing to pay for experimental treatments for AIDS, Harrington said. They would only pay for FDA-approved drugs, not any costs that came with joining clinical trials.

**9.** *"The Orphan Drug Act must be amended so that products developed at public expense are priced fairly, that sponsors open their books, that* *products are licensed to competing licensees, and that Orphan Drug status is revocable if a drug becomes unexpectedly lucrative."*

Harrington reminded the audience that the initial impetus for the Kefauver amendments of 1962 were hearings on outrageous prices charged for new drugs. ACT UP was founded, he said, as a reaction to AZT's incredible price.

**10.** *"The community-based trials network, NIAID, NCI, FDA, and other drug development entities must be granted the staff, funding, and facilities necessary to wage a successful war on AIDS."*

Community-based research, especially, lacked the money to reach its potential, according to Harrington. At a fraction of the cost of NIAID trials, the CRI in New York and the San Francisco CCC did the research on aerosol pentamidine that led to its approval by the FDA.

**11.** *"An accurate, up-to-date, accessible and international registry of clinical trials and promising experimental treatments for AIDS and AIDS-related opportunistic infections must be established."*

**12.** *"Recognizing that Treatment IND and Compassionate Use have failed to fulfill their promise, a new nationwide distribution program for promising experimental drugs for HIV and opportunistic infections, accessible to all without regard to income or location, must be established."*

Exhausting and exhaustive was Harrington's testimony. It was the finale for Harrington and for ACT UP at the Lasagna committee hearings. The message from ACT UP was simple—something new must be created. For the first time, Washington began to listen.

# ..9..
# Financing the Fight

It was a guerrilla attack, a small-scale action against the biomedical research establishment. Joe Sonnabend and Mathilde Krim organized it and when it was over, American medicine was forever changed.

The first grass-roots, community-based drug trial took place in 1984. Sonnabend provided the drive, chose the drug, and enrolled many of the patients. Krim provided the connections and arranged for the cash. The American Medical Foundation provided the organizational framework.

Four years after the first symptoms of the AIDS epidemic showed up in Los Angeles and New York, not a thing was being done. The Reagan administration was still fighting Congress over every penny spent on research for what it considered "only" a gay disease. The NIH didn't have a single trial going testing a prospective AIDS drug. Scientists who were working on the disease were chasing its etiology, which was all to the good. But meanwhile, people were dying.

Joe Sonnabend could see that they were not dying of AIDS per se, just as people don't die of old age. His patients were being killed by specific opportunistic infections that developed as AIDS crippled their immune systems. *Pneumocystis carinii* pneumonia alone was killing practically half of his patients. What was needed were drugs to fight these specific infections as well as drugs to boost the body's overall immune system.

Sonnabend knew how to get them. He and other private doctors could do their own research on their own AIDS patients. Who knew more about the disease, anyway? Doctors and their patients were already experimenting with drugs to see which, if any, worked. Sonnabend believed these patients and doctors were reservoirs of data. All he had to do was organize and channel that information.

Besides, Sonnabend had already proved that simple research could be done; back in 1982 his "sluts" work had shown a correlation among promiscuity, frequency of sexually transmitted diseases, and suppressed immunity. Now he wanted to show that local doctors could conduct sophisticated clinical trials on human beings. He wanted to prove that he, Joe Sonnabend, and his fellow practitioners could do research as good, if not better, than NIH and university-based researchers. No one had ever tried this before in the United States. No one had ever dared challenge the power of the big-time researchers.

Sonnabend and Krim picked isoprinosine as the drug the AMF should sponsor in its first community-based clinical trial. Isoprinosine was an immune modulator. It had been around for years, although not widely used, and was already proven safe for people. Sonnabend figured that since AIDS hurt the body's immunity, anything that bolstered it would help. The logic was clear to both Sonnabend and Krim. They were trained in the European medical tradition, where immune modulators were a popular field of study. The field was in favor in Japan as well. But American medicine had generally ignored it. It wasn't "hot."

Sonnabend was the principal investigator on the isoprinosine trial. He was joined by three other doctors. All four used their own patient base for enrollment. It wasn't hard to find volunteers. Practically everyone put his hand up. The only treatment people with AIDS were receiving at that time were the few drugs that their own community doctors were dispensing. Nothing else was being done for them. Of course they volunteered.

Then Michael Callen offered a suggestion that changed everything. Why not include people with AIDS in the design of the isoprinosine trial? he asked. Why not include people with the disease in the decisions that go into their own treatment? he said. It was a revolutionary step for American medicine. It was the first time patient and doctor would collaborate at the experimental drug level in developing new treatments for a disease.

Callen's suggestion was also a logical outgrowth of the empowerment movement within the AIDS community that had begun with the Denver Principles. People fighting for their lives against the epidemic *should* participate in their medical treatment, according to Callen. Callen believed the very fight prolonged life. It had prolonged his. He had seen how other "survivors," PWAs who lived far longer than the average year or two after diagnosis, were also fighters who took major roles in their own medical treatment.

Callen specifically suggested that PWAs join the isoprinosine trial's Institutional Review Board. The IRB reviewed all trial protocols and monitored the safety of the patients. It was a key institution derived from the Nuremberg trials, where it was revealed that Nazi doctors had performed experiments on concentration camp prisoners. IRBs consisted of all kinds of people, not just scientists. It was the perfect place to start empowering PWAs in their own treatment. Krim loved the idea. Sonnabend said it made sense.

At this time, Krim was a trustee of the Hastings Institute, a center for bioethics. She was able to persuade Carol Levine, a medical ethicist, to sit on the AMF's first IRB. Two PWAs then joined the IRB, Callen, who was then working as an assistant to Sonnabend, and Richard Berkowitz. They joined Vanessa Merton, a lawyer, and Arlene Carmen from Judson Memorial Church in the Village. Sonnabend couldn't be on it since the IRB was going to review his research proposals for the isoprinosine and future drug trials. But he was a silent member. "We didn't make a move without Joe," says Callen.

The clinical trial went smoothly. Krim was able to persuade Newport Pharmaceuticals, which owned isoprinosine, to finance the test. Two outside labs were used to do the technical analysis. The trial results showed that isoprinosine was a promising drug. It was safe and there were indications that it might help against AIDS. Sonnabend and Krim concluded that it had possibilities and probably should go on to a big Phase II trial.

It was a good deal all around. The community-based trial cost just a fraction of what university-based researchers demanded to test a pharmaceutical company's drugs. The AMF staff was very small, with little overhead. Newport Pharmaceuticals got a bargain.

The trial also got patients fast. Over the past two decades, enrollment in drug trials at academic medical centers had been taking longer and longer, costing drug companies more and more. There really wasn't any mystery about this trend, although it did evade the ivory tower scientists. Academic researchers were completely cut off from the people with the disease under study, the people they were trying to enroll. They designed their trials in a vacuum and patients increasingly didn't like them. For starters, half of all those enrolled always received a placebo, which meant no treatment. Then there were the long distances many had to travel to get to the medical school hospitals. Enrollment had long been a problem in cancer. It would soon turn out to be a very serious problem in AIDS.

For its part, Newport reimbursed the doctors handsomely. The AMF got a share of overhead money, just as Stanford or Harvard or any other sponsoring organization would. The sum of money was small and it was a bargain for Newport, but it still meant a great deal for the tiny AMF.

The biggest benefit, however, was that Sonnabend, Krim, and Callen proved that privately funded, community-based clinical research was not only possible, but efficient. They showed that local doctors could keep good, clean records, keep to a protocol, and analyze the data. They also opened beachheads in trial design and medical ethics by including PWAs on iso-prinosine's IRB. No placebos were used in the trial. Everyone received some drug, some treatment.

It was great. "Everybody got something in this little trial," says Krim. "We became convinced that it was perfectly feasible to do community research. Sonnabend led the way."

Then Krim dumped Sonnabend for Liz Taylor.

It all began with Rock Hudson's will. After he died of AIDS in the fall of 1985, Hudson's former live-in lover, Marc Christian, sued the estate for millions of dollars. He claimed that Hudson had deceived him about the deadly disease and had therefore threatened his life.

One item in the will that was not challenged was the $250,000 the actor had left to his doctor, Michael Gottlieb. Hudson instructed Gottlieb to set up a foundation that would support AIDS research and spread information about the disease. By this time, Gottlieb was already an established figure. In 1981, he'd authored the first paper on AIDS. At the time he was a young assistant professor in the immunology department at UCLA. He had a friend, Joel Weisman, who had gay patients. It was Weisman who first perceived the strange occurrence of *Pneumocystis carinii* pneumonia in his Los Angeles practice and made the connection with a decline in the patients' immune systems. He sent his patients to Gottlieb, who ran the tests. The two wrote the first paper on AIDS, but Gottlieb was first author so it became his great claim to fame.

Responding to Hudson's bequest, Gottlieb put together a glitzy, Hollywood board of trustees for the new AIDS foundation. AIDS was devastating the movie industry. Rock Hudson was just one of thousands of actors, producers, directors, and writers who were gay and very sick. Elizabeth Taylor, a close friend of Hudson's, agreed to be the head of the foundation.

But then Gottlieb met with Mathilde Krim, who said, "Michael, this is ridiculous. We are not going to create two competing foundations. This is a national problem. We should be one national foundation. Let's merge."

Gottlieb agreed and the two entered a period of serious, complicated, and very nearly disastrous negotiations. Krim and her board had been operating for three years at this point, financing AIDS research by Joe Sonnabend, Michael Lange, and other community doctors. Krim felt very protective of what she had created—a grass-roots research organization with very close ties to the patient community. In fact, Michael Callen had made sure that patients not only were represented at the AMF, but had real power. Nothing like that existed in Gottlieb's group on the West Coast. It was far more traditional, with no bows toward PWA empowerment. The match between the two organizations was not exact by any means.

Gottlieb went into the negotiations assuming his foundation would simply take over Krim's AMF. He didn't know Mathilde Krim very well. The first big fight was over a new board. Gottlieb wanted a big one weighted toward the West Coast. Krim, ever the pragmatist, wanted a small one to get things done. She wasn't about to cede control of the board, either. In the end, Krim and Gottlieb compromised. Both the East and West Coasts would contribute one-third each from their existing boards to the new board. Then Krim and Gottlieb would appoint an equal number of fresh faces to complete the governing body.

The conflict grew worse, and more personal. Gottlieb made it clear that he wanted, he expected, to be head of the new foundation. Krim refused. It infuriated her. Her AMF had been in business for three years, amassing a wealth of experience fighting AIDS. Gottlieb's group didn't even have its office set up yet. Krim went to the wall with Gottlieb. "Absolutely not," she said. "You are not going to be chairman. Either I am chairman or we are cochairmen. But you are not taking us over." When the legal papers were signed for the new nonprofit American Foundation for AIDS Research, or AmFAR, there were two cochairs at the top of the organizational chart. Win number two for Krim.

In many drawn-out, rough negotiations, even a successful completion often leaves a bitter residue behind in personal relations. This was so in AmFAR. Tension permeated the Krim-Gottlieb relationship. When she said one thing, he would say the opposite. While Krim was firmly in favor of continuing the community-based research pioneered by Sonnabend in the isoprinosine trial, Gottlieb was dead against it. His constituency back in Los

Angeles, doctors with private practices, were afraid of legal liability. Gottlieb was dismissive of the whole idea of doctors doing their own research. He told Krim it was all "nonsense." Research was supposed to be done in big research centers, like the NIH and big medical school hospitals. Gottlieb's attitude was terribly insulting to Krim. "When I was advocating community research," says Krim, "Gottlieb would dismiss it by saying that I was not a doctor, so what did I know? I was just a biologist, a Ph.D., not an M.D., so what was I talking about, ha?"

Gottlieb wouldn't budge on this one. He'd lost twice and wasn't going to lose again. Krim had to give in. In 1985, she sacrificed Joe Sonnabend to make AmFAR work. Krim the pragmatist did battle with Krim the scientist and friend. In the end, she did what had to be done to set up AmFAR. She compromised, something Sonnabend could never do. The new foundation would support AIDS research by giving grants to scientists in established laboratories and by informing the public about AIDS and its treatments, but it wouldn't do any clinical trials of its own. That was over. It would no longer support Sonnabend's research.

Sonnabend was crushed. He felt betrayed by Krim and by the AMF. After all, it had been created in the first place to fund and support him and his kind of patient-focused research. He felt rejected and abandoned.

Sonnabend believed that one of the main reasons he was dumped was his multicausal theory of AIDS. Just a few months earlier, HHS Secretary Margaret Heckler had gone before a bank of TV lights to announce that Dr. Robert Gallo of the National Cancer Institute had discovered the cause of AIDS—a retrovirus. Since then, the general public, and the gay community in particular, had become convinced that this AIDS retrovirus was the sole cause of the disease. There was almost a sigh of relief at the announcement. At last, the cause of this dreadful disease had been found. It was the official wisdom and it affected AmFAR. "One of the realities of fund-raising at the time meant that the AIDS virus was not to be disputed," Sonnabend explains. "There was only one cause of AIDS and the AIDS virus was it." Certainly Gottlieb believed this was the truth. So Sonnabend was out: "I really couldn't stay there with the views that I held. I made way for Michael Gottlieb. He replaced me."

In exchange for Sonnabend and his ground-breaking community research, Krim got Elizabeth Taylor and Barbra Streisand, two celebrities with immense fund-raising capabilities. It was a practical, necessary choice, but it still left her very uneasy. True, big money began flowing into AmFAR once the Hollywood star circuit took up the AIDS cause. True, this money went into AIDS research. Yet Krim felt guilty about Sonnabend. "We had to compromise," she says with a what-could-we-do shrug of her shoulders.

Sonnabend thought he was being exchanged for Gottlieb over a scientific issue. The reality was that he was traded by Krim for Liz, glitz, and L.A. millions.

The dream did not die, however. Sonnabend wouldn't quit. He wouldn't let go.

Even though he was deeply hurt by Krim, Sonnabend continued to lobby her for help in setting up a second community-based research effort. He knew Krim agreed with him on principle because she had told him of her fights with Gottlieb. So he kept hammering away at her, for nearly two years.

Sonnabend had a way of getting around Gottlieb, he told Krim. If the new AmFAR didn't want to do clinical drug trials itself, Sonnabend argued, why not simply fund a completely new organization that would do it? AmFAR was in the AIDS research funding business, wasn't it? Sonnabend told Krim that the AMF's IRB still existed on paper. Indeed, even the old AMF itself existed because people had bequeathed it money upon their deaths. Sonnabend could simply resurrect it and AmFAR could support it.

It was a practical solution and Krim loved it. It appealed to her sense of negotiating play, to her pragmatism. She told Sonnabend to go ahead and try to set up another grass-roots research organization. She would lobby for money back at AmFAR to support it. But first, Krim warned Sonnabend, this new thing must really exist and apply for funding before she could do anything. Sonnabend had to create it.

Sonnabend, Callen, Krim, and a fourth person, Tom Hannan, began to meet every week to discuss the organizational structure of a new community-based research organization. At first they met at Judson Memorial Church in the Village. Then they moved to meeting in their own apartments. The best place to get together, of course, was in Mathilde Krim's townhouse on Manhattan's East Side. There was no name on the door, just a buzzer and a butler who answered up. A long, winding staircase rose five stories. The four usually met on the first floor in Arthur Krim's study, where built-in wood bookcases lined the wall, an Oscar for humanitarianism shared shelf space with Saint Thomas Aquinas, and cigarettes lay scattered over every empty table space. Mathilde Krim, "Matild" to Sonnabend and Callen, was a fierce, defiant smoker.

The structure they wanted to create was basically a copy of the old AMF model, but with a difference. This time, PWAs would be present at each and every level of decision making, not just the IRB. The new organization would be a testament to self-empowerment.

There was one other difference. Sonnabend wanted the new community research group to have its own clinic where it could do the research. A clinic would provide essential services to doctors participating in the research, such as monitoring their patients, collecting data, and analyzing the information.

Sonnabend persuaded about half of the original AMF Institutional Review Board to join the new one. Dr. Bernard Bihari, an original participant in the early AL 721 days, joined both the IRB and the board of directors. So did Krim and Callen. Joe Sonnabend too went on the board. Tom Hannan was chosen to be the first administrator and run the place. The CRI, the Community Research Initiative, was born.

On paper it looked great. Sonnabend had been hoping that by the time the CRI was organized, Krim would have found the money to support it. She hadn't. Krim was trying her best, but "Michael Gottlieb just didn't like the idea," she told Sonnabend.

The CRI had to find another sponsor, an umbrella organization that would provide some cash and perhaps facilities. Sonnabend knew Michael Callen was a founder of the People With Aids Coalition, or PWAC (pronounced "Pee Wack"). Why not try to put the new CRI under PWAC? thought Sonnabend.

Sonnabend proposed the idea to Callen, who went to the PWAC board, but they were cool to it. Sonnabend then went to a board meeting himself and told them that drug companies would pay real money to get their drugs tested. He said they would, of course, pay overhead expenses that PWAC could use for its newsletter or for anything else. Since Callen wrote the *Newsline,* which provided treatment data for people with AIDS, he pushed extra hard for Sonnabend and the CRI. "They weren't terribly enthusiastic," Sonnabend remembered later, "but they bought the idea."

The PWAC board, of course, wanted a written proposal to consider and told Sonnabend to write one, but paperwork was not one of Sonnabend's strengths and he procrastinated. He couldn't bring himself to actually sit down and write out all that bureaucratic crap necessary to get something important done. The CRI was self-evidently important, he thought. Why did he have to write out a ten-page proposal?

It was Sonnabend's quirky personality at work again. He'd run into trouble before because of it, even at such friendly places as the AMF with friends like Mathilde Krim. In the lab, with patients, doing what he wanted to do, he was decisive, quick, in control. But get him close to anything that smacked of bureaucracy and he turned from Jekyll to Hyde, a complete monster. He couldn't help resisting, fighting the paper pushers, even such benign bureaucrats as the PWAC board of directors. It was a childish rebelliousness that Sonnabend should have grown out of long ago. Had it not interfered with such important issues as doing critical AIDS research, it wouldn't have mattered. But at times it did.

Finally, after weeks of delay, Callen and Hannan blew up and screamed at Sonnabend to just *do* the damn thing! He gave in, came out of his rebel-with-a-cause mentality, and wrote the proposal for a community-based research outfit. Sonnabend put both Callen's and Krim's names on it. Callen brought it over to PWAC and the board approved it. It was late fall, 1986.

CRI's first quarters were a rented room on the ninth floor of a Manhattan building. It had been used as a storeroom, had no windows, and pipes stuck out all over the place. There was never any air or light in it. "Matild" often stopped by and so did Bernie Bihari, offering his advice. Sonnabend's patients, or friends of his patients, were usually crowded in, asking questions on treatment or just trying to find a comforting word after being tested seropositive.

The main business, however, was to come up with a number of operational objectives for the CRI. Callen especially wanted to be specific about how this community-based research organization was going to be different from Tony Fauci's NIAID clinical trials system. It was mid-1987 by this time and it was already clear that the government testing effort was going to focus on AZT and other nucleosides almost exclusively. It was also clear that all the trial slots were filled. There was nowhere for the growing number of people with AIDS to go for treatment.

After weeks of talk an agreement was reached on the CRI's four major priorities. First, the CRI would emphasize opportunistic infections in its drug trials. It would focus on testing drugs that might prevent specific OIs as well as those that might treat them as they developed. The CRI narrowed down the dozens of OIs to *Pneumocystis carinii* pneumonia, fungal infections, CMV infections, and MAI, the "slimming" disease. MAI was becoming more and more threatening as people with AIDS lived longer. It killed through malnutrition as people suffered from diarrhea, loss of appetite, and eventually loss of weight.

Opportunistic infections had a relatively low priority at NIAID, which emphasized antivirals, or rather antiretrovirals, almost to the exclusion of other drugs. As Iris Long of ACT UP would soon show, 80 percent of the people enrolled were in trials using AZT. Very few were in trials designed to test drugs for treating the killer infections.

Next, the CRI would test drugs that built up the body's immune system. Sonnabend and Bihari believed that if they could enhance immune function, they could help PWAs ward off infections long enough for the hotshots at the NIH to come up with the big breakthrough.

The CRI would also test underground drugs in use in the community. People with AIDS themselves had often been way ahead of the research scientists in Bethesda in finding drugs that appeared to help. They had had no success in getting NIAID—or more pointedly, the drug selection committee of the ACTG—to listen to them. The CRI would make it a matter of principle to take very seriously what the PWAs were saying about drugs. In 1987, the one drug everyone was taking was bootleg AL 721. It would be the first tested.

Trial design would also be a major CRI focus. Krim, Sonnabend, Bihari, and Callen all wanted to make it an important point of policy that trial design be directed at the patient, not the scientist. They knew, as the big-time researchers did not, that the reason NIAID was having trouble getting people to enroll in their trials had to do with their design. Placebo-controlled experiments meant half the people received nothing, no treatment. NIAID's design also called for recruiting people into trials slowly, over a period of two or three years. There wasn't any hurry—or at least the scientists weren't in a hurry. But AIDS could be a quick killer and PWAs dealt with death in terms of months, not years.

CRI was going to design trials that did not have placebos. People would not have to die to prove a point. Comparisons could be made by measuring low, medium, and high doses of a drug against one another. Historical data could be used as a baseline as well for comparison. The guiding principle would be that everyone would get treatment. "We've got to take into account what the AIDS patients want," said Bihari. "What will attract them to trials? What will make sense *to them?* What will help them? They will not enter trials for the sake of humanity. You enter a trial because it offers you something you don't have access to. It increases your chances of survival."

The first drug Sonnabend wanted to test was aerosol pentamidine. Since late 1986, he'd been spending many of his days over at Memorial Sloan-Kettering Cancer Center, Mathilde Krim's old camping ground. Dr. Donald Armstrong, an old buddy of Sonnabend's, had his lab there and was doing an incredibly exciting experiment.

Sonnabend had been a pioneer in giving his AIDS patients anti-PCP drugs to ward off the deadly pneumonia. Ordinarily, he prescribed Bactrim or Septra, but the sulfa drugs were far from perfect. They had serious side effects for about half the people taking them. Severe skin rashes and anemia could occur. Since the AIDS virus attacked bone marrow and also caused anemia, Sonnabend and other community physicians found themselves taking patients off Bactrim even though they knew it was effective against PCP.

Another drug, pentamidine, had been used against the same disease. Originally, pentamidine was developed to fight sleeping sickness in Africa. Then it was found to work against *Pneumocystis carinii* pneumonia. But there were problems. Originally, to fight PCP, pentamidine was given intravenously. That, unfortunately, led to serious complications. Only a tiny amount of the drug actually got to the lungs to fight the PCP. Most of it was absorbed by the liver, kidneys, and spleen, where it was very toxic.

Armstrong came up with a brilliant plan to get pentamidine directly into the lungs: turn it into an aerosol mist that would go straight to the lungs when breathed. For two years he tried to get NIAID to do a clinical trial of aerosol pentamidine. It was like poking a marshmallow. Nothing happened. Tony Fauci's clinical trials network couldn't get its act together enough to get a trial of this drug going, even though everyone knew by that time that PCP alone accounted for 60 percent of all deaths from AIDS.

Armstrong went out and found a little financing from a small private drug company called Fisons. He then imported a number of ultrasonic, hand-held nebulizers from West Germany, which he called "the green machines." By the time Joe Sonnabend began visiting Armstrong in the fall of '86, Armstrong had about a hundred people with AIDS inhaling a fine mist of aerosol pentamidine fifteen to thirty minutes every other week.

None of them died from PCP. Not a one. That's what amazed Sonnabend. Delirious joy didn't come naturally to the British-trained South African, but he couldn't help thinking that this aerosol pentamidine was just fantastic! He put many of his own patients on the green machines, including Michael Callen. The word spread to other community doctors in

New York. And on the West Coast, San Francisco's Pacific Presbyterian Medical Center began a study as well.

Sonnabend decided that his new CRI should do its first clinical trial on aerosol pentamidine. Armstrong agreed. It was perfect. The NIH didn't have one trial going on a safe drug that clearly was working against the number one killer of PWAs. The community would then do the testing.

The CRI began negotiations with Fisons, the company that supported Donald Armstrong's research at Sloan-Kettering. Sonnabend wanted enough money to do a modest clinical trial of aerosol pentamidine. But Fisons wouldn't commit; it looked as though the whole effort was about to collapse, when another small drug company, LyphoMed of Rosemont, Illinois, offered to finance the trial. "We jumped," says Callen. It was late '87. They set up a clinic, hired four nurses and a small administrative staff.

Callen then learned that CRI wasn't alone. He gave a talk on the West Coast and said that CRI was the only community-based research organization in America. Very quickly, a letter arrived from the County Community Consortium of Bay Area HIV Health Care Providers (CCC) begging to differ. It had been formed under the auspices of none other than Paul Volberding to channel information on AIDS from academic hospital researchers to local doctors treating the disease. Dr. Donald Abrams was the CCC's first chairman. He was the assistant director of the AIDS Division at San Francisco General Hospital and assistant clinical professor at the Cancer Research Institute of the University of California at San Francisco. The letter said that the CCC was already in operation, thanks to—guess what?—LyphoMed. It was running a clinical trial of 440 patients out of San Francisco General Hospital.

The CCC was a very different model of community organization from the CRI. The CCC used San Francisco General Hospital's IRB and facilities. The CRI had its own IRB and its own freestanding clinic. Thanks to Callen, PWAs held responsible positions throughout the CRI. Patients had power. The CCC was more hierarchically organized. Information flowed down from hospital researchers to doctors in the field, not up from the community. People with AIDS didn't sit on any committees, either.

But the CCC did share some important values with its East Coast cousin. It didn't believe in placebos, for example, at least not when it came to PCP and pentamidine. And it didn't use the usual double-blind format either. Instead, they compared different dose ranges. Each patient, therefore, received some kind of treatment. No one got a sugar pill. The CCC had written a protocol for an aerosol pentamidine trial and received an IND from the FDA several months before the CRI got into the act. That trial design attracted a very large number of volunteers. At a time when NIAID was having severe problems filling its trials, the CCC was able to get its trial enrolled within days.

Sonnabend and Bihari decided to adopt the CCC's entire protocol in the belief that with the same IND, they would have a better chance of getting their data accepted by the FDA. It was a long shot, though. Neither doctor could remember a time when the FDA had accepted data as legitimate from a trial that didn't include a placebo. But Sonnabend and Bihari hoped that they could show such amazing results with aerosol pentamidine that the FDA would have no choice but to break with standard operating procedure.

It worked. The CCC provided data to the FDA on the efficacy of aerosol pentamidine, but its toxicity work wasn't done in a totally reliable way. The data came from many different doctors' offices and there was no real consistency. At the CRI, the data was collected centrally, from 232 people seen at the clinic. Pulmonary function studies were performed by one doctor always using the same machine, allowing the FDA to make a judgment about toxicity that it couldn't make on the basis of the CCC data. The CRI information proved critical; the FDA wouldn't have approved aerosol pentamidine without it.

On June 15, 1989, the FDA approved the commercial sale of aerosol pentamidine for the prevention and treatment of PCP. It was the first time ever that a drug had been approved based on grass-roots research. It was the first time that the FDA had approved an AIDS drug that had been tested without a placebo. This precedent-setting move was a major victory for the CRI. Death would no longer be the only satisfactory measurement of the success or failure of a drug in a life-threatening disease. For the FDA, this was a revolutionary step that would affect all drug approval, all medicine.

Even before the FDA gave its okay, its staff visited the CRI and commended Sonnabend and Bihari on the quality of the organization's case record forms. Their forms demonstrated how well the science was being performed, how thorough the data, how organized CRI was. "They said publicly at that meeting," Bihari remembers, "that they were very pleased with the quality they saw in our data."

This was critical for the future of community-based research. Sonnabend and Bihari at CRI, and Don Abrams at the CCC in San Francisco, had shown that they were capable of doing serious science, science by the rules, "science as good as the science the medical schools are doing," says Bihari. They showed the FDA, the NIH, and the all-important pharmaceutical industry that community-based researchers were not just a bunch of crazy quacks. "If we did bad science, then people would have been happy to write us off," says Bihari. "Doing good science allowed us to establish our credibility. Then and only then did people look at the other things we were talking about—the different drugs that should be put into trials, the need to include minorities and IV users in trials, the ability to design protocols that did not include placebos so that all the patients got some kind of treatment. [Doing] good science . . . was crucial."

The FDA approval was just what the CRI needed for legitimacy. Once it got the Good Housekeeping Seal of Drug Approval from the FDA, drug companies began lining up at CRI's door. CRI was able to show it could test drugs faster and cheaper than either NIAID's giant clinical trials system or the PIs at the big academic hospitals. After all, what new drug had ever come out of the ACTG? Nothing. What were they forever testing? Burroughs Wellcome's AZT and AZT analogues such as ddI and ddC. Bihari and Sonnabend told the drug companies they would test any compound that could possibly work against AIDS.

But even that paled in importance compared with what else the CRI had proved. It had shown the pharmacutical industry that *it had the patients!* Control of the AIDS patient population had shifted away from the PIs and the NIH, the biomedical establishment, over to the community-based researchers. This was a critical move in the history of medicine and research. The ability to deliver patients for testing had always been the primary concern in drug research. The CRI and the CCC showed they could enroll patients quickly and cut testing costs. It made their reputation. "We got put on the map by LyphoMed and the aerosol pentamidine trial," says Callen. "At that point, DuPont got serious with the CRI about financing a clinical trial of its drug Ampligen. They had been in on-and-off negotiations for quite a while, but after the FDA accepted the pentamidine data, DuPont committed. So did Ortho and Johnson and Johnson. The others came rolling in."

The CRI was extraordinary. A new alliance between private drug companies and local, grass-roots research organizations was created. A new collaboration between patients and doctors to test out drugs for their own treatment appeared. Patients were actually making decisions on drugs and trial designs that affected their own health. *Their* interests were taking precedence, not the scientists'. *Their* health was the priority, not the careers of academic researchers. A new medical underground was being created with the CRI, an alternative drug development track. Nothing like it had ever been done before in the United States.

And why? Because the government effort to develop drugs for AIDS was a fiasco, an out-of-control fiasco. It was too slow, too restricted, too expensive. The government, through Tony Fauci's NIAID, had lost control of the patient population it was supposed to be helping. Control was passing instead to the CRI and the new medical underground that was offering PWAs an alternative way of getting experimental treatment. No placebos, just drug treatment for everybody. The pharmaceutical companies saw the switch in power. They saw how the CRI was able to do low-cost, fast drug testing and they jumped to support it. Mainstream financing of the medical underground began to take place. Soon the CRI would have a dozen drugs under way, funded by a whole series of drug companies. Soon there would be a dozen CRIs. It was a message the PIs didn't want to hear. It was a challenge to their authority and their power. It was a threat.

# PART THREE

# MEDICAL SCIENTISTS: LESS ARROGANCE, BETTER RESEARCH

Montreal on this quiet summer night in 1989 was delivering on its promise to be very special. The air was balmy, the streets were filled with people strolling slowly home, reluctantly returning from parties or from feasting on rich French restaurant food. Larry Kramer was taking it all in as he walked Molly, his shaggy-haired dog. The past weekend had been very busy. ACT UP and other AIDS activist groups had met Saturday and Sunday to thrash out policy and strategy. There had been a lot of shouting, a lot of disagreement. Now, the night before the official June 4 opening of the Fifth International Conference on AIDS, Kramer was letting himself be pulled along behind the ever-sniffing Molly.

He was walking away from the Palais du Congrès convention center, where the conference was scheduled to take place. As Molly was doing her business, Kramer looked up and who should be coming down the street directly in front of him but Tony Fauci, the director of NIAID. With him was his assistant, James Hill.

Kramer froze. It had been a year since he had penned his infamous "Open Letter to Dr. Anthony Fauci" in the *Village Voice,* accusing him of being a "murderer" for having remained silent about his need for more people and space to do AIDS research. Kramer had compared Fauci to Adolf Eichmann.

So here were Fauci and Hill standing right in front of Kramer and Molly. Kramer braced himself. Fauci moved very close and raised his hand. But instead of belting Kramer in the face, he threw his arm around his shoulders and smiled. "How are ya, Larry?" he said.

Kramer was stunned into silence, an unusual state of being for him. Finally he said, "You're a real gentleman, Tony. If anyone had said about me what I said about you, I would not be throwing my arms around him."

To Kramer's surprise, Fauci continued to be very friendly. He suggested that they walk a ways together. Kramer agreed, of course. Here was a chance to chat up the most important player in the NIH AIDS game.

But it wasn't going to be all that easy. Fauci's assistant Hill was terrified that Fauci would say something he shouldn't and that Kramer would use it against him in the press. So Hill kept trying to insert himself between Kramer and Fauci as they walked the Montreal streets. Molly got all tangled up in everyone's legs as the men jockeyed for position. Hill kept trying to interrupt Kramer by identifying all the sights along the way. He pointed to the ugly, concrete, bunker-shaped convention center and said, "This is where we're going to meet tomorrow." Then he pointed out the street that had all the chic stores and then the street with good restaurants. It drove Kramer nuts.

Through it all, however, Fauci was talking on and on about the "parallel track." Once Kramer tuned Hill out and Fauci in, he couldn't believe his ears. This was the first time anyone at the NIH had mentioned the term since Jim Eigo of ACT UP and Marty Delaney of Project Inform had suggested it in their testimony to the Lasagna committee as a way of speeding up access to experimental drugs for people with AIDS. That was back in January, six months ago. What was going on here? thought Kramer.

Eigo in particular had argued that only a tiny percentage of people with AIDS could get into any clinical trial and thereby get medical treatment. Why not open a second, parallel track to give safe but experimental drugs to any PWA who couldn't qualify for enrollment in a regular clinical trial, he suggested. At the moment, thousands of individuals who couldn't stand to take AZT, who lived far from the big academic hospitals, or who were taking Bactrim or other drugs prohibited in particular trial protocols were frozen out. A parallel track would open drug treatment to them.

But what the hell was Fauci doing talking about it? thought Kramer. Was this the same Fauci who wouldn't even listen when he and Michael Callen begged him back in 1987 to simply advise doctors about aerosol pentamidine, a drug community doctors were successfully using to prevent PCP? The Fauci in front of him was talking, in the dead of night, as if he had invented the concept of parallel track. He was offering it up to Kramer as the solution to the community's need for great treatment access. Kramer

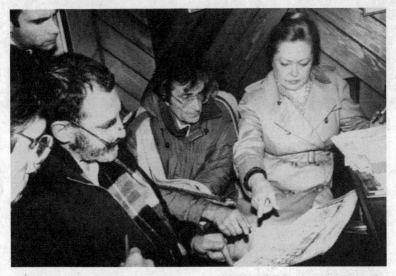

*Mathilde Krim was the force behind the establishment of the Community Research Initiative, along with Michael Callen, Tom Hannan, Joe Sonnabend, and Bernard Bihari. It was launched from a tiny cramped room in the GMHC. No one complained about Krim's ever-present cigarette.* (© Jane Rosett)

*The drug aerosol pentamidine may have saved more lives than AZT. It was not tested by the NIH but by two small local groups in New York City and San Francisco — the CRI and CCC.* (© Jane Rosett)

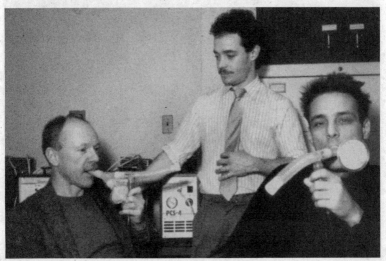

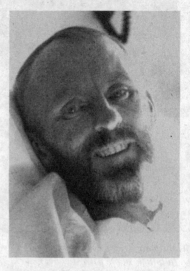

*Bobbi Campbell was a man of many "firsts": first in San Francisco to go public as a Person With AIDS; first to begin an AIDS support group; first to conceive of the PWA self-empowerment movement.* (© Jane Rosett)

*West Coast John James (left) amd East Coast Michael Callen fought over AZT, testing for AIDS, and the secret clinical trial of "Compound Q."* (© Jane Rosett)

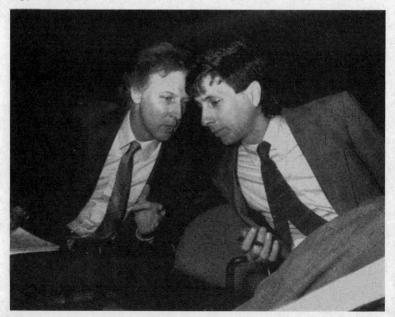

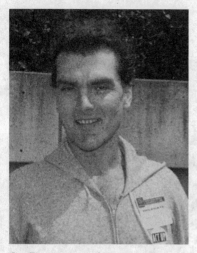

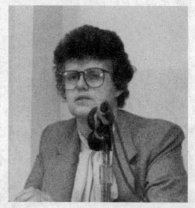

Jim Eigo was one of Iris Long's pro-
tégés. His ability to speak to the medical researchers in their own language
gained him — and ACT UP — entrée
into the secret world of the FDA-NIH.

Iris Long wandered into an ACT UP
meeting and transformed the organization into an instrument of change for
medical science. A shy person, educated as a pharmaceutical chemist, Long
trained a cadre of ACT UP members
who knew more about drug development than most medical researchers.

Mark Harrington of ACT UP's Treatment and Data Committee blasted the
NIH and the FDA in his testimony at
the Lasagna Committee hearings. His
analysis of their shortcomings triggered
major changes. (© Jane Rosett)

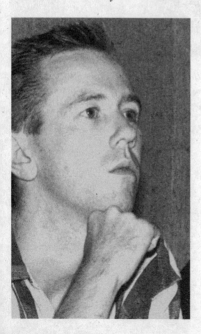

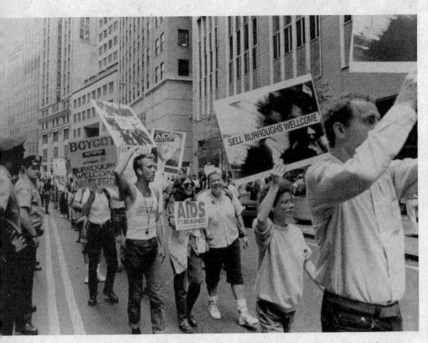

*ACT UP demonstrated against the NIH, the FDA, and the pharmaceutical compa-
nies to cut the price of AZT, speed up drug development, and increase access to
treatments for PWAs.* (© Lee Snider / Ph. Images)

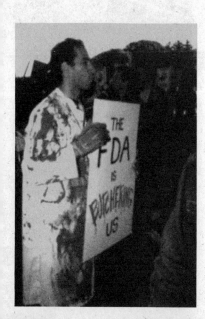

*The FDA had to be pushed screaming and kicking to change its rigid adherence to placebo testing — which guaranteed that sick people would die.*
(© Jane Rosett)

*Ronald Reagan refused to say the word "AIDS" until his friend Rock Hudson died of it.* (© Jane Rosett)

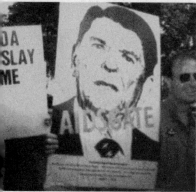

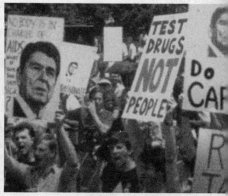

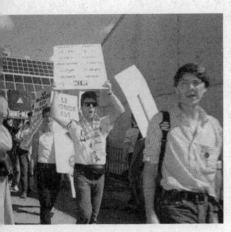

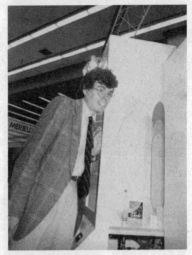

ACT UP took control of opening cere-
monies at Montreal to protest the kind
of medical research being done on
AIDS. Its serious message got lost in
the theatrics on stage. (© Jane Rosett)

Blowing up condoms to illustrate their
size and strength was a major commercial effort at the Fifth International
AIDS Conference in Montreal. It was
also a source of gleeful delight to the
conference participants. (© Jane Rosett)

"It was a love-in," said Mathilde Krim, describing the three day CRI-CCC confer-
ence on community-based research held at Columbia University. Left to right:
John James, Stuart Nightingale, "Bopper" Deyton, Mathilde Krim, Michael Callen,
Tony Fauci, Sam Broder, Donald Abrams, Burton Lee. (© Jane Rosset)

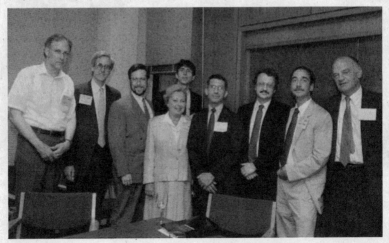

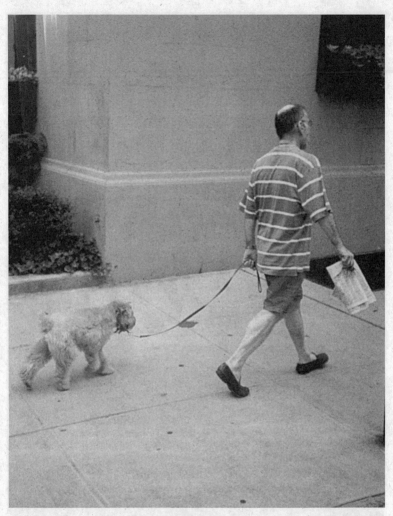

*Larry Kramer was walking his dog Molly in Montreal at the Fifth International AIDS Conference when he ran into the NIH's Tony Fauci. Kramer had just called Fauci a "murderer" in print. Instead of belting him, Fauci threw his arm around Kramer and said, "How are ya, Larry?"* (© Jane Rosett)

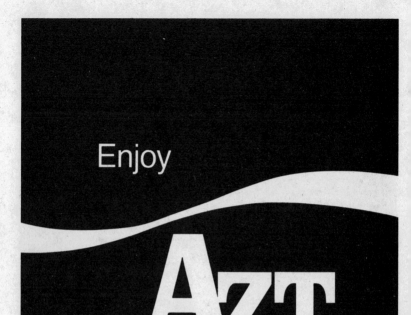

Enjoy

AZT

Trade-mark

The U.S. government has spent one billion dollars over the past 10 years to research new AIDS drugs. The result, 1 drug–AZT. It makes half the people who try it sick and for the other half it stops working after a year. Is AZT the last, best hope for people with AIDS, or is it a short-cut to the killing Burroughs Wellcome is making in the AIDS marketplace? Scores of drugs languish in government pipelines, while fortunes are made on this monopoly.

## IS THIS HEALTH CARE OR WEALTH CARE?

STORM THE N.I.H. MAY 21. INFO: 212-989-1114

*A brilliant use of graphics gives ACT UP's serious critique of medical research added persuasive power.*

was confused, but he recognized an easy lob when he saw one coming. In his usual style, Kramer rushed in with a blitzkrieg of questions. How can we get the drug companies and you and us into a room next week? he asked. Can you do it on Monday? How about Tuesday? We gotta move fast on this, Tony, he said. Real fast.

Startled, Fauci's bureaucratic conservatism recaptured him for a moment. "Wait a minute, Larry. You're moving too fast for me." But Kramer's emotionalism captured him. He practically shouted, "Why? Why am I going too fast? We need to get this going, Tony. This is very important." Allowing Fauci to take credit for the parallel track idea and stroking him at the same time, Kramer then said, "You've got a terrific idea here. The time has come for parallel track. You're very courageous for suggesting this. It won't be easy for you. Let's run with it."

The words came splattering out. But even as Kramer gushed all over Fauci, he was wondering what in hell the guy was up to. It was a complete about-face. The enemy of the AIDS community was now coming on as a friend. A defender of conservative scientific research was now posturing as a total revolutionary. Why, Fauci could almost belong to ACT UP with *that* kind of attitude, thought Kramer.

The day after the midnight stroll with Fauci, Kramer had the *Village Voice* play a minor role in a major AIDS drug policy shift. He called a meeting of all the members of ACT UP's Treatment and Data Committee, who had come to the convention. Iris Long, Jim Eigo, Mark Harrington, and others joined Kramer at the Meridien Hotel for lunch. Kramer was covering the convention for the *Voice,* and he put the ACT UP lunch on his expense account. Thus the *Voice,* and its owner, Leonard Stern, who made his millions with Hartz Mountain pet foods, paid for a crucial meeting in the history of AIDS research.

Before anyone could start eating, Kramer rushed out with, "Okay, Fauci's tossed us the ball. Let's choose a list of drugs and go after them, one at a time." The group then debated which drug would be the best to push for a new parallel track; ddI, an AZT cousin that was supposed to have fewer toxic side effects, kept coming up.

As different people spoke, it became clear that a coalition of forces could be put together to promote this particular drug for fast-tracking. Sam Broder, at the NCI, loved ddI because it came out of his lab, said Kramer. Broder's right-hand man, Robert Yarchoan, was presenting data on ddI at the Montreal conference that promised to show good results against AIDS with the drug. Jerry Groopman, one of the original PIs on the AZT Phase II trial, liked ddI. And Fauci himself was anxious to get going with his new idea, of a parallel track, so he too climbed aboard.

Best of all, ddI was scheduled to go into Phase II trials in just a couple of months anyway. The timing was perfect. The Treatment and Data members decided that Kramer should write a letter to Bristol-Myers, the pharmaceutical company that held the license for ddI, suggesting they put their drug into a new trial system, the parallel track. Agreed. This was science by political coalition building.

Later, activists on both coasts would chuckle over Fauci's attachment to parallel track. One major organizer on the scene has said, "Sure, it wasn't an original idea of Tony's. He took it on and we decided to let him have credit for it. Why not, if it gets drugs out to people faster?"

He then recalled how impossible it had been to get Fauci to answer phone calls in the past. It hadn't been just Fauci, either. Scientists had cut themselves off from the people with AIDS and community doctors who treated them. ACT UP's whole *raison d'être* had been to force the NIH and the FDA to speed up its drug approval process through loud, embarrassing, persistent protest. Antagonism was ACT UP's major strategy for change.

Now, one of the main targets of that protest had walked along in the Montreal night with one of the angriest founders of ACT UP, talking, listening, asking questions, and promoting a most revolutionary concept. It was the beginning of what was to become a sudden rapprochement between radical AIDS advocates and the Washington biomedical research establishment. Not the entire establishment, parts of it.

Over the next four months, through the summer and fall of 1989, Martin Delaney would spend many days talking with FDA Commissioner Frank Young about how to relax the rules of drug regulation. Mathilde Krim would bring Sam Broder, who had already become almost like a son to her, even closer to radical policy positions. Broder had already expressed his revulsion at the FDA's bureaucratic control of drug development during the Lasagna hearings. He would soon come out in favor of the Community Research Initiative and give modest support to the parallel track idea. He was critical of the ineptitude shown by NIAID's clinical trials system, although he was politic enough never to discuss it publicly. Through it all, however, he remained Mr. AZT.

Fauci himself would begin going to ACT UP meetings. He began appointing Jim Eigo and Martin Delaney to AIDS committees in NIAID.

He appointed Dr. Lawrence "Bopper" Deyton, a gay man, to head NIAID's newly formed community-based clinical trials network, funded with $9 million from Congress. So taken was the Watkins commission on AIDS with Joe Sonnabend's and Michael Callen's CRI in New York, that it had strongly recommended that the NIH finance its own community research effort. Congress mandated it and Fauci implemented the orders. By choosing a gay man to do the job, Fauci was clearly reaching out to the community for support.

No one in the gay community missed the irony in all of this. Sonnabend had started the CRI precisely because Fauci's own clinical trials network had failed to test the dozens of drugs available in the underground thought to be effective in treating AIDS. Fauci's system was obsessed with only a single drug, AZT, and had missed aerosol pentamidine entirely.

Fauci had spent hundreds of millions of dollars building a drug-testing network that didn't work. Congress was turning on him, telling him what to do. In an attempt to salvage his reputation, if not his career, Fauci was now ready to change tack and adopt the AIDS medical treatment agenda of ACT UP and the CRI. Kramer, to his astonishment, discovered on that warm June night in Montreal that he was to be Fauci's vector.

# ..10..
# The Drug Underground

It was America's first medical drug underground, an organized network of private "buyers clubs" that sold treatments not approved by the FDA to people with AIDS. Just as the Community Research Initiative threatened the medical status quo by gaining control over patients and by offering the pharmaceutical companies an alternative drug-testing option, so too did the underground challenge powerful principal investigators and their institutions. If people with AIDS, indeed if people with cancer or Alzheimer's for that matter, were able to gain access to experimental drugs without going through the PIs, their dominance of the nation's biomedical research facilities would be challenged. This is precisely what happened.

Stephen Roach started it all—by chance. Roach was a graduate student in chemistry at Columbia University in November 1985 when the *New England Journal of Medicine* appeared with a letter on AL 721. The letter described AL 721 as a "novel compound . . . that inhibits HTLV-III [AIDS] infection of human peripheral blood lymphocytes [T-4 cells]." The letter went on to say that the compound wasn't toxic and "this factor makes AL 721 a promising new candidate for clinical investigation in the treatment of AIDS and AIDS-Related Complex." It was signed by several people, including the famous Dr. Robert Gallo. Roach took it seriously.

The information had special relevance to Roach. He had recently tested seropositive himself—he had the AIDS virus. The clock was ticking inside his own body.

Over the course of 1986, Roach became an AIDS drug maven, according to Suzanne Phillips, in "Surviving and Thriving with AIDS, Volume Two." He hung out at the Gay Men's Health Crisis lounge in New York, where

PWAs gathered to trade gossip about possible unauthorized treatments for their disease. Nothing was coming out of the government, so people felt they had to treat themselves. Some of the treatments struck Roach as weird. As a chemist, he had a more scientific approach to the search than many of the other desperate men who came to the GMHC ready to try anything to save their lives.

In the summer of '86, Roach read a fascinating story in the *PWA Coalition Newsline,* one of the earlier sources of AIDS drug information. Michael Callen had set it up and ran it. The story was by Michael May, who wrote about his experience with AL 721 in Israel. May had been a young conductor, but his music career came to an abrupt halt with AIDS. In a breathless style, May described how an Israeli friend told him about work being done at the Weizmann Institute on a drug called AL 721. May had left New York in a wheelchair. His Israeli doctor, Yehuda Skornick, treated him with AL 721 spread over a slice of bread every day for several weeks. In the *Newsline,* May said he gained weight, felt better, and believed his AIDS had gone into remission. He returned to New York ready to conduct an orchestra again.

Roach read all this and remembered the Gallo letter in the *NEJM.* He got in contact with May, who gave him the specifics about the Weizmann Institute and the scientific papers published about this new drug. Roach then tracked down these papers and read up about lipid chemistry and cell membrane fluidity.

At this point, Roach was invited by a friend, Kevin Imbusch, to meet Imbusch's personal doctor, Joseph Sonnabend. Sonnabend thought AL 721 had possibilities. It was safe. It appeared to be antiviral. And it had a good pedigree. Sonnabend knew from his experience years ago in Israel that the Weizmann Institute was a world-class science academy. Over lunch, Roach, Imbusch, and Sonnabend discussed how they might obtain AL 721 for the gay community. The effort would require organization, not one of Sonnabend's strong points. It was not one of Roach's either, so he suggested that Sonnabend meet one of the best organizers Roach had ever known, his lover Tom Hannan. A short time later, they met and Sonnabend was impressed with Hannan's boundless energy. Hannan couldn't stop talking. Sonnabend, Hannan, and his lover Stephen Roach began the drive to build the first AIDS drug buyers club—a club built on a foundation of AL 721.

In December 1986, Roach and Hannan held a series of weekly meetings in their apartment on Perry Street in the Village. The group, which included Sonnabend, gave themselves the name of Ad Hoc Group for a Community Treatment Initiative.

During the winter months, attempts were made to get Praxis Pharmaceuticals, which held the licensing rights on AL 721, to provide it to the community. Intense pressure was put on Arnold Lippa to go over-the-counter with the compound and not wait for the FDA to approve it as a drug. On one occasion, Sonnabend asked Michael Callen and the People With Aids Coalition to help. Callen called. "I begged Lippa to do the moral thing," says Callen. He told Lippa that there was a major demand for AL 721 by people who were desperate. "I beg you, please make it available," Callen repeated.

Lippa replied that he couldn't release AL 721 over the counter as a food supplement because his company had applied for an IND from the FDA. The FDA would turn down its request for a clinical trial if the company simply gave it to people without regulatory approval, Lippa argued. Callen became incensed. It could take years to get the FDA to act, he screamed. People are dying now every day. Callen then accused Lippa of deliberately trying to sell AL 721 as a drug and not a food in order to reap huge profits. Finally, Callen ended the conversation with a threat. "If you don't make it available, *we will*. We will get it bootleg!"

Tom Hannan tried his hand at getting Praxis to release AL 721 to the community. He visited its uptown laboratory where it rented space at City College. He went with Roach. Hannan didn't have any better luck than Callen in getting the company to release the drug, but he was able to get help in making it. Claire Klepner, at Praxis, told Hannan she didn't have the power to make AL 721 available, but she would show Steve Roach how he might make it in the kitchen. Klepner warned them that there was a good chance the "bathtub" AL 721 would not be as effective as the factory-made compound because the processing would have to be different, but it was the best she could do. Roach and Hannan took notes, thanked her, and left.

In the end, Larry Kramer and a friend from the GMHC also tried to get Lippa and Jacobson to release AL 721. All the AIDS activists argued that people were dying. Waiting for the FDA and testing was criminal. They pleaded with Lippa and Jacobson to work with them. And both said no. The government was going to test AL 721 very soon in its new ATEU system and it would be available.

It was a terrible tactical mistake for Lippa and Jacobson to oppose the gay community over AL 721. They did not know it at the time, but community activists, especially ACT UP, would come to play a major role in drug development. They would force the FDA and the NIH to accept drugs that neither would have ever dreamed of passing. They would force major changes in the drug development process itself, transforming it to allow access to experimental drugs by the ill. AL 721 might have joined aerosol pentamidine, successfully pushed by the CRI, if Lippa and Jacobson had not antagonized community doctors and PWAs with their obstinacy.

True, there appeared to be legitimate reasons for them to wait. At this point in time, in late 1986 and early '87, both Lippa and Jake Jacobson honestly believed that it was only a matter of a few weeks or a couple of months before the NIH would test AL 721 in their new clinical trials system. That's what Ellen Cooper at the FDA had said, so why question her? Their drug was finally about to be given a priority rating by the new drug selection committee of the NIAID AIDS Program, two years after the Gallo article on AL 721 in the *NEJM*. Once they got the rating, the government would get AL 721 into trial. Or so Lippa and Jacobson thought.

They did not know that Mathilde Krim had been calling Tony Fauci around that time, only to find out that his new clinical trials system wasn't going anywhere. They didn't know that NIAID didn't have enough people to write protocols, so trials weren't taking place. They couldn't be aware that AZT would soon put AL 721, and virtually all other potential anti-AIDS drugs, on the back burner once the code of the Phase II Burroughs Wellcome trial was broken.

Lippa and Jacobson believed their drug would soon be tested by the NIH, and if it proved effective, as they believed it would, the FDA would give the go-ahead to sell it commercially. That's the way drug development was supposed to happen. Neither Lippa nor Jacobson had any direct experience in the administrative and regulatory side of the drug development process. They were naive, a personality trait not afflicting Wellcome's David Barry. AL 721 was ill-served by this naiveté. But Lippa and Jacobson, entrepreneurs with an exciting new drug, were ill-served by the whole government research system. The NIH and FDA, explicitly set up to develop new treatments for diseases, delayed and blocked the development of AL 721. Lippa and Jacobson were naive, but the scientists and bureaucrats serving the American public were something much worse. They were, in ways they could not comprehend, blinded by an institutional conflict of interest.

In January 1987, frustration within the gay community over AL 721 was boiling over. No one could pry the drug away from the company that owned it. So Sonnabend, Hannan, and Roach put forth an agenda for action, an eleven-point program for making AL 721 available to people with AIDS that included (1) putting political pressure on Lippa to quickly release the drug as a food supplement and not wait for it to be approved by the FDA; (2) contacting manufacturers to produce generic AL 721—egg lipids; and (3) helping to develop underground kitchen laboratories to produce bathtub AL 721 using a scaled-down method.

Sonnabend, Hannan, and Roach explored different ways of making AL 721. Imbusch, James Perez, a grad student, and Suzanne Phillips, a medical student who was soon to become a major force in ACT UP, tried making the sticky stuff themselves. They shopped Canal Street in Manhattan, looking for generators, vacuum pumps, and pressure cookers. Five-gallon drums of acetone were dragged up five flights of stairs to Perez's apartment on East Ninety-sixth Street. Each of them took turns stirring pots of highly flammable acetone and egg yolks by hand. Unfortunately, the whole process yielded very little. Klepner had told them that AL 721 was difficult to make. Experienced scientists could do it on a very small scale in their labs, but large quantities could probably only be made by big pharmaceutical companies.

By March 1987, Tom Hannan had found a distributor that said it could sell him large quantities of generic egg lipids, much of it manufactured in Germany by Lucas Meyer, a big lecithin producer. It wouldn't be produced by the acetone process but it would work. At least that is what was promised. Hannan also knew of a lab that would do QC, quality control, to check for purity and make sure the 7:2:1 ratio of the drug was met.

It was time for action. Sonnabend and Hannan were convinced that once they began to sell this AL 721 knockoff, all hell would break loose. Lippa and Jacobson would probably sue for circumventing their rights to AL 721. The FDA was almost sure to get into the case and close them down. Selling unapproved drugs was forbidden under the law.

Sonnabend and Hannan figured they would get only one chance to distribute the drug. They hoped the publicity would generate enough interest to get a private pharmaceutical company to sell tons of the stuff as a food supplement. They had a second goal—shaming the government to finally test AL 721 and make it legally available to PWAs who wanted it.

But first they needed TV and press coverage. They needed a big public splash with the distribution of the drug. Neither Sonnabend nor Hannan, however, was particularly knowledgeable about or skillful with the press. Michael Callen, however, was a performer. He was used to getting up in front of an audience. And he looked good on TV. So Sonnabend began pressuring his protégé to join the underground effort. It wasn't easy.

Callen was down, at that time, with yet another opportunistic infection. He wasn't feeling great. He was also trying to cut a new album called *Purple Heart*. In addition, Callen was writing the second edition of *Surviving and Thriving with AIDS*. The first, published by the People With AIDS Coalition in 1985, had gone into three printings and sold thirty thousand copies. It was one of the earliest attempts to provide PWAs with advice on drugs, on telling their parents about the disease, on coping with depression, friendships, and relationships, on preventing *Pneumocystis carinii* pneumonia, on having sex in the AIDSies, and so on. *Surviving and Thriving* also contained a number of articles on AL 721, including Michael May's testimonial, and home formulas for bootleg AL 721. Callen had dedicated the book to several people, including Bobbi Campbell.

The second edition would be double the size of the first and had chapters called "So, You've Just Been Diagnosed with AIDS," "Treating OIs & AIDS Itself," and "Emotional Responses to Diagnosis." It was also dedicated to many people, including Michael May.

Callen had even more burdens to cope with when Sonnabend asked him to help out with the first shipment of bootleg AL 721. He was still editing the *Newsline* and he was sitting on the New York State AIDS Advisory Council. "I told [Sonnabend] I just couldn't handle another thing," he remembers. "I had to be dragged kicking and screaming into the buyers club."

Sonnabend guilt-tripped Callen mercilessly. "Don't you care? Here is a possible treatment. You've got to help," he said. Sonnabend asked Callen just to see Hannan. Callen said no. Sonnabend really turned it on. "You're abandoning people with AIDS," he said. "There's a demand for this product. People need it. What's more important than treatment? If you say that you really care about people with AIDS, you've got to help." Okay, Callen said. He would meet with Hannan.

He did, in Sonnabend's office. Callen remembers that "Tom was really hyper. He was speaking a mile a minute. He was bouncing off walls." Callen was put off by Hannan's personality and he was skeptical about AL 721 itself. "This stuff can easily get contaminated with bacteria," he said. Callen said he wouldn't do it.

But Sonnabend continued to lobby. He got Callen to meet with several

PWAs who had traveled to Israel for AL 721. These firsthand accounts of recovery really impressed Callen and he began to soften. He asked Hannan point-blank, "Why do you want me, why does this have to be something I'm involved in?" Hannan said, "Look, I'm not good on camera, you are. I'm a behind-the-scenes guy. You have great credibility. You can handle the camera."

Soon after that, Hannan filed papers with New York State for a not-for-profit organization. He and Callen chose the name People With AIDS Health Group in the hope that the name would generate sympathy and deter Lippa and Jacobson from suing them for knocking off their product. "Who could sue a group with that kind of name?" says Callen with a smirk. "Or so we hoped."

The PWAHG was set up to act as a bridge between individual PWAs and drug wholesalers. That way it was nonprofit. Callen and Hannan collected twenty-five thousand dollars from several hundred individuals who really wanted AL 721 or, failing that, a similar compound. They placed the order. Then they went over to Judson Memorial Church and asked if they could park a refrigerated truck outside and pass out the bootleg AL 721 inside the church. The answer was yes. Callen hit the phones at this point and did all the media work, arranging for TV and press coverage of the big event.

The evening before five hundred people were scheduled to go to the church and get their drug, Sonnabend called Hannan. "We can't do it," he said. "We ran the tests on the first shipment and the ratios were off." They were far from the expected 7:2:1. It might not work.

Callen was at a recording studio that night spending sixty dollars an hour rehearsing a song, "Love Don't Need a Reason," which would become his signature ballad when he performed onstage in the future. Hannan called with the bad news. Callen then called Sonnabend: "How can you do this to me? How can I call all these people and say don't come?" he cried, referring to the dozens of media people he had contacted in the previous weeks. Sonnabend told him that if the 7:2:1 ratio wasn't just right, it wouldn't work. Callen argued that they weren't really sure which ratios worked. Besides, there were two or three people he knew who were near death. This was their last chance. Why not tell the people that the ratios were off and give them the choice of taking the bootleg AL 721 or not? Sonnabend refused. That night, Sonnabend, Hannan, and Callen called hundreds of people and the press and told them not to come.

Several weeks later, on May 4, 1987, a second batch of bootleg AL

721 arrived. Again it was tested and this time fell within the 7:2:1 ratio. The drug was passed out to five hundred PWAs at the church. "It was very exciting," Callen remembers. "You can imagine the excitement!" Then he held a press conference, went public with the news, and waited for the ax to fall.

And nothing bad happened. They weren't sued by Lippa. The FDA was strangely silent. And the PWA Health Group became the first buyers club in the country to offer an alternative supply of an anti-AIDS drug to the gay community. In the first year of operation, the PWAHG sold $1 million worth of bootleg AL 721. At its peak, in the summer of '87, the buyers club was selling several hundred kilos of the knockoff a month. All kinds and qualities of bootleg AL 721 rushed in to satisfy the booming demand for the drug.

Unfortunately, AL 721 was not easy to manufacture. It spoiled very easily unless refrigerated properly. The compound could become contaminated, the last thing a person with a weakened immune system needed. In 1987, literally tons of bootleg AL 721 flooded into the gay community and people received compounds of varying ratios, varying colors, varying consistency. Much of it didn't even look like the AL 721 produced in Israel. The Weizmann AL 721 was made with an acetone process that appeared to be essential to its efficacy. It was a difficult process with only a 10 percent yield of pure AL 721. Nearly all of the bootleg drug used a different extraction method. That made the product cheaper, but may also have made it ineffective. Indeed, when Fulton Crews, one of the original authors of the *New England Journal of Medicine* letter on AL 721, tested out most of the bootleg products, he found that they didn't do what AL 721 was supposed to do—leach out cholesterol from cell walls, thereby preventing the AIDS virus from attaching itself to, and infecting, T-4 cells. They didn't fluidize the cell membrane walls of the virus and curb the progression of AIDS.

But no one with AIDS was willing to hear this news. They wanted to believe. They had no choice, either. The "pure" AL 721 was unavailable, thanks to Lippa and Jacobson, who were playing the drug development game. People facing death, desperate people, wanted to try anything that might help. They did.

For its part, the PWAHG expanded its inventory and in 1988 began selling dextran sulfate and a dozen other drugs. By 1989 it had two thousand clients. Some two dozen buyers clubs sprang up in all the major cities of the country, creating the foundation for an alternative drug supply for people with AIDS.

The FDA could easily have closed down the first buyers club from the beginning. Its legal status was murky at best. It pretended to act as a mere go-between, pooling individual contributions and buying drugs wholesale. But it wouldn't have been difficult to convince the authorities that the PWAHG was going beyond what FDA regulations actually permitted. The FDA, under tremendous pressure to do something about AIDS, chose to look the other way.

Lippa and Jacobson were both within their rights to sue. But whom would they sue? Their own potential customers? It wouldn't work politically. So they turned a blind eye. Besides, they were expecting FDA approval at any moment. At the time, they saw the bootlegging as a short storm that had to be weathered. But the decision left an opening for the growth of the medical drug underground. The net result was the widening of a fissure in the nation's biomedical research system. A new source of drugs and treatment was built by a patient population taking power into its own hands. The launch of the first buyers club was the clearest example to date of the power of self-empowerment.

Stephen Roach died on January 9, 1988, at home of AIDS. Tom Hannan was at his bedside. Joe Sonnabend was at his bedside. Tom Hannan and Suzanne Phillips washed and bathed his body, as they had done for so many others.

What Sonnabend, Callen, Hannan, and other AIDS activists didn't know as they established the medical drug underground was that Lippa, Jacobson, and everyone else associated with AL 721 were going through the most acute personal and professional torture. They were so close, they thought! So very close. Everything appeared lined up: the science, the need, the market, the product. So close.

Lippa was cruisin'. He had Bob Gallo's imprimatur on his drug. He had published in the prestigious *New England Journal of Medicine.* By the summer of 1986, he had great data on safety and efficacy from the small St. Luke's trial. His friend, Fulton Crews, had even shown that AL 721 worked on a whole family of unique viruses that had similar membranes, or envelopes. Crews called them "envelope viruses" and they all had particularly high levels of cholesterol in their membranes. To his surprise, Crews found that herpes was one of them. AL 721 might work not only against the AIDS virus but against the many herpes viruses, such as CMV, that ravage people down with the disease.

With all this, Lippa thought that accolades from his peers were just a matter of time. He could taste the Nobel Prize.

But first, the research on AL 721 had to be aired in scientific forums. The most prestigious scientific meeting coming up was the Interscience Conference on Antimicrobial Agents and Chemotherapy. Scheduled for September 28, 1986, in New Orleans, ICAAC was perfect.

In August, Lippa called and found a wall of opposition. His old enemy, Sam Broder, was running one of two sessions on AIDS. Lippa asked him for a mere ten minutes to present his data. Broder refused. He suggested that Lippa talk to a friend and colleague who was running the only other session on AIDS, Martin Hirsch, a well-known researcher from Boston. Lippa called. Hirsch was even more abrupt. No, absolutely not, he said. There was no time on his program either. Lippa insisted that this was very important. Please, he pleaded. He had fresh data. Hirsch rudely cut him off. "No."

Of course, what Lippa didn't know was that by this time, both Broder and Hirsch were deeply committed to AZT. Hirsch was one of the PIs on the Burroughs Wellcome Phase II trial, which was already under way when Lippa called. On the NIH campus, Broder was being called Mr. AZT behind his back. By August, the safety panel of the Phase II clinical trial was already seeing signs of what it considered efficacy in the drug. By early September, it would be convinced; the code would be broken and the trial ended. Broder and Hirsch wanted to talk at ICAAC about AZT, not some weird egg-based compound. Neither one had any inkling that thousands of people with AIDS were desperately trying to get AL 721 for treatment. Neither had heard of Michael May. They didn't know and they didn't care. Broder and Hirsch had AZT. AZT was the one.

The rejection sent Lippa into a frenzied paranoia. His fantasies about a Nobel were destroyed. His dream of getting rich was shattered. What if he never got recognized by the research establishment? What if they ignored him no matter how much of a genius he was, no matter what marvelous drug he developed?

Desperate, Lippa decided to put on an alternative conference in New Orleans. He turned to the company's public relations person to organize an adjunct symposium and she did, on the other side of town from ICAAC. Two hundred scientists were invited to hear the data on AL 721. About a dozen showed up. Another dozen people walked in off the street, attracted by the open buffet.

Lippa was the introductory speaker. Then Fulton Crews got up to talk about how AL 721 takes cholesterol out of the AIDS virus's cell membrane, and the membranes of all envelope viruses. David Scheer read a short paper on the anti-AIDS test run by Prem Sarin in Robert Gallo's lab. Michael Grieco then presented the clinical data of the St. Luke's trial. His report was balanced but generally positive toward AL 721. Later, he would turn on the drug and write an extremely negative paper about it. Why he did this was never made clear: perhaps because he was also one of the original PIs on the AZT Phase II trial. He was monitoring patients taking AZT in New York during the time he was presenting the paper on AL 721. When the AZT results were announced, all of the PIs received tremendous recognition. Loyalties changed rapidly. You were either pro-AZT or anti-AZT. Grieco chose to be pro.

By the time Lippa got up again to close the discussion, he was losing it. He stood there facing all the empty seats, wooden, withdrawn, fighting for control. Once the presentations were over, he bolted for the door. He tried to rent a car to drive down to the bayou but couldn't. He then walked around New Orleans in a sweating, eye-darting daze. Finally at five in the morning, Lippa returned to his room, shivering.

The press didn't cover Lippa's alternative conference. The scientific establishment didn't confer its blessings either. Later, Lippa would say that "the demons were there, sticking knives in my eyes."

Then the stock of his company collapsed. Trading had been heavy in the month before the ICAAC meeting. Rumors about what would be revealed about AL 721's effectiveness had washed through the OTC market, and shares had been run up sharply to $11.50.

Lippa and Jacobson had invited a number of Wall Street investors to their conference. These investment bankers, from Merrill Lynch, Morgan Stanley, and Salomon Brothers, did show up, but they didn't like what they saw. The scientific presentations were first-rate, but it was clear to them that there was a problem with the management of the company. They couldn't even pull off a small meeting, much less the successful marketing of a new drug.

A number of them were invited to dinner that night. Arnold Lippa, president and resident guru, was supposed to be there schmoozing it up with the money people. He wasn't. He was off somewhere in the night. The investment bankers didn't like it. "We acted like schmucks," says one participant. "These guys didn't like what they saw." The next day the stock fell like a stone: science in America, circa the mid-eighties.

While Sonnabend and Callen hammered away at Lippa and Jacobson throughout 1987 to get them to release AL 721, they had no idea how the government was acting to stop the same two men from getting their drug out. For that matter, Lippa and Jacobson also were in the dark; they didn't have a clue how incompetent the NIH and FDA were in fostering anti-AIDS drugs. They naively accepted every promise of fast action made by the government bureaucrats.

After the ICAAC fiasco in the fall of 1986, it was clear to Lippa and Jacobson that it would be very difficult raising the tens of millions of dollars necessary to finance a Phase II clinical trial for AL 721. Wellcome was a huge pharmaceutical company. Praxis was tiny and out of favor for the moment with the investment community.

Lippa had hired a private company called Oxford Research to run the St. Luke's Phase I safety trial. Oxford was experienced at doing all kinds of clinical work for drug companies, including start-ups such as Praxis. Lippa asked Oxford Research to write a series of protocols for trials that would prove the drug's effectiveness once and for all. One protocol called for AL 721 to be tested directly against AZT. Another called for a dose comparison of AL 721, with no placebo.

Lippa then called Donna Mildvan, the head of infectious diseases at Beth Israel Medical Center. She knew Michael Grieco. Like Grieco, she too was a PI on the Burroughs Wellcome's Phase II trial of AZT.

Mildvan believed that the safety of AL 721 had already been proven in Israel and at St. Luke's. She wrote up an efficacy protocol for a big Phasae II clinical trial. It was sent to Ellen Cooper and rejected. Cooper said that the maximum allowable dosage of AL 721 had not been established at St. Luke's. Instead of 30 grams a day, what if the max were 50? She was parroting the same old cancer chemotherapy argument. Standard operating procedure was to test until the maximum allowable dosage was attained. It had been done this way in cancer for decades. The same procedure was expected with AIDS drugs.

Unfortunately, community doctors were already showing that *reduced* doses of certain drugs were the most effective in the case of AIDS. Years later, NIAID and the FDA would agree.

But not in 1987. Cooper rejected the efficacy protocol. She demanded a dose-ranging trial first to find out how much AL 721 could be put into humans. She didn't even want to hear about the nonplacebo trial. "Everybody dies," she told Oxford when it complained that doing a placebo trial with AL 721 would kill people needlessly.

At this point, Cooper also recommended that Lippa wait for the new clinical trials system that Tony Fauci was building. It would be just a few months before it was finished. A short time.

Jacobson and Lippa welcomed the news. They didn't have the money on hand to start a big Phase II trial. Even if they could raise it, they stood to save a fortune if the government did the testing, they thought.

This decision was the kiss of death for AL 721. When Cooper first suggested that Lippa and Jacobson put their drug into the new NIAID trials network, AL 721 was near the top of the list of drugs to be tested first. It was on the government's short list. But when AZT was proclaimed effective against AIDS, the short list went out the window. Practically all the slots in the new NIAID trials system filled up immediately with AZT experiments. A number of drugs, including AL 721, dropped way down the list. In the fall of 1986, AL 721 was seen as a promising drug. After AZT was proclaimed king, it became a rather stupid lipid concoction to Tony Fauci and Maureen Myers, as well as to Ellen Cooper. It got worse. Much worse.

Once AZT was given the stamp of approval by the FDA and the NIH, the PIs who ran the Phase II became heroes to the scientific world. They became virtually identified with a single drug. These were the supposedly unbiased researchers who even did a Burroughs Wellcome video extolling the virtues of AZT. Their careers rode AZT to the top.

These same people also took control of the government's entire anti-AIDS effort. It wasn't a revolution, it was a coup. They were asked to take over when the initial attempt by Maureen Myers to set up a clinical trials network ended in total failure. Dan Hoth was brought in from the National Cancer Institute and he asked the AZT PIs to join the NIAID effort. They ran all the major committees, including the AIDS Clinical Drug Development Committee, the ACDDC, which voted on every single potential anti-AIDS drug. In effect, scientists who had bet their professional careers on one drug, AZT, were put in positions to vote on other drugs that might compete with AZT in the marketplace, not just the scientific marketplace but the commercial marketplace. It was a clear institutional conflict of interest and not a single voice was raised inside the world of research, inside the NIH or the FDA, against it.

The ACDDC gathered in February 1987 to take a stand on AL 721, a full two years after the *New England Journal of Medicine* letter on AL 721. A medical drug underground was growing based on AL 721's professed antiviral activity against AIDS. Thousands were using bootleg AL 721. Yet the drug didn't stand a chance of being approved. There were sixteen ACDDC members present on the day AL 721 came up for rating. A high rating would have sent it to the top of the list of drugs scheduled to get into government trials. A low rating would normally kill it.

The scientists and NIAID bureaucrats sitting around the room made for an interesting collection of judges for AL 721. Dr. Henry Masur, the chairman of the ACDDC, walked into the room believing that AL 721 was no better than laetrile, the compound that many cancer patients turned to despite the objections of their doctors and that in fact turned out to be a phony. The word "laetrile" was on the minds of most of the people voting that day and was spoken more than once during the meeting.

The FDA's Ellen Cooper was there. Like virtually everyone at the NIH, she became extremely uncomfortable talking about AL 721, almost emotional. Cooper recalls that at the time, "because people were buying this stuff and using it, there was a lot of pressure to study it and have NIH study it." This "stuff."

To one degree or another, Martin Hirsch, Thomas Merigan, and Fred Valentine had all hitched their career wagons to AZT or to an AZT nucleoside analogue. They were either PIs on the original Burroughs Wellcome Phase II trial or were about to join the club. Merigan was planning shortly to begin a trial on ddC, a cousin to AZT. Hirsch was an original member of the Gang of Twelve, the original PIs on the Phase II trial. He'd had a cold exchange with Arnold Lippa just a few months back when Lippa pleaded to present late-minute data from St. Luke's at Hirsch's session at ICAAC. Hirsch had refused. In addition, Hirsch's colleague, Michael Grieco, who ran the St. Luke's AL 721 trial with Michael Lange, was now bad-mouthing AL 721 as another laetrile. Grieco, of course, was also a PI on the AZT Phase II trial with Hirsch. Maureen Myers had no respect for AL 721 whatsoever. Paul Volberding was a member of the ACDDC but he wasn't present at the AL 721 meeting. He, too, was a PI on the original Phase II AZT trial and had become known as an "AZT man." He was also on the Burroughs Wellcome video for AZT. Paul Lietman, another member voting on AL 721, believed the compound would be thoroughly digested before it had any chance of working against the AIDS virus. His mind was already made up. Lietman didn't see any conflict between his sitting on the ACDDC and being supported by Burroughs Wellcome. Lietman was the Wellcome Professor of Clinical Pharmacology at Johns Hopkins. He held a Burroughs Wellcome–financed chair. But it wasn't the "company," it was the Wellcome Foundation, the charity, the other part of Burroughs Wellcome, so where was the conflict of interest? No one else in the room saw any conflict of interest either. And since they made the rules . . . Clifford Lane was there that day. He worked in Tony Fauci's lab and shared Fauci's condescension toward the drug, if you could call something made out of eggs a drug. Neither Lippa nor Jacobson was invited to speak in support of AL 721 at the ACDDC meeting on February 28, 1987.

So, at 8:08 A.M. the ACDDC meeting began. There was a lot of business to attend to before the actual voting on drugs, the first being a discussion about conflict of interest and confidentiality. Each member's policy was recorded in two ways: in a written statement, to be kept confidential by the executive secretary, Judith Feinberg, M.D., and orally, at the beginning of the agenda. Strange to have this kind of discussion without anyone seeing any conflict of interest in his own being there at that time. But scientists were used to making their own rules without being accountable to any "outside" authorities.

Four other drugs in addition to AL 721 were scheduled to be reviewed on that cold winter day. They were isoprinosine, ribavirin, Imuthiol, and Ampligen. All were well known and had been used for years among people with AIDS. Joe Sonnabend had done the first community-based trial on isoprinosine back in 1984. Ribavirin had first been smuggled in from Mexico in the early eighties. It had been around even longer than AL 721.

The ACDDC on that day gave a high priority rating to ribavirin and said, according to the minutes of the meeting, that it "should be studied with a placebo control." Isoprinosine and Ampligen received medium ratings. For isoprinosine: "Some biologic activity has been shown, but is it significant, particularly in AIDS?" For Ampligen: "It may have both antiviral and immunomodulatory effects that are promising." They had been promising three years earlier.

AL 721 received a low priority rating, which meant "absolutely no trial." The members of the committee refused to buckle to all those thousands of people with AIDS out there. Their attitude was, these are sick people, what do they know? Cooper and Myers had said it many times: You can't approve drugs on the basis of testimonials, can you? Michael May's experience meant nothing. For AL 721, the minutes read: "Immunologic data presented do not support a claim for immunomodulatory activity at doses tested so far."

In the end, Tony Fauci interceded. As head of NIAID, he was not as insulated from popular and political pressures as the members of the ACDDC. Fauci told the ACTG to do something with AL 721, anything. "It was *me* that said put it into trials, even though it was given a low scientific priority," Fauci later said, "because I wanted to *debunk* it. Because there were so many people who were using it by making it in their bathtubs. In my mind, this was keeping them away from a potentially promising drug by wasting their time with that," he said. "So I said to the committee, even though you gave it a low priority, let's put the thing into trial and get it over with once and for all." Wow. How's that for objective, balanced scientific research? AL 721 was a "thing" that had to be debunked. If there was any chance for a fair test for AL 721, it wasn't going to come from Tony Fauci's clinical trials system, the government system that was supposed to evaluate the best drug treatments for the AIDS virus.

Given Fauci's tone, no one in the NIAID network wanted to touch the drug. It was the kiss of death. But Donna Mildvan had shown interest in it and now she was basically told to be a good sport and take care of the problem. No one said "bury it," but that message was clearly in the air. Fauci had used the term "debunk." Mildvan was part of the AZT team. She was a trusted PI. So in November 1987, just a few months after Donna Mildvan appeared as host on the Burroughs Wellcome video *A Ray of Hope*, promoting AZT, she launched ACTG protocol 022, a dose-ranging study of AL 721.

Praxis had to provide the drug. This time, it went to a large, established pharmaceutical company, Abbott Laboratories. A lot of AL 721 was needed. Abbott made a clean batch of AL 721 and charged Praxis about $150 a kilo. That was much higher than the bootleg AL 721 being sold on the streets of Los Angeles or New York but the supply was manufactured using the more expensive acetone-extraction method.

Mildvan ran a standard-operating-procedure trial right out of the cancer chemotherapy cookbook. She had people eating 50 grams of AL 721 twice a day. That's very close to eating a full cup of butter twice a day. Mildvan didn't announce the results until June 1989, at the Fifth International Conference on AIDS in Montreal.

In the abstract presented at Montreal, Mildvan said that "AL 721 was well-tolerated, even at high doses, over eight weeks and resulted in modest weight gain." She added that "disease progression was not noted in this short-term study. No consistent trends were observed in T-cell quantitation or HIV AIDS virus cultures."

So according to Mildvan's NIAID trial, AL 721 was safe, but it was still unclear as to whether it was effective or not. AIDS didn't get worse in the patients taking AL 721 but there were no clear trends in T-4 cell counts. It was a mixed bag of indicators. Five years had gone by since the St. Luke's trial, four years since the Gallo letter in the *New England Journal of Medicine*, and still no definitive answer was forthcoming about a potential treatment for AIDS. This trial did not "debunk" AL 721.

At the same time, AL 721's owners were undermining the drug through their own inadequacies. Once it became clear that the NIH and the FDA were going to button up their drug for years, Lippa and Jacobson desperately tried to raise money to run their own efficacy trials. The October '87 stock market crash made everything worse. Interest in small biotech start-ups disappeared overnight. Money managers were scared to take risks. Cash became king to investors. What had been hot was not any longer.

In February 1987, Jacobson hired an investment banker in Los Angeles, Fred Roberts of F. M. Roberts and Company to help generate financing for Ethigen. He was paid $140,000 over the next twelve months to set up meetings between Wall Street investors and Jacobson and Lippa. Roberts appeared to be successful; Lippa estimates he went to nearly fifty "dog and pony shows," as they are called on Wall Street. These were essentially presentations to moneybags showing that AL 721 could make them all rich.

Unfortunately, Roberts didn't succeed in raising any real money. Deutsche Bank was especially interested in putting client money into the company, but it never happened. Financing for private clinical trials always stayed just around the corner.

Lippa and Jacobson got along extremely well at first, but by early '87 they were at each other's throats. Neither one was particularly strong on management. Quality control of the product was a sometime thing. Until the switch to Abbott Labs, batch after batch of AL 721 was ordered only to find that it was impure or not the right consistency or not in the correct ratio. No one took quality control seriously.

Then Lippa and Jacobson began fighting over who was at fault for the failure to bring in new financing. Lippa believed he was holding up his end by putting on a great performance for the investors, only to have Jacobson flop when it came to closing the deal. He also complained very loudly that Jacobson was often late in paying people. Bernie Bihari, who was the first person to show that AL 721 might work against AIDS by giving it to one of his patients, often complained that Jacobson owed him money. In fact, Lippa felt that Michael Grieco eventually became embittered against AL 721 because he wasn't paid fully by Jacobson for the St. Luke's trial.

Jacobson, in turn, thought Lippa was not paying attention to detail, not focusing on the product. Quality control was Lippa's job and he couldn't do it properly. Which was true. "You had a nonconformist and a poor businessman in one small company and they couldn't agree on anything," recalls one person who was in on most of the negotiations during those years. "Their entire personal relationship dissolved at this time." It got ugly.

Inevitably, their personal dispute came down to a fight over control of the company. Lippa felt that Jacobson could never run a start-up and that *he* should take over. Lippa began telling people on the outside that only *he* could make it work, that only *he* could arrange the financing. Lippa believed that Jacobson only wanted to do small private placements through his own contacts. In fact, Lippa persuaded the banker on the AL 721 account at Deutsche Bank that without his being in total control, the drug would never be developed. She decided to finance it only if Lippa were made CEO.

In October of '87, Lippa made his play. There was a board of directors meeting of Praxis in Beverly Hills. It was a very small board, composed of six people, including Jacobson, his uncle Lester, and Lippa. Lippa went in and said he wanted to be made CEO: "I want you to vote for me now. I want control. Jake can stay as chairman but I want to be CEO."

The board members were astonished. They looked at each other in silence. No one had expected this move. Lester Jacobson then got up and asked Lippa to go outside into the corridor. Jacobson was seventy-seven years old at the time and walked a bit slowly. When they stopped, Lester Jacobson leaned over to Lippa and said, "If you don't like it here, why don't you get the fuck out?"

Lippa stood there frozen. Somehow, he had persuaded himself that taking control and becoming CEO were inevitable. Didn't everyone see that only *he* could save the company? Wasn't it obvious?

Lippa walked back into the boardroom and was silent for the rest of the discussion. The vote came and the board voted not to make him CEO. Lippa's power play was over.

The next day, the board made Lippa sign a piece of paper saying he would no longer have any operational control in the company. With that, Deutsche Bank backed away from any financing of AL 721 and the drug never did get a big clinical trial to test its efficacy.

What happened to AL 721 is a sad, sad story—saddest, of course, to the people with AIDS. Little Praxis could not compete against the Burroughs Wellcome behemoth. Arnold Lippa and James Jacobson were no match for David Barry. The two had no substantial experience in running a start-up company and let their egos get in the way of business. This was especially true of Lippa, an exceptional scientist but an erratic manager, at best. Neither one of them had any experience negotiating with the FDA, either.

But perhaps it is too easy to blame these men for failure, especially when the consequences are so severe. It is true they had in their hands a potential treatment for the epidemic and they failed to bring it out. It is also true that they made serious political mistakes in alienating the gay community by not bringing the drug out sooner over the counter. There were too many dreams of fame and fortune for such a pint-sized company.

Yet Jacobson did finance the development of AL 721 in Israel and did bring it to the United States. Lippa did get the drug tested for safety at St. Luke's, did get Robert Gallo to show its efficacy in his lab, and did publish a letter on AL 721 in the *NEJM*. These were all significant steps in the development of any drug. Had they been able to work together and raise millions of dollars, had the October 1987 Wall Street stock market crash not occurred, the question of whether AL 721 works against AIDS might have been answered. It never was.

The fault lies as much outside Lippa and Jacobson's company as within it. Institutional conflicts of interest among scientists played a significant role in denying AL 721 its potential place among AIDS treatments. PIs wedded to AZT, NIH officials depending on AZT, FDA bureaucrats under heavy political pressure also tied to AZT, acted to stomp AL 721 into the ground. Prejudice against any drug that was not a nucleoside was very real. Extreme prejudice against an egg-based natural compound among scientists was palpable. Finally, incompetence within the NIH, especially within Tony Fauci's NIAID clinical trials system, was every bit as great as that within Praxis.

The fact is that the people Americans look to for health protection blew

263

it. They fouled up on a spectacular scale. The sad story of AL 721 is but a small part of this terrible drama. If the government biomedical research apparatus had been functioning properly, AL 721 would have had an even chance no matter how clumsy Lippa and Jacobson were. An open, fair drug approval system would have pushed AL 721 right to the top of any list of compounds to be tested.

Instead, AL 721 to this day has never been properly evaluated. People with AIDS, for the most part, are convinced the drug doesn't work. But their perception is based on bootleg AL 721 that may not have been biologically active.

Scientific research continues to show efficacy. Jeffrey Laurence at the Cornell Medical School has shown that AL 721 stops the replication of the AIDS virus in macrophage cells, a sort of vacuum cleaner that sweeps diseases out of the body. The AIDS virus, it was found, can hide in macrophage cells for up to a decade before some trigger activates it, causing it to spill forth destroying the entire immune system. AL 721 apparently keeps macrophages in an inactivated state. AZT cannot do this.

The Israelis continue to do research at the Weizmann and show the drug's efficacy against AIDS, dementia in older persons, and drug addiction. Each of these afflictions is characterized by an unusually large amount of cholesterol in cell membranes.

Ironically, American scientific research has recently changed its focus from inside the cell to the outside cell wall. It is now fashionable to talk about preventing the AIDS virus from attaching itself to the T-4 cell wall, or membrane. A new compound, CD4, is very hot, partly because it is backed by Robert Gallo but also because it is said to be able to stop the AIDS virus from attaching itself to body cells. It connects to the sites on T-4 cells where the AIDS virus normally attaches itself, thereby replacing the AIDS virus.

Of course, AL 721 works in a very similar way, by leaching out cholesterol from virus walls and changing their shape so that they can't connect to normal human cells. While AL 721 is still considered a "laetrile" by practically all NIH researchers, the same condescending scientists now gush over CD4. Amazing.

The irony is probably lost on the one hundred and sixty thousand people with AIDS in America. The million or so individuals infected with the virus but not yet suffering from its symptomatic opportunistic infections can't be expected to be highly amused either. The nation's medical system is killing them. Despite the good intentions of everyone involved, the established institutions aren't working. It should be no surprise that PWAs started taking things into their own hands; they felt they had been misused in the hands of the professionals.

Their first step was to build alternative, underground organizations for medical treatments and for research. These grew rapidly, taking control over patients and drugs away from principal investigators, academic hospitals, the NIH, and the FDA. But alternative medical institutions were not enough. Reform of the NIH and the FDA themselves was the next step. Reform of the entire drug development and approval system was essential if hundreds of thousands of PWAs were going to have a chance at living long lives. Buoyed by their successes at creating the Community Research Initiative and the PWA Health Group, AIDS activists prepared to storm the ramparts. Literally.

# ..11..

# $300 Million and No Drugs

This was the first hearing on AIDS for Patsy Fleming, but for her boss, Congressman Ted Weiss of Manhattan, it felt like the hundredth. Both of them had been busy in recent weeks, talking to their sources in the NIH and in the gay community about progress on treatments for AIDS. Patsy had been especially impressed by the ACT UP people. They knew their science and they knew what was wrong with the system. So did the PWAs from the Community Research Initiative in New York and Martin Delaney from Project Inform out of San Francisco. Fleming hadn't expected such detailed technical knowledge from political activists. They helped structure the line of questioning that Ted Weiss was now about to begin.

The room was crowded at 9:30 on the morning of April 28, 1988. There was a long list of speakers scheduled; so long, in fact, that each person was allocated just five to ten minutes for his or her oral statements. They were allowed to submit to the Human Resources subcommittee any and all written documents they deemed important.

The subject at hand was "Therapeutic Drugs for AIDS: Development, Testing, and Availability." The goal was a reality check. After fighting terrible battles with David Stockman's OMB, Congress had finally wrestled away from the Reagan administration a significant sum of money for AIDS research. It now wanted to see how that money was being spent by the NIH.

In his opening remarks, Weiss went right to the heart of the problem. "Since 1981, sixty thousand Americans have contracted AIDS and more than thirty-three thousand have died. Since 1981, many millions of dollars and many thousands of hours have been spent trying to find safe, efficacious drugs that can deliver us from the deadly AIDS virus and the opportunistic

266

infections it invites into our bodies. As the AIDS epidemic continues to flourish we are frustrated."

By mentioning opportunistic infections, Weiss hinted from the beginning where the hearings were going to go. The National Institute of Allergy and Infectious Diseases had for the most part neglected the OIs that did the actual killing of people with AIDS. Meanwhile, thousands of PWAs were dying from *Pneumocystis* and other opportunistic infections. Despite their entreaties, very little research was being done on developing treatments for these killers. The private investigators in the field strongly resisted doing research on what they considered mundane opportunistic infections. They preferred the more glamorous work of antiviral experimentation. That's where there was glory in science. Only community doctors such as Joe Sonnabend and Barbara Starrett were focusing on drugs for the infections that were killing their patients. But no one at the NIH was listening to them.

Weiss went on to say that NIAID had been the focal point for the government effort to develop AIDS drugs. He said that there were many dedicated public servants who had worked tirelessly to make the NIAID operation succeed. Then the warning lights began to blink. "But the process has been slow, sometimes due to bureaucratic inefficiency, at other times due to political reasons," he said.

Weiss went on to point his verbal finger directly at the Reagan White House. Weiss: "Historically from the time that we held our very first hearing, one of the problems that we have identified is that the professionals, both inside and outside of the federal government, have always been on top of the situation as far as knowing what their budgetary needs were. They are always inevitably overridden by the policymakers, the Office of Management and Budget . . . or someplace higher which makes policy judgments."

But that attack was a feint by Weiss. The real target of that morning's hearing was not Ronald Reagan. It was Tony Fauci. After countless battles with the Reagan administration, big money had begun to flow in late 1985. Fauci's institute had had two years to build a clinical trials system to churn out AIDS drugs. But not a single new drug was yet available, only AZT, a Burroughs Wellcome drug boosted by Sam Broder at the National Cancer Institute. After putting in hundreds of his own hours fighting for AIDS research funds, Weiss was angry that nothing was coming of it. Where was the money going? Why hadn't there been progress?

Mathilde Krim knew precisely why. She believed that Tony Fauci was over his head from the beginning. Broder was her favorite. Broder had quietly provided Krim with information on AZT long before the final data was released, permitting her to lobby for the early termination of the Phase II trial. She and Fauci had even been on TV a week before they broke the code, debating the merits of AZT. Fauci was cool to the drug but Krim, armed with information provided by Broder, said it was very effective. Besides, Krim liked Broder because he was a tough survivor, a street kid who got by on his wits. He was the child of concentration camp survivors, and that touched her deeply.

But Krim's early wariness about Fauci did not prepare her for what she saw back in 1986 and 1987 when he was trying to build a new clinical trials system for AIDS drugs. No matter how many resources Fauci received, things just didn't get done at NIAID. Remembering her private telephone talks with Fauci and his complaints about the lack of people to write protocols, then the lack of time to interview people to write protocols, then the lack of desks to put people to write protocols, it all seemed endless to Krim. During those years she felt she was forever on the phone to Senator Weicker or Congressmen Waxman or Weiss trying to get *something* for Fauci.

For what? Not a single new drug had yet appeared at the end of the long and expensive NIAID drug approval pipeline. So on April 28, she publicly told the Weiss hearing the truth. Krim said that responsibility for conducting clinical trials in AIDS was given to NIAID only because AIDS was shown to be a viral infection, not because the institute was the best place for the research. Krim went on to say that NIAID then created "an ambitious plan to develop its own protocols for all AIDS-related trials, to obtain its own INDs from the Food and Drug Administration, and to sponsor trials to be conducted—following its own protocols—in a network of the most expert clinical research centers."

Krim then said: "There was little that was wrong with this concept or these plans, except that they proved overambitious for an institute that, unlike the National Cancer Institute, had little or no experience with the logistical complexities of multicenter clinical trials and one that lacked sufficient staff and facilities to set the large machinery rapidly into motion."

Krim didn't level all the blame at Fauci. She told Weiss that a clear mandate from President Reagan had never been forthcoming on the fight against the epidemic. "Federal agencies such as the Office of Management and Budget, the General Services Administration, and the Office of Personnel Management obviously did not share the sense of urgency felt by the public and by the NIH itself."

How much responsibility Fauci should bear for the fruitlessness of NIAID's labor was a question that PWAs, their doctors, their friends, and their political representatives would argue over for many years to come. On the one hand, it was clear in the eighties that conservative politicians and their bureaucratic knife-wielders went out of their way to curb the anti-AIDS fight. Both homophobia and fiscal conservatism played a part in the efforts of the Reagan administration to keep spending on AIDS to an absolute minimum.

Yet all managers operate under a condition of resource scarcity and no one ever feels that he or she has enough to do the proper job. The more skillful managers learn to hide job slots from their superiors, shifting them around under different names or under different covers. They learn how to call meeting rooms "offices," how to give needed employees different job titles. The ability to do that kind of bureaucratic subterfuge is, in many ways, the mark of a capable administrator, one who gets the job done. Anyone who has ever worked in a big organization, in an office, knows this to be true.

In the Washington political context, congressmen expected NIH institute directors to quietly call to complain on the sly about administration harassment or political difficulties and to request more money or people or space. It was all part of the game, a game that some clearly excelled at and others did not. To Krim, who was as good a player at this game of pragmatics as anyone living, Tony Fauci had proved he was not first-string material.

Tony Fauci followed Krim and used his prepared remarks to put an upbeat face on his faltering clinical trials system. "What has been accomplished to date by the AIDS Clinical Trials Group?" he asked rhetorically. "At present, approximately thirty protocols have been started involving approximately thirty-five hundred volunteers. Although AZT has been the primary drug studied, approximately sixteen others have entered clinical trials, including five antivirals, five drugs for opportunistic infection, four immunomodulators, and two antineoplastic drugs. While much has been achieved, we are never completely satisfied."

Weiss looked at Fauci skeptically. His own sources within the NIH had told him that Fauci's sanguine view of progress was all smoke. By this time Weiss had become adept at pulling the truth from reluctant scientists and administrators. From the very first hearings back in the early eighties, Weiss had been able to discern a pattern of obfuscation by NIH officials. Fear of getting their budgets cut by the OMB or even of being fired by the Reagan administration had led to a constant stream of disingenuous testimonies.

Administrators desperately in need of resources to fight AIDS were afraid to tell Congress how the OMB's stranglehold was hurting their efforts. Without that information, Weiss couldn't fight back against the White House. It was a terrible Catch-22, alleviated only occasionally by leaks. Leaked information helped the congressman prepare questions for public hearings, such as the one being held that day, that would force the bureaucrats to admit under oath how they were hurting and what they really needed. The whole process was a bizarre game of politics and it took a bit of courage on the part of bureaucrats to make it work. It hadn't with Tony Fauci.

Congressman Henry Waxman then took over the questioning. He addressed Fauci on the progress of the trials. Fauci had been given hundreds of millions of dollars, mostly through the efforts of Weiss and Waxman as well as Senator Lowell Weicker. The money was supposed to set up a system of drug testing for AIDS.

Waxman: "Dr. Fauci, many people have complained that the NIH drug development process is too slow to put volunteers in trials. Thirteen months ago your own drug selection committee said that aerosolized pentamidine, to prevent the deadly pneumonia in AIDS patients, was a very high priority for research. You have three protocols designed, but as best I can discover, no patients yet. Why are no trials under way?"

Fauci: "We have just started. The fact is, with all of the obstacles that got in the way of getting that drug into a protocol . . . it would have taken a person on our staff full-time doing nothing else but trying to push aerosolized pentamidine through. And unfortunately, we just didn't have the staff to take someone and say, 'The only thing you're going to do for the next X number of months is aerosolized pentamidine,' because, as you know, we have all these other things to do."

Waxman darkened visibly. He was furious. He practically levitated out of his chair. He then said, almost growling: "Pneumonia costs us millions of dollars in Medicaid dollars. Why can't we hire one full-time person to [get] this study under way?"

The angry outburst took Fauci by surprise. Instead of receiving sympathy, he was getting blasted. He was getting blamed. Fauci immediately began to backtrack. He explained that "We had asked for 127 FTEs that we thought were necessary, and we got 11 of those. So we have a significant shortfall in the number of FTEs to work with these clinical trials." Fauci's opening remarks about "while much has been achieved" suddenly became transformed into "we have a significant shortfall." He looked stupid.

Nearly a year and a half to the day after Fauci quietly complained to Mathilde Krim about his lack of personnel to write protocols, he was being forced to go public with his organizational inadequacies. Indeed, it appeared that whatever else Krim and Senator Weicker had quietly done for Fauci, it hadn't been enough. Fauci had refused for all these years to go to Waxman and Weiss, to complain personally about the stranglehold OMB was placing on AIDS research. Fauci didn't want to risk getting reprimanded, if not fired, for secretly talking with the Reagan administration's "enemies." He chose silence. Later, Fauci complained that he really had spoken to anyone who would listen about his staff shortage. But no one could remember his complaining that way. Certainly not Mathilde Krim.

It was Weiss's hearing, and by this time he wanted a piece of Fauci too. Weiss: "On page three [of your testimony], where you say that, after referring to all the things that you've done, 'while much has been achieved, we are never completely satisfied,' it seems to me that you have to be saying that as far as drug development is concerned very little has been achieved and you still have a long, long way to go and you need a tremendous amount of assistance to help you move from where you are. Wouldn't you say that that's a more accurate representation as to where you are with drug development?"

Fauci was in deep trouble. These were his supporters, his financial mentors, his political protectors from an administration that was so ideologically antagonistic to the very existence of the NIH that at one point it had suggested the whole thing be privatized. Yet Weiss and Waxman were clearly gunning for him. Fauci realized that the entire hearing was a setup to show his personal shortcomings.

The coup de grace came from Congresswoman Nancy Pelosi, a Democrat from California. Pelosi read a question by Waxman, who had to leave for a House vote. Pelosi: "Assume you lived in San Francisco, that you had AIDS and that you have had pneumonia once. You know the theory behind aerosol pentamidine to prevent pneumonia is strong. You know that the aerosol pentamidine was evaluated by the NIH as highly promising. You know that many studies in San Francisco recommend it routinely and that it is available. You know, as of today, that the delays in NIH trials are a problem of personnel that may not be solved this year. You know that your second or third bout of pneumonia will kill you. Would you take aerosol pentamidine or would you wait for a study?"

Fauci replied: "If I were an individual patient, I would probably take aerosolized pentamidine if I already had a bout of *Pneumocystis.* In fact, I might try, even before then, taking prophylactic Bactrim."

Silence. There was dead silence in room 2154 of the Rayburn House Office Building. People at the hearing just stared at Fauci and at one another. Here was the head of the NIH effort against AIDS publicly admitting that he personally would not follow the government's own guidelines and recommendations. Here was a top government scientist basically admitting that the government effort should be circumvented by people with AIDS. Here was Tony Fauci openly calling for the prophylaxis of *Pneumocystis carinii* pneumonia while his own clinical trials system did not have a single preventative drug in trial. It was a truly mind-wrenching admission. Fauci himself was calling into question the very foundation of the government's entire research effort against AIDS.

The furies ran wild in Larry Kramer when he read Tony Fauci's testimony. Over the past two years, while Fauci was getting millions to put together his AIDS network, Kramer was watching friends die. Some had starved to death, grown men shriveling up into sixty-pound skeletons. Others became demented and lost their minds before they died. It was too horrible. Nothing had ever prepared Kramer for this carnage. Nothing could.

When he read about the NIH delays, the ineptitude and perhaps the moral cowardice behind them, Kramer lost control. In a rhetorical flash of heat and light, he asked the questions and said the things that went unsaid in the decorous, proper congressional chambers. In vein-popping prose on May 31, 1988, he screeched in the *Village Voice* directly at Tony Fauci:

> I have been screaming at the National Institutes of Health since I first visited your Animal House of Horrors in 1984. I called you monsters then and I called you idiots in my play *The Normal Heart* and now I call you murderers.
>
> At hearings on April 29th before Representative Ted Weiss (D.-N.Y.) and his House Subcommittee on Human Resources, after almost eight years of the worst epidemic in modern history, perhaps

to be the worst in all history, you were pummeled into admitting publicly what some have been claiming since you took over some three years ago.

You have admitted that you are an incompetent idiot.

Over the past four years, $374 million has been allocated for AIDS treatment and research. You were in charge of spending much of that money.

It doesn't take a genius to set up a nationwide network of testing sites, commence a small number of moderately sized treatment efficacy tests on a population desperate to participate in them, import any and all interesting drugs (now numbering approximately 200) . . . and swiftly get into circulation anything that remotely passes muster. Yet after three years you have established only a system of waste, chaos, and uselessness.

It doesn't take a genius to request, as you did, 126 new staff persons, receive only eleven, AND THEN KEEP YOUR MOUTH SHUT ABOUT IT.

Now you come bawling to Congress that you don't have enough staff, office space, lab space, secretaries, computer operators, lab technicians, file clerks, janitors, toilet paper and that's why the drugs aren't being tested and the network of treatment centers isn't working and the drug protocols aren't in place. You expect us to buy this bullshit and feel sorry for you? YOU FUCKING SON OF A BITCH OF A DUMB IDIOT, YOU HAVE HAD $374 MILLION AND YOU EXPECT US TO BUY THIS GARBAGE OF EXCUSES!

For 36 agonizing months you refused to go public with what was happening (correction: not happening) and because you wouldn't speak up until you were asked pointedly and under oath by a congressional committee, we lie down and die and our bodies pile up higher and higher in hospitals and homes and hospices and streets and doorways.

The gay community has for five years told the NIH what drugs to test because we know and hear what is working on some of us somewhere. You couldn't care less about what we say. You won't answer our phone calls or letters, or listen to anyone in our stricken community. What tragic pomposity!

How many years ago did we tell you about aerosol pentamidine, Tony? That this stuff saves lives. And WE discovered it ourselves. We came to you, bearing this great news on a silver platter as a gift, begging you: Can we get it officially tested, can we get it approved by you so that insurance companies and Medicaid will pay for it (as well as other drugs we beg you to test) as a routine treatment, and our patients going broke paying for medicine can get it cheaper? You monster.

We tell you what the good drugs are, you don't test them, and YOU TELL US TO GET THEM ON THE STREETS! You continue to pass down word from On High that you don't like this drug or that drug—WHEN YOU HAVEN'T EVEN TESTED THEM! You pass word down from On High that you don't want "to endanger the life of the patient." THERE ARE MORE AIDS VICTIMS DEAD BECAUSE YOU DIDN'T TEST DRUGS ON THEM THAN BECAUSE YOU DID!

Whose ass are you covering, Tony (besides your own)? Is it the head of your Animal House, the invisible Dr. James Wyngaarden, director of the National Institutes of Health (and may a Democratic President get him out of office fast)? Is it Dr. Vincent DeVita, head of the National Cancer Institute, another invisible murderer who lets you be his fallguy? Or Dr. Otis Bowen, Secretary of the Department of Health and Human Services, no doubt the biggest murderer on this list: George Shultz and Caspar Weinberger would never take the constricting bullshit from the Office of Management and Budget that Bowen wallows in. All you "doctors" have, continuously, told the world that All Is Being Done That Can Be Done. Now you admit that isn't so.

WHY DID YOU KEEP QUIET FOR SO LONG?

I don't know (though it wouldn't surprise me) if you kept quiet intentionally. I don't know (though it wouldn't surprise me) if you were ordered to keep quiet by Higher Ups Somewhere and you're a good lieutenant, like Adolf Eichmann. . . .

# ..12..
# Winning

The six-story yellow condom swayed gently in the wind against the clear blue sky of Montreal. Across the street was the Palais du Congrès packed with 11,600 scientists, 1,300 reporters, 1,000 gate-crashers, and an unknown number of hookers. The Fifth International Conference on AIDS was set to begin. It was the summer of 1989 and an extraordinary series of changes in America's medical system was about to take place. They were quiet changes, at the high end, in the biomedical research arena, but they would affect the whole spectrum of medicine, from cancer to Alzheimer's, from treating infections to transplanting organs.

But first the condom fetish. In a huge exposition hall within the convention center, 102 booths hawked the wares of corporations from around the world. It was more medieval fair than scientific symposium. Burroughs Wellcome had the largest stall and anyone walking within five feet of it was inundated with pamphlets extolling the virtues of AZT. But the defining element of this bazaar was the condom.

Preaching the gospel of safe sex, a dozen companies had set up shop to peddle their prophylactics. The Japanese were out trying to break into the market by emphasizing the "quality" of their products. One company gave away five thousand condoms an hour, hour after hour. Others also passed out condoms, so that the quarter-sized, shiny articles were everywhere, in bulging shirt pockets, falling out of stuffed AIDS literature, on the floors.

There were Rough Rider "studded" condoms, Panther brand condoms, and the old favorites, Trojans. Ramses rigged up a machine to show

275

that its condom could contain much more fluid than any competitor's without bursting. It had an air compressor blow up condoms and measure its capacity in liters. The Ramses brand blew up into an enormous balloon that exploded at 45 liters. Other, weaker condoms blew at 20 or 30 liters. The explosions could be heard all day long throughout the exposition hall. So could jokes about having "45 liters' worth."

Brian Mulroney, the Canadian prime minister, was scheduled to open the conference the evening of June 4. He had to wait. Just before the opening speech, three hundred ACT UP protesters swept into the building, bringing with them perhaps another five or six hundred conference participants already on their way in to hear the opening remarks. It appeared as though a thousand people were storming the main hall, chanting, "The whole world is watching," carrying placards reading SILENCE = DEATH in both French and English.

The ACT UP members moved quickly past the Mounties who were there to protect the prime minister and seized the dais. One protester with a bullhorn announced that "this conference is going to be different. It's going to be led by people with AIDS." Then he proceeded to welcome the audience to the AIDS conference. Cheers rose from the ACT UP members, who by now had commandeered chairs from conference organizers. PWAs were opening the conference: not scientists or politicians but people with the AIDS; not passive victims or patients but self-empowered individuals demanding a role in their own treatment. This was a rowdy way of making the point, but TV made sure it was effective.

It was all "very ACT UPish," very high drama, with all the elements of an ACT UP demo: lightning-fast action, colorful media props, and a confrontation with the authorities as cameras rolled, cameras flashed, and tape recorders recorded. Beneath the theatrics, however, was, as always, a serious ACT UP message. This time it was more than a simple demand. They offered a sixteen-page document entitled "A National AIDS Treatment Research Agenda," in which Iris Long, Jim Eigo, Mark Harrington, and other members of ACT UP/New York's Treatment and Data Committee presented a critique of the NIH and FDA's inept and incompetent efforts against AIDS. It was the best-researched, most detailed and scientifically based paper ever produced on the subject outside the hallowed scientific halls of Bethesda and Rockville. ACT UP had done a brilliant job.

Onstage at Montreal, different members of the organization took turns reading out loud, in both English and French, the new agenda's twelve principles. Essentially, they were identical to those outlined by Mark Harrington at the Lasagna committee hearings sponsored by the National Cancer Institute at the beginning of 1989. In introducing the speakers, Harrington said that "There is a vacuum at the heart of the U.S. research and regulatory effort. The U.S. is ignoring the opportunistic infections that afflict people with AIDS, which is focusing too much effort on expensive and often toxic antivirals." He went on to criticize Tony Fauci for failing to provide new drug treatments for PWAs after three years' effort and half a billion dollars in taxpayer money. "Dr. Fauci likes to say the pipeline is full of AIDS drugs," Harrington told the audience. "The pipeline is full," he said. "It is utterly clogged with AZT. More than 80 percent of people in federal AIDS trials are on AZT, which has been approved for two years. We need new, cheap, nontoxic drugs, and where the U.S. government cannot take action, AIDS activists will."

Then ACT UP members on the stage began reading out loud the twelve principles. They demanded including PWAs in the design and execution of drug trials; establishing a master strategy that would ensure that all promising anti-AIDS drugs were quickly tested and distributed; refocusing resources on opportunistic infections as well as the AIDS virus itself; ending the exclusion of minorities, IV drug users, women, the poor, and children from trials; opening trials to the AZT-intolerant, 50 percent of PWAs; designing trials for the real world, which meant permitting PCP prophylaxis, avoiding placebos, and not using death as the end point; supporting community research projects; establishing an up-to-date, accessible registry of all clinical trials; opening a parallel track to make safe but unproven drugs available to people with life-threatening diseases.

The official ACT UP stage show at Montreal ended with the reading of the twelve principles. The document, however, went on to suggest "Five Drugs We Need Now," "Seven Treatments We Want Tested Faster," and a series of "Guidelines for Research." They were specific, detailed, and logical. The new research agenda discussed new models for clinical trials that would speed up drug testing and development, including curbing the endless search for the "maximum" tolerated dosage, which wasn't working in AIDS the way it was supposed to in cancer.

The document ended with a quote from Louis Lasagna, the head of the Lasagna committee. "The time is ripe to proclaim and implement a new mission for the FDA—to speed the public's access to important new drugs. No change in the law is needed to do this—simply acceptance of the fact that past approaches have not served the public well enough." By including this passage, ACT UP joined a strange coalition composed of Lasagna, Sam Broder and the NCI, plus the deregulatory forces of the Republican Bush administration and the editorial page of the *Wall Street Journal,* which had been blasting the FDA for nearly a decade. The AIDS epidemic was making for strange bedfellows. But then so does every social crisis.

Then came self-destruction. Upon completing the reading of their twelve principles, most of the ACT UP members left, turning control back to the Mounties and the conference organizers. But not all. About sixty of the more radical members remained, shouting slogans, continuing to disrupt the meeting. When the original contingent marched into the hall, more than half of the people sitting in their seats had risen with applause at their action. An hour later, their patience worn thin, the audience began to clap in unison, expressing their impatience at the remaining group of self-absorbed protesters.

It was ACT UP at its adolescent worst. The intellectually mature and scientifically sophisticated were replaced by a bunch of me-me-me egocentrics whining at the top of their voices. Their tantrum lasted yet another hour, which meant that when Mulroney finally appeared, people had been forced to wait two hours.

It didn't end there, either. The sixty ACT UP people heckled the speakers throughout the evening, booing and laughing at everyone. The worst came when the Barbadian delegate to the UN, Nita Barrow, got up to speak about how AIDS was devastating the Caribbean. She spoke movingly and emotionally of the people being destroyed by the disease, of a woman left to raise twelve grandchildren because her six children, four sons and two daughters, had all been killed by AIDS. She told the audience that the church had refused to allow the woman's children to be buried in its graveyard. She had the graves dug behind her own house.

Barrow ended her speech with a plea for the "victims of this disease." All hell broke loose. The small contingent of protesters remaining began screaming at her, hissing and booing. Barrow had sinned by using the word *victim,* a forbidden piece of language on ACT UP's shit list of politically unacceptable terms. The word police were at it again. Ms. Barrow, looking confused and hurt, simply looked at the young men in front of her in astonishment. In the end, the extreme behavior of an irresponsible few served to dilute the impact of ACT UP's important AIDS research document. Attention was focused on them, not on the analysis of what was wrong with the country's biomedical research system.

And yet so cogent and powerful was ACT UP's "A National AIDS Treatment Research Agenda," that it couldn't be dismissed. Just the reverse happened. It became the bridge into the NIH and the FDA for ACT UP and other AIDS activists. It showed the scientists in Washington, D.C., that PWAs could understand the scientific world in its own terms. The scientists began to take Jim Eigo, Mark Harrington, Martin Delaney, and others very seriously. After Montreal, a dialogue quickly opened up between the two camps.

Tony Fauci in particular shifted position dramatically. After the Weiss hearings back in April, Fauci surely recognized that he was politically exposed, vulnerable. He had been tarred with an "incompetence" brush by the very people who were his major support in the past. It was time for a complete change of strategy for Tony Fauci. If he was to continue receiving financial support for AIDS research from Congress, if he was to continue being the head of NIAID, he had to reinvent himself. He did, and his transformation became a major factor in the key victories ACT UP, Project Inform, and other AIDS activist groups began achieving in their fight to change the nation's medical research system. It was Fauci more than anyone who gave these activists a seat at the table of biomedical power that summer, the summer when the number of people with AIDS reached 100,000 and the number of AIDS deaths passed 60,000. It had taken a decade to arrive at 100,000. It would be only fifteen months before it would double to 200,000.

Tony Fauci has a story he tells anyone who asks about his sudden conversion from staunch defender of the traditional scientific method and NIH orthodoxy to change agent for AIDS activists. Many people have heard it, and they all agree that as Fauci describes it, his San Francisco meeting takes on the patina of a religious experience, an enlightenment. It goes like this: At a Project Inform conference in mid-June, right after the Fifth International Conference on AIDS in Montreal, Fauci met a thirty-three-year-old schoolteacher. The man had been diagnosed just five months before. His name was Terry Sutton and he taught emotionally disturbed children in San Francisco. He also worked with Marty Delaney at Project Inform when he could.

During the conference, Sutton told Fauci his story. Each person with AIDS, according to Michael Callen, has a "story." Sutton's was even more horrendous than most. He was being forced to choose between blindness and death.

Sutton explained to Fauci that he had come down with cytomegalovirus (CMV) retinitis, a herpes-type infection of the retina that up to a third of all PWAs eventually develop if they escape the clutches of PCP, as nearly all of them were now doing in San Francisco, thanks to aerosol pentamidine.

The drug being used in the underground community against CMV retinitis was ganciclovir, or DHPG. Luckily for Sutton, the developer of DHPG, Syntex, a Palo Alto–based company, had made the drug available through the FDA's Compassionate Use program at no cost to the patient. About thirty-six hundred people were taking it and the number was growing quickly. But the drug had one major drawback. It was toxic to bone marrow and therefore severely suppressed the body's immunity. Just like AZT.

Sutton told Fauci that he was already taking AZT to combat the AIDS virus itself. Since AZT had the same toxicity as DHPG, a PWA could take either AZT or DHPG, but not both. It would kill him. So Sutton now had to choose between a drug that would save his eyesight and a drug that could prolong his life. He could continue to live but only by going blind.

But, Sutton told Fauci, there was another drug, Foscarnet, that worked against CMV retinitis and could be taken with AZT. It wasn't toxic to bone marrow. But Sutton wasn't being allowed to take Foscarnet because of a bewildering series of bureaucratic rules, government regulations, and private industry decisions. He was literally going blind because of red tape in America's biomedical research system.

Sutton told Fauci that there was only one way at present for him to get Foscarnet and that was to enroll in a tiny, fifty-nine-person FDA-approved trial being run by Astra, the Swedish company that owned the drug. But the study protocol wouldn't allow anyone to enroll who had ever taken DHPG. That was because the FDA insisted on receiving only "clean" data. The FDA believed that any past use of DHPG would taint that data. This was, according to Sutton and all the community doctors he had consulted, ridiculous; DHPG would be flushed out of the body over time. But those were the rules. Fauci looked dumbfounded as Sutton finished up his story. He knew things were bad in the Washington drug approval bureaucracy, he said, but not *this* bad.

What Sutton did not tell Fauci at the time was the reason Astra had decided not to release Foscarnet under the FDA's Compassionate Use protocol and instead to limit access to only a few dozen people.

Under Compassionate Use, a company can offer a drug to anyone at cost if the drug has tested out for safety and has shown some promise of efficacy. The FDA put this policy into effect in the mid-eighties, under heavy pressure from Congress and AIDS activists to speed up the drug approval process.

Syntex did take the FDA up on its offer and made its drug, DHPG, available under Compassionate Use. As far back as 1985, researchers had noted that DHPG sharply curtailed CMV retinitis. When the drug was offered to thousands of people with AIDS, community doctors saw immediately that it was clearly effective in preventing blindness.

The FDA, however, disagreed. Syntex took the patients' records to the FDA and offered them up as evidence to obtain an NDA, New Drug Application, to sell DHPG commercially. The FDA refused to accept the data. Ellen Cooper said at the time that the data did not have any information on "control efficacy"—a coded way of saying that Syntex had not done placebo-controlled testing on DHPG and didn't have the requisite "clean" control data. The FDA was suggesting that a company do a double-blind trial in which people literally went blind to prove the effectiveness of the drug.

After eight months of lobbying by AIDS activists and Congressmen Waxman and Weiss, the FDA compromised. It said NIAID should go ahead and do placebo testing of DHPG but that those who did not receive the drug would be monitored. If their CMV appeared to be making them blind, the patients would be told and they could drop out of the study and take DHPG.

In announcing this compromise, the FDA touted it as an example of how flexible it had become. Most community doctors considered the posturing ridiculous. They already believed through their own experience with DHPG that the drug worked effectively against CMV retinitis. Additional testing was simply a waste of time. Moreover, since they knew that DHPG was effective, they asked how any scientist could ethically allow a disease to worsen. Community doctors believed that the earlier a patient received treatment for an AIDS-induced disease, the better the chance of prevention or recovery.

The FDA's rejection of Syntex's original patient data made Compassionate Use a dirty word within the pharmaceutical industry. No company wanted to find itself without the right kind of "clean," placebo-controlled data for a commercial license after treating thousands of patients at cost. Astra was one of them. After what had happened to Syntex, Astra preferred to follow the FDA's old-fashioned rules and go by the book, hence a tiny fifty-nine-person trial at NIAID.

After Sutton explained his situation, he asked Fauci why the crazy rules couldn't be changed so he didn't have to make a Hobson's choice between blindness and death.

Fauci says he was a different man after this San Francisco meeting. Instead of being a defender of the scientific method and all its rules and regulations, he became, in effect, an AIDS activist himself. For the rest of 1989, on issue after issue, he accepted virtually the entire ACT UP program and championed it against status quo forces within his own institute and in the FDA. In fact, the FDA quickly became the "enemy" in the months following the Fauci conversion.

When he got back to Washington, Fauci called FDA Commissioner Frank Young to lobby for the release of Foscarnet on behalf of Terry Sutton and other PWAs in the same fix. The FDA, under pressure for months on its handling of DHPG and Foscarnet, relented and loosened its policy.

Fauci transformed himself in the summer of 1989. He became an aggressive advocate for speeding up testing and approval of drugs for all life-threatening diseases, not just AIDS. His testimony at the Lasagna committee hearings had been tepid. While Sam Broder had publicly criticized the FDA for "excessive micromanagement and interference" in NCI studies, Fauci had been virtually silent. Broder had leveled blast after blast at the FDA during the January hearings, with nary a nod to the conventional bureaucratic niceties that normally define such occasions. Fauci, in comparison, appeared cowardly.

But now, just a few months later, Fauci was telling people that AIDS was really just the beginning of a major overhaul of the entire system. The FDA had to change. Medical programs for all diseases, from cancer to Alzheimer's and stroke, affecting tens of millions of people, would have to change, he said. They would be modeled on the new system Fauci himself was now trying to build, a system that consisted of greater access to drugs at a much earlier stage in the testing game.

In this, Tony Fauci of NIAID joined Sam Broder of the NCI in an alliance against the FDA. In fact, a fierce behind-the-scenes rivalry was soon to bloom between Broder's lab and Fauci's NIAID on just who was the bigger advocate of change in the NIH, over just who should get the credit for those changes. In the summer of '89, Fauci came out in support of releasing ddI, an analogue to AZT with less toxicity, on a new parallel track of drug development. The parallel track, pushed by ACT UP in New York, would give PWAs early access to drugs proven safe but not yet proven effective by the FDA. ACT UP negotiated a parallel track release of ddI directly with Bristol-Myers, the company that held the license for the drug. As Fauci was receiving credit for his liberal position on ddI, Broder's lab speeded up publication of a story in *Science* magazine about the drug's safety. Broder's lab at the NCI had done the Phase I safety trial for ddI, as it does for many AIDS drugs. Why did they want to get into print early? Robert Yarchoan, Broder's right-hand lab man, boasts that "ddI's *our* drug. *We* have the patent for ddI and licensed it to Bristol-Myers."

Fauci's conversion smacked of opportunism. Broder's did not. For one thing, Fauci adopted virtually the entire ACT UP program at once and as a whole. It was the kind of flip-flop that comes with a true religious conversion. It was so startling that it appeared as if Fauci had found the light, had an epiphany, and transformed himself into another being.

In addition, Fauci's change of position followed close on the heels of his disastrous performance at the Weiss hearings, where he was pilloried by one and all for ineptitude. Moreover, his turning against the FDA followed Sam Broder's outspoken criticism of the agency. Fauci could see that it was okay to be anti-FDA: the Bush administration loved it; the AIDS activists loved it; Congress applauded it; and Broder had paved the way. Being anti-FDA was a safe position within the NIH bureaucracy.

Broder was different. For one thing, he was much more conservative. He did attack the FDA for overmanaging drug development because it interfered with his own lab work. Broder was nothing if not fast in latching on to drugs, testing them, and shoving them out the door. Suramin and AZT were just two examples of that. They were also examples of Broder's getting drugs out the door perhaps too fast.

Nonetheless, Broder had the courage to go after the FDA before anyone else at the NIH did it. In that he allied himself with ACT UP, the CRI, Project Inform, and Mathilde Krim's AmFAR. He would also, in the weeks ahead, come out in support of community-based research in general. But Broder refused to adopt the entire activist program. He continued to favor placebo testing in many cases, even when Tony Fauci rejected it. Broder wasn't excited about the parallel track idea of getting experimental drugs out to PWAs before they were approved by the FDA for efficacy. And he wasn't too keen on having people with AIDS or any other disease sitting on committees with scientists making decisions on trial designs and testing priorities. That really made Broder uneasy. But Fauci was suddenly advocating practically all of these revolutionary medical concepts.

Finally, Broder continued to push AZT with all the enthusiasm he could muster. At the Fifth International Conference on AIDS, he gave a charming speech, opening in halting French, moving on to jokes in English, in which he ascribed the growing longevity of PWAs directly to AZT. It was a scientifically feeble assertion. The prevention and treatment of *Pneumocystis carinii* pneumonia, the greatest AIDS killer, with Bactrim and aerosol pentamidine probably saved many more lives than AZT. Both came up from the community doctor level, not down from the NCI. Since AZT, aerosol pentamidine, and Bactrim came into widespread use in 1987–88, and since most PWAs took a combination of drugs to fight AIDS, it was impossible to say that AZT by itself contributed anything to longevity. Perhaps it did; perhaps it didn't. Broder was more propagandist than scientist in Montreal, and in that sense hardly a friend of the CRI or ACT UP or Project Inform. Unlike Tony Fauci, Sam Broder was not a quick convert.

Right after Montreal, Larry Kramer went to work on getting ddI on the new parallel track that Tony Fauci was now advocating, thanks to their long evening stroll together on the streets of Montreal. The week Kramer returned to New York, he was on TV with ex-Senator Lowell Weicker talking about AIDS and the need for speedier drug approval and wider access to drug treatment, essentially parallel track. When he was in the Senate, Weicker had proved himself effective in battling Stockman's OMB to generate resources for AIDS research. Kramer, like virtually all AIDS activists, was sad that Weicker was no longer there to help. They had lost an important ally in Washington when Weicker lost his seat in 1988.

After the TV program, Kramer asked Weicker about Bristol-Myers, which held the license to ddI. It was, after all, a Connecticut-based company, Weicker's home state. How should Kramer approach Bristol-Myers? What should he say in a letter? Weicker, it turned out, actually knew Richard Gelb, the chairman and chief executive officer of the company. Weicker had met Gelb many times and he told Kramer that Gelb was a good guy. His own family had experienced cancer in recent years. Perhaps most important, Gelb was a Yale man. So were George Bush, Burton Lee—and Larry Kramer.

Kramer wrote Gelb, dropped Weicker's name, mentioned Yale, enclosed several articles on ACT UP, making sure to include a few about their "zaps" and demos against pharmaceutical companies, and said he would like to have a meeting about making ddI the first drug available on the new parallel track. Kramer said he would give a call the following Monday.

A few days before that Monday, Kramer received a call from Tom McCann, head of corporate communications, the latest euphemism for public relations in corporate America. McCann was very upbeat on the phone. "I think you'll find support for your notion here in the company," he said. There wasn't any sense of ACT UP pushing Bristol-Myers against the wall, forcing them to meet. It was all so cordial. McCann suggested meeting at their headquarters at 345 Park Avenue in Manhattan.

Kramer went over with Jim Eigo and Mark Harrington. They met with Dr. Jerry Birnbaum, who was introduced to them as the company's chief scientist and the person most responsible for dealing with ddI. Birnbaum was normally based in Wallingford, Connecticut, where Bristol-Myers's major labs were located.

It was a historic meeting. This was the first time that a drug company had ever sat down with people suffering from a disease to plan clinical trials of the drug intended to treat them.

Eigo talked in detail about the parallel track. He knew that the most important worry for drug companies about the parallel track idea was not getting enough patients into the regular clinical trials. If people could get their drug outside the normal channels, why should they enter the company-sponsored trials? And if they didn't enter the trials, how could Bristol-Myers ever convince the FDA to allow it to market the drug commercially? From the company's point of view, would it be committing profit suicide to go into the parallel track?

Harrington weighed in with a detailed scientific discussion. He tried to show Birnbaum that only people who could not qualify for the regular clinical trials would go into the parallel track open trials. There would be no loss of patients for clinical trials. Eigo was in his regular uniform—T-shirt and ponytail. Harrington looked more "respectable" in a shirt and tie—so respectable, in fact, that he was mistaken for something other than a young ACT UP radical by the Bristol-Myers scientist. During a break, Kramer went to the bathroom and soon found himself with Birnbaum. The Bristol-Myers scientist turned to Kramer and asked, "That Mr. Harrington, that's *Dr.* Harrington, right?" Kramer laughed and said, "No, but he knows his science and his pharmacology so well that people often mistake him for a doctor."

The conversation that morning was really a debate, with Eigo and

Harrington on one side arguing for ddI to become the first parallel track drug and Birnbaum on the other side playing defense. Kramer kept quiet, which for Kramer was an extraordinary feat.

Birnbaum, a man in his mid-forties, was the classic scientific bureaucrat. He listened intently but didn't give anything away. He was new at Bristol-Myers, having arrived there just two years ago. This was the first time he was dealing with the AIDS activist community. Birnbaum told Eigo and Harrington that the Phase II study of ddI scheduled for July was being postponed to September. That didn't make them terribly happy. But Birnbaum went on to say that he didn't know of any reason why ddI couldn't be made available to the community somehow in September, whether it was called parallel track or something else.

This was what the ACT UP trio were waiting for. Birnbaum could not have made that statement without checking with Washington. And Kramer secretly knew that Birnbaum had done just that. The Thursday before this meeting at the Bristol-Myers headquarters in New York, Tony Fauci had gone out to San Francisco to attend a big meeting set up by Marty Delaney and Project Inform. This would be remembered as a very important moment in the annals of AIDS because it was there that Tony Fauci went public for the first time with "his" suggestion that a parallel track be opened up for people with AIDS. Delaney was with Fauci in Fauci's hotel room when he noticed a stack of phone messages. On top was a call from Dr. Birnbaum in New York—please call right away. Delaney called Kramer later that day to tell him that Birnbaum had been in contact with Fauci, just as Fauci was putting NIAID publicly behind the parallel track idea.

The first part of the meeting between ACT UP and Bristol-Myers went well. Birnbaum listened and didn't say no. In fact, he held out the promise that all would go well for releasing ddI sometime in the early fall.

Then Kramer spoke up for the first time and went into his "bad-cop" routine. He said that he hoped Bristol-Myers would come through with ddI because if it didn't, this was what was going to happen: The AIDS medical underground would flood the community with bootleg ddI. The drug was already available at quite a high price, a thousand dollars a month, to anyone who could afford it. The buyers clubs would purchase so large a quantity that the price would fall sharply and *all* the people with AIDS would be able to get it. Enough ddI was already being secretly imported into the country to worry the FDA. In June they interdicted and seized a shipment of the drug out on the West Coast. "Your trials are going to be worth shit," Kramer warned. "If you don't hurry up and get this stuff out there and get these trials going, you won't have any trials and your drug will be worthless."

Birnbaum froze. He and company officials had just heard the same thing from a different source. They didn't know where or how the black market underground was getting ddI, but they did know that other promising drugs, such as AL 721 and HPA-23, had been crippled as commercial products by the AIDS underground buyers clubs. The same thing could easily happen to ddI, costing the company tens of millions of dollars in profits.

Kramer wasn't finished. He told Birnbaum that Bristol-Myers would be picketed by ACT UP and the radical organization would create a public relations nightmare for the drug company. "For the first time," Kramer said, "the community is powerful and active." Montreal was still burning brightly in the collective memory of Eigo, Harrington, and Kramer. By taking over the opening speech of Canadian Prime Minister Mulroney, ACT UP had been able to project its own agenda of needed AIDS research to the whole assembly as well as to millions of people watching news reports of the convention. It was an enormous triumph for ACT UP and they were feeling very strong.

Kramer's threats were too much for Birnbaum. He was only a scientist working for a big drug company. He didn't know how to handle it. He became visibly nervous. Birnbaum began getting up from his chair to make phone calls. First he said he had to call his son. Then he said he had to call his boss. Finally he announced that he could only stay until one o'clock. Then he bolted for the door, saying, "I've got to go back, my boss will be wondering where I am." It was strange. Presumably his boss knew exactly where Birnbaum was since his boss had sent him to the meeting with ACT UP. Kramer, Eigo, and Harrington left wondering what had happened. Until Kramer spoke up, everything had moved smoothly. Maybe I shouldn't have come on so strong, Kramer asked himself.

It didn't matter, as it turned out. Bristol-Myers's CEO, Gelb, decided to take a chance with ddI and permit it to be the first drug used under the new parallel track program. His Yale friends in Washington had cogently explained that the new trials system would not compromise the company's efforts to gain FDA approval for the drug.

\* \* \*

GOOD INTENTIONS

It was never part of his formal speech. In fact, it hadn't even been written down. But when Tony Fauci went out to San Francisco to speak at a large Project Inform conference on AIDS, he ad-libbed himself into history.

Fauci was now implementing full force his new stragety of making alliances with the AIDS activists, especially ACT UP on the East Coast and Project Inform on the West. As part of that effort, he was building personal relationships with a handful of people he was going to let "in," allow to sit at the table of power in the biomedical research world. The rest would be excluded. Joe Sonnabend and Michael Callen, for example, were not invited to the party by Fauci. This was going to be a very deliberate, thought-out strategy of co-optation. If successful, Fauci might even split the AIDS activist movement into the ins and outs. As one top official at NIAID put it: "Tony is being very proactive about establishing a dialogue with selected individuals in some of these groups to enhance communications and to break down a lot of the antagonism that has developed."

Jim Eigo and Mark Harrington were clearly among the anointed by Fauci. So was Martin Delaney. That's why Fauci was in San Francisco in late June attending a Project Inform conference. When he got up to speak, Fauci announced he was in favor of the idea of a parallel track of drug trials for people with AIDS. He said that at the end of Phase I safety trials, just as Phase II efficacy trials were about to begin, another track could be opened where patients could get the drug if they weren't eligible for the controlled trials. Fauci was vague about who would qualify for the new parallel track. He left it as a broad concept, very open-ended.

When Fauci mentioned parallel track in San Francisco, the first thing that came to mind was AZT resistance. In Montreal, there'd been a whole panel addressing the growing problem of resistance to AZT. PWAs had taken to AZT much earlier out on the West Coast than in the East. But the AIDS virus was mutating in their bodies and resisting whatever positive effects AZT was having on them. For those taking the full-strength dosage originally recommended by the FDA, 1200 milligrams a day, resistance was showing up very quickly, three months into the drug therapy. For those PWAs who, with their community doctors, had decided to cut the dosage in half or more, resistance appeared later. Now, even people using relatively small doses of AZT were having trouble with resistance. Those who could tolerate it and who survived the onslaught of opportunistic infections had been on the drug for up to two years by the summer of '89. Unfortunately, many of them had little bone marrow left as AIDS and AZT ate it away.

A substitute drug was needed and fast to replace AZT. There wasn't time to wait. The sense of urgency became translated into a community buzz about ddI. It was a nucleoside analogue, a cousin of AZT, but was said to be much less toxic. The Phase I safety trial was finishing up and the drug looked relatively safe. The Phase II efficacy trial was scheduled to start in July. The PWAs in San Francisco couldn't wait a year or two for the results. They would be without an antiviral drug very soon. So ddI and parallel track became synonymous at the Project Inform conference.

Tony Fauci became the key NIH proponent of the parallel track concept. In a number of congressional hearings, at scientific conferences, in front of the media, Fauci proselytized for it. "It doesn't make any sense to deprive those people of the choice of whether or not they want to take a chance on a drug that isn't yet proven to be effective," he said time and again. "As long as it doesn't interfere with the clinical trials, as a scientist I think it is an appropriate thing to do. We will get people into trial who are more motivated into getting into trial rather than just getting a drug." It was almost verbatim from the speeches, testimony, and written demands issued by ACT UP. Fauci was becoming the point man for ACT UP's Treatment and Data Committee.

Tony Fauci did his best proselytizing in front of the FDA. In mid-August, the FDA's Anti-Infective Drugs Advisory Committee met to discuss the parallel track concept and make its recommendation to the FDA. The meeting was held in Bethesda, Maryland. Fifty members of ACT UP/New York attended and, with cheers and hisses, made their presence felt. Jim Eigo, Mark Harrington, and Larry Kramer were in the contingent.

The only real concern of the FDA committee was patient control. Principal investigators had universally testified that they feared patients would not join clinical trials, with all their rules and regulations, if they could get into parallel track trials. For the PIs, control over the patient population was always key. It was one of their major sources of power in the scientific community. They were terrified of losing it. For that reason alone, practically all of the PIs involved in AIDS research opposed the parallel track idea.

Jim Eigo stood up and refuted the PIs' accusation that the parallel track would deplete the pool of people for their clinical trials. Eigo told them that clinical trials were chronically underenrolled because the PIs didn't know how to design them. He said the PIs refused to listen to PWAs and their doctors when writing protocols. They never left their ivory towers in universities to visit the neighborhoods, talk to the people. As a consequence, protocols were never realistic. "Trials are underenrolled when they're not designed with people in mind," said Eigo. The parallel track had nothing to do with it.

Then Tony Fauci got up to defend the parallel track idea. He told the committee that it was possible to maintain the integrity of the clinical trials system while opening up a new parallel track of trials for those unable to get into the formal protocols. At the end of Fauci's presentation, Larry Kramer jumped up and yelled, "President Bush was right! You *are* our hero, Dr. Fauci!" The audience was quite aware that during the televised Presidential debates between Bush and Michael Dukakis, Bush had listed Fauci as one of the nation's heroes. It was also well aware that Kramer had just a year before called Fauci a murderer and compared him to the Nazi war criminal Adolf Eichmann.

In the end, the committee lifted the language right out of the two-page letter on parallel track that AIDS activists had written in Mathilde Krim's townhouse just a week before. In clear, declarative sentences, the Anti-Infective Drugs Advisory Committee recommended the parallel track concept to the FDA.

It was head-spinning for the people of ACT UP and Project Inform. Not only was Washington listening to them now, they were beginning to write the rules and regulations for drug development! What an incredible change since May, since the Lasagna committee hearings. They were being let inside the tent of biomedical research. After nine years.

In the end, it wasn't called parallel track. The conservative forces opposed to the idea of freer access to treatment drugs saw to that. The PIs and many of the mid- and lower-level bureaucrats at the FDA and NIAID worked against it. Maureen Myers at NIAID hated the idea, and Ellen Cooper at the FDA just gave lip service to parallel track. But their opposition wasn't strong enough to derail the political momentum behind the concept. The language was fudged, but the Department of Health and Human Services did in fact open access to the drug ddI in a precedent-setting way. At the end of September, the HHS announced that the FDA had accepted the recommendation of its advisory committee, for AIDS and perhaps for other diseases.

Five trials were approved for ddI. There would be three traditional clinical trials, two comparing ddI with AZT and the third comparing different doses of ddI. Then instead of a new parallel track, the FDA said it would authorize a Treatment IND and a Compassionate Use trial. Together, they would make the drug available to anyone who couldn't get into the regular clinical trials. It was a very complicated way of proclaiming a parallel track without naming it that.

The fact that the press release announcing the new de facto parallel track trials came out of the Department of Health and Human Services indicated how political the whole process of drug development and treatment had become. In the past, no public announcement would have appeared on such a mundane thing as drug protocols. If one had come out, it would have been released by the FDA or NIAID or the pharmaceutical company running the trials. But not this time. There was too much politics involved.

Congressman Henry Waxman had made sure that was true. In late July he held a hearing on the parallel track, generating just the right pressure to keep the momentum from faltering as the concept wound its way through the Washington bureaucracy. Waxman got all the heavy hitters in AIDS public policy to come to his hearing. James Mason, the assistant secretary for health and head of the Public Health Service, sat right in front of Waxman. He was flanked by Anthony Fauci from NIAID, Sam Broder from the NCI, and Commissioner Frank Young from the FDA. Seated one row behind them were Martin Delaney from Project Inform and ACT UP's Jim Eigo.

Waxman started off with a speech that put the issue in clear focus. "Thousands of Americans find themselves without useful approved treatment and with steadily declining health. A handful can get into controlled trials, but most can just read about drugs they cannot get.

"During the course of the epidemic," he explained, "this rationing has been scientifically and morally justified as necessary to the conduct of trials and appropriate for quickly meeting the needs of future Americans with AIDS. We have lived with a policy of limited distribution today so that we will have adequate information for tomorrow.

"But now many people—patients, their families, and researchers—are questioning this policy. They argue that scientific trials do not require that everyone else be denied access to potential therapies; indeed they say the trials are better conducted with willing volunteers rather than desperate ones. And, they continue, it is therefore morally wrong to withhold promising drugs from patients with nothing else to turn to."

Waxman ended his opening remarks by saying that the changes proposed—parallel track—went far beyond the fight against AIDS. "This is an important proposal. It could change ground rules on research, clinical care, markets, and insurance. It could also provide access to drugs—the good ones and the worthless ones—long before data are available. If it works, it could revolutionize drug development. If it fails, it could cripple AIDS research for some time."

Mason then spoke into the mike. He supported the idea of parallel track, not only for AIDS but for cancer and other diseases. It was the first time any Bush administration official publicly came out for parallel track. It was a major victory for ACT UP and Project Inform just to have Mason say he favored parallel track.

That hearing was a month ago. Now Health and Human Services was issuing a press release that said that the combination of Treatment IND and Compassionate Use was "consistent with the parallel track concept and [is] an interim measure to make a promising investigational therapy available for people with AIDS who do not have satisfactory treatment options." The ACT UP and Project Inform radicals had won.

They weren't the only winners in that summer of '89. Mathilde Krim at AmFAR pulled off one of the major coups in modern medical research. "It was a love-in!" says Krim, describing her three-day conference on community-based research held at Columbia University. "Can you imagine? At the head table at the dinner Friday night was Dr. Broder, Dr. Sonnabend, Dr. Fauci, Don Abrams from California, Dr. Burton Lee—a very straitlaced Republican who is physician to President Bush—and a nice guy from the FDA, Nightingale. Who was presiding in the middle of the table? Michael Callen! Can you imagine Michael and Joe Sonnabend sitting inches away from Dr. Fauci, Dr. Broder, and the FDA? After all that has been said on both sides? Oh, it was so funny."

It was so funny because it was so incongruous. As at most peace conferences, bitter enemies were now smiling at each other, nodding and agreeing over good food and wine, with flowers on the table. It was July 7, 1989, and they were all at the Columbia University School for International Affairs, an appropriate setting for the forging of a new peace treaty, a new consensus between adversaries over how AIDS—indeed, how all diseases—should be fought.

Ostensibly, the conference was called to celebrate the growth of community-based research throughout the United States. It was officially sponsored by the Community Research Initiative of New York and the County Community Consortium of San Francisco. Krim's American Foundation for AIDS Research picked up the bill. In fact, Krim had set the stage for the whole shebang seven months earlier at Carnegie Hall.

The stars were out at Leonard Bernstein's concert on the first day of December, 1988. Isaac Stern and Placido Domingo performed onstage. Meryl Streep, Paul Simon, and Steve Martin made special appearances. The celebrity chairpersons for the night, First Ladies all, included Lady Bird Johnson, Betty Ford, Rosalynn Carter, and, of course, Nancy Reagan.

Lady Bird was an old friend; Mathilde's husband, Arthur, was a former finance chairman of the Democratic National Committee and the Krims were very close to Lyndon and Lady Bird. Rosalynn Carter was an old friend too; she had been on the board of directors of the American Medical Foundation, the predecessor to AmFAR. Although Betty Ford was not a particularly close friend, Krim regarded her as warmly as she did Rosalynn Carter. That left Nancy. . . .

It was billed as a "Serenade: A Musical Tribute to Mathilde Krim," and it helped transform the idea of community-based research into a national movement. Krim wanted it that way. Bernstein had just wanted to raise money to honor her. When Krim asked if it would be okay to use most of the proceeds to seed local research operations around the country, Bernstein said, "Great idea. Sure. Wonderful." Krim beamed.

It was a perfect way to circumvent Michael Gottlieb's near veto over any AmFAR money going to community-based research. *This* money was under Krim's control. She was going to spend it where she knew it was needed.

Krim had been able to squeeze a small amount of money out of the AmFAR board for the Community Research Initiative and the San Francisco County Consortium—small seed grants to develop or expand programs to test AIDS treatments on the community level. The CRI received thirty thousand dollars and the CCC got fifty thousand.

But this was peanuts and Krim knew it. The Bernstein concert could raise big bucks. It did. "We made a million dollars," says Krim proudly. All of it was committed to community-based research. When the commitment was announced, Dr. Burton Lee was on the staff of Memorial Sloan-Kettering Cancer Center and a member of the president's AIDS commission. The commission, of course, had come out strongly in favor of community-based research. In its final report, Lee wrote that "Community-based clinical trials serve an important purpose—they are faster and there is less bureaucratic red tape." He added that "There is no evidence of slippage in quality in these clinical trials because many of the people who are on the advisory boards are the same people who are doing research in the academic institutions."

AmFAR set about parceling out the new money just as it did with all its other research projects. It sent out a request for proposals to set up community-based research organizations, then set up a panel of experts to read the proposals and make recommendations to the board. The reviewers scored the applications, and the board went down the list until it ran out of money.

In April of 1989, AmFAR announced it was awarding $1.4 million to sixteen community-based AIDS research centers. Money went to groups in Atlanta; Austin and Houston; Boston; Los Angeles; New Haven; New York (CRI); Portland, Oregon; Redwood City, California; San Francisco (two groups, the County Community Consortium and the Community Research Alliance); Santa Fe; Springfield, Virginia; and Westwood, New Jersey.

Krim had done something extraordinary. She'd financed a revolution in medical research and basically done it by herself. With Joe Sonnabend back in the early eighties, Krim had helped develop the very concept of community research. Then, along with Sonnabend and Callen, she'd set up the AMF. Michael Gottlieb had forced her to jettison Sonnabend and community research as the price for uniting their two AIDS foundations, but Krim never lost the dream. Instead, she discovered an alternative funding mechanism outside Gottlieb's control—Leonard Bernstein's personal, musical tribute to her—and used it to establish a community-based system throughout the United States. It was a breakhtaking venture and a magnificent success.

Now Krim was trying something else. Although the Columbia conference was called to celebrate community-based research, a second agenda was to bring together all the major players in the AIDS drama in one contained space, to get them to talk privately and intimately for three days and reach a consensus on the future of all AIDS research.

To that end, six people from the FDA attended, including Ellen Cooper, who stayed Friday and Saturday and attended all the sessions. Drug companies sent over a dozen representatives, including Sandra Nusinoff-Lehrman from Burroughs Wellcome. No one knew exactly how many people from ACT UP were attending since so many of the younger persons in the CRI, AmFAR, and other groups were quietly members of ACT UP as well. Jim Eigo was there in his ponytail, SILENCE = DEATH T-shirt, and shorts, as was Iris Long—the Treatment and Data crowd.

"There were about a hundred people there at any one time," recalls Bernie Bihari, who was the director of research for the CRI at the time and who became executive director a few months later. "You really got to know one another. The community groups spent a lot of time having meals with people from the NIH, the FDA, and the pharmaceutical industry. People ate dinner and breakfast and lunch together. A real sense of community developed over the weekend. A sense of common purpose developed."

That sense began Friday night with the speeches. Michael Callen got up first and gave the opening speech. Instead of blasting Fauci, as he had done many times in the past, often to his face, or Ellen Cooper or Burroughs Wellcome, "I deliberately decided to put it positively," he says. Rather than dwell on the deficiencies in the fight against AIDS, "I made nice. I said we can now sit down and talk to each other. It was time to call a truce."

Now Callen and everyone else at that head table were perfectly aware that the mere existence of the CRI, the CCC, and all the other community-based research groups that AmFAR was nurturing was inherently a sharp criticism of Tony Fauci's clinical trials system, the FDA, the old-boys network of PIs, indeed the entire U.S. biomedical apparatus that had been around for decades.

But Callen made no reference to that criticism, and neither did anyone else at the head table as they came up to the podium to read their prepared speeches. Everyone agreed to call a truce. Everyone virtually gave his or her support to the community-based research movement and to the principles for which it stood—participation by people with AIDS in all modes of decision making, increased access to drug trials as treatment, parallel track, use of surrogate markers instead of death as end points in drug trials, increased testing of drugs for opportunistic infections, etc. It was practically the entire AIDS activist program.

Broder stood up and came out foursquare for community-based research and for using surrogate markers rather than death to mark progress in clinical trials. On this last issue he was taking ACT UP's side against the FDA. Broder said that scientists already had laboratory markers—an increase in T-4 cell counts and a decrease in p24 levels—that clearly showed whether or not a drug was working against the AIDS virus. "We know if a drug is biologically active and is a good antiviral today. We have the markers. We don't need to wait any longer." Ellen Cooper fumed quietly at the table. She hated the idea. She hated almost every one of the ideas for changing the established scientific method and the bureaucratic rules of behavior in research. She saw herself as a very careful, conservative scientist. Period.

Broder went further and took a direct potshot at the FDA, continuing his Lasagna committee attacks. "We must make sure that our government apparatus can develop drugs to help people and *then get out of the way,*" he said. "We need to quickly reach the point of knowing what is good and bad about therapies, communicating this to physicians . . . and then letting those physicians and patients make the crucial decisions about treatment on an individual basis, with as little interference from central kinds of authority as possible."

Tony Fauci rose and said, "What I see in community-based research is totally compatible with the mission of the National Institutes of Health." Fauci went on to say that the "parallel track" program would "allow individuals who were otherwise disenfranchised to get some form of therapy."

Ellen Cooper then got up, and sounded the only sour note of the evening. She said that Fauci's public talk about a "parallel track" had raised expectations within the patient community "unrealistically" and that they were going to be deeply disappointed when it finally went into operation. Cooper did grudgingly say that the FDA would begin to look at a wider range of laboratory and clinical surrogate markers in evaluating drug efficacy. Death wouldn't be the only measurement.

Burton Lee ended the round of speeches that Friday evening by joining in on the attack on the FDA. "I hope you bring down a large part of this drug regulatory system that has been built up over the last thirty years," he said. "I love to see power going back to the people."

At the end of three long days and nights, the conference appeared to establish a broad consensus among the players. ACT UP, the CRI, and AIDS activists in general wanted increased access to drug trials for treatment. The pharmaceutical companies wanted the same thing. There were nearly seventy drugs that showed promise against AIDS or its infections that weren't in trials. Tony Fauci's clinical trials system was going nowhere. It was clogged up with AZT. There was no way to test all the drugs now available in the government system. Private clinical trials at the traditional academic hospital sites were beginning to cost a fortune and the PIs were having a terrible time enrolling patients with their outdated trial designs. The new community-based groups had the loyalty of the people with AIDS. They had shown in the aerosol pentamidine trial that they could also do precise science, adequate enough for the FDA. The drug companies were on board. Tony Fauci was about to announce his own community-based network, mandated by the Watkins commission and Congress. It was his way of saving face. So Fauci was in favor of the community-based research concept. And Broder was on board, too.

A broad coalition had been built by Krim behind the radical biomedical research agenda proposed on both coasts by ACT UP, CRI, Project Inform—the entire radical antiestablishment AIDS movement. It had been a remarkable exercise in tact, strategy, patience, and managerial expertise. It had taken nearly a decade. But Krim had done it. There were still major pockets of opposition. The PIs were furious. The FDA's Ellen Cooper was a reluctant fellow traveler. And who really knew what Tony Fauci was thinking? He shifted with each change of the political winds. But there was no doubt that Mathilde Krim had masterminded a sea change in the way medical research was performed in America. She had set the stage for a faster, better, cheaper way of developing drugs. She had increased access to treatment. It was all done in the name of AIDS, but it had the potential for transforming the way all major diseases were treated as well.

# ..13..
# Betrayal

Michael Callen was pacing his kitchen with a remote phone in his hand. He was distraught and couldn't stand still. Dressed in black Levi's, a dark green shirt, an old blue sweater, and drinking a Classic Coke, he paced back and forth talking into the phone. "No. Don't worry. No. No one will know. No one."

The inside source was calling with the news and she was worried about being discovered. Callen was furious, and he had to reassure her that he wouldn't mention her name when he called the press with his side of the story.

The woman had called with the list of organizations to get funding from NIAID's new $9 million community-based research program. The CRI wasn't on it. Callen just couldn't believe it. He kept repeating over and over again that the CRI was the model for community-based organizations. It was the oldest, the biggest, and the most experienced. How could they do this? he asked rhetorically. How could they do this?

The betrayal Callen felt went very deep. Just a couple of months ago, he was sitting at the same dinner table with Tony Fauci, director of NIAID. It was the July conference, sponsored by Mathilde Krim's AmFAR. Everyone had been there—Fauci, Sam Broder, Ellen Cooper, Burton Lee—to celebrate the concept of community-based research. There were all those speeches in support of it plus all those behind-the-scenes private talks about working together on AIDS treatment, burying the hatchet, ending the long animosity between AIDS activists and the government. Was it all a joke? asked Callen. Were they being set up? What had happened?

"Fauci is clearly sending a signal," said Callen. But what? Am I being

298

paranoid? he asked himself. Everybody in the AIDS movement was paranoid, but so many times their worst fears had turned out to be true. Now Callen wondered whether *his* paranoia was real or not.

Callen attributed blame first to himself, then to the CRI, then to homophobia and politics. Most of all he blamed himself. He felt that Fauci was getting even for his trip down to Bethesda back in 1987 when he begged Fauci to issue consensus guidelines to doctors recommending aerosol pentamidine. Fauci had refused and Callen later testified publicly that Fauci's decision was responsible for the deaths of nearly seventeen thousand people with AIDS from PCP. It had humiliated Fauci in front of Congress.

Callen and Joe Sonnabend had been critical of Fauci and his AIDS Clinical Trials Group from the beginning. They had said time and again that NIAID was obsessed with AZT, that most of the trials and people with AIDS involved in the trials were on just that one drug.

Callen felt so guilty. He'd hurt the CRI. "I want to be clear on this. CRI, the organization, has not been all that critical of the NIH. Joe Sonnabend and I, however, have been extremely critical of the NIH." He felt the failure of the CRI to get any government funding from Fauci's NIAID was payback.

He couldn't believe it no matter how many times he played it through in his head. The presidential commission on AIDS, the Watkins commission, had singled out the CRI as being a terrific model for community-based research. Burton Lee, then on the commission, personally commended the CRI for helping bust up the FDA's monopoly control over drug development. The CRI had even made the first cutoff for the NIAID funding in June. There hadn't been any confusion as to what "Bopper" Deyton, head of the new NIAID community-based clinical trials program, wanted from them. The Request For Proposals said that applicants had to be able to do two things: enroll minority AIDS patients and be able to conduct proper scientific research.

The CRI's record on research was there for everyone to see, according to Callen. Look at the success of aerosol pentamidine. There were now nearly two hundred community doctors linked up through the CRI. Ten anti-AIDS drugs either had been or were in the process of being tested. The drug companies loved the CRI's efficiency, low cost, and quick patient enrollment. So Callen believed that the research part of the application couldn't have been the problem.

Two-thirds of the CRI application had to do with setting up scattered sites in the Bronx and Brooklyn to involve people of color. So the emphasis on getting minorities into AIDS drug trials was addressed as well. CRI had been pushing that issue for years now, said Callen, while big academic hospitals continued to enroll white, middle-class gay men. "I have no doubt that the CRI's proposal was the most carefully planned effort to do community outreach of any of the proposals."

It was true that federal auditors had come to discuss the proposal's budget, said Callen, but all their questions were answered adequately. It was also true that the NIAID review panel had several other questions after the June cut, but the CRI answered those as well. So what had happened?

That Bopper Deyton was in charge of these new NIAID community grants made the hurt even more personal to Callen. "I fixed Bopper up with his lover, Jeff Levi. He's a Washington lobbyist for gay rights. I'm a yenta when I'm not doing this stuff. I set them up. I feel so hurt. If I were Bopper, I would resign in protest. But he won't. Bopper has to say the process was impeccable."

So it had to be revenge, said Callen. He couldn't be sure but his gut had no doubts. Callen had heard a story making the rounds of AIDS activists some months before about Fauci. It went like this: The principal investigators had been complaining about everything Fauci was doing. They hated his idea of a parallel track. They didn't want to stop using placebos. They were furious at Fauci's idea of letting a handful of ACT UP people sit in on their committees. And they weren't happy at this damn new NIAID community-based clinical trials system. The PIs didn't give a damn that the Watkins commission recommended it and Congress mandated it. Nothing that Fauci was doing was any good. And the PIs said so to Fauci's face again and again.

The story goes that Fauci took it and took it until one day recently he got really angry. He warned a group of PIs that "what goes around comes around." Fauci then threatened the PIs by reminding them that their contracts with NIAID for testing AIDS drugs was coming up for renewal. Maybe, Callen speculated, Fauci was doing the same thing to the CRI. "What goes around comes around," that's what Tony Fauci said.

What really happened was very simple. Michael Callen may have been paranoid, but it was, in fact, justified. Yet again the worst nightmare had come true in the AIDS community.

Peer review is sacred in the world of science. Scientists are supposed to analyze each other's proposals so that only the very best are chosen for funding or for publication. Politics and personal animosities are supposed to be circumvented. It's a wonderful ideal that does work at times. Not this time.

The peer review panel established by Tony Fauci to screen proposals for the new government-financed community-based research group was run by the PIs doing AIDS research at NIAID. The only criterion for choice, according to Tony Fauci, was the ability to bring some expertise to the review panel.

The review panel had a lot to do. Of the eighteen proposals that did receive NIAID funding, eleven grants went to brand-new start-ups that had never done any testing. Seven grants went to more established organizations that were able to begin enrolling people with AIDS for trials immediately. CRI entered its proposal into this competition, inasmuch as it had already run the aerosol pentamidine trial, which the FDA considered just fine.

Margaret Fischl was chosen to be chairperson of the review panel for the second group, the panel that rejected the CRI. Margaret Fischl, of course, was the chief PI for Burroughs Wellcome's Phase II AZT trial. She was also a very powerful force within NIAID's clinical trials system.

Now Joe Sonnabend and Michael Callen were both well known for their criticism of that Phase II AZT trial as being a poor example of scientific research. Sonnabend had made his criticisms known in print. Furthermore, both men had criticized Fischl by name many times. In addition, both had come out against AZT as a therapeutic drug. Sonnabend wasn't even sure that the AIDS virus, AZT's target, was the sole cause of AIDS. Callen, his patient for nine years, had never taken AZT and strongly recommended against taking it. Sonnabend and Callen had condemned the old-boy network, which Fischl was part of, as focusing almost exclusively on AZT-type drugs to the exclusion of less glamorous treatments for the opportunistic infections that actually killed PWAs. Both had attacked again and again the principal investigators of the ACTG clinical trials network for designing trials that were so ill-constructed that few PWAs would join. They were also against placebos, which Fischl continued to use in her trials.

The list of Sonnabend's and Callen's complaints about Fischl was as long as an EKG readout. And it wasn't any secret. Everyone in the AIDS research field knew about it, including Tony Fauci and Maureen Myers.

So how did a person who had a history of antagonism with the founders of the community-based research movement come to review a funding proposal sent in by that organization? Just standard operating procedure, according to one high NIAID official. "The institute has standing committees that are involved in doing peer review for initiatives that the institute puts forth," says the person. "Depending on the work load and timing, you sometimes have to have ad hoc committees set up in addition. When you do that, you have a couple of people from the standing committee sitting on the ad hoc. This was an ad hoc review because it was critical that the reviewers be people who were sensitive to and aware of the issues being presented in the proposals. Margaret was selected as a person from the current standing committee because of her knowledge and expertise. She, being an ACTG person, knew about clinical trials and logistics that would contribute to the review panel."

That was the opinion of the NIH, Burroughs Wellcome, and the scientific establishment. Fischl's prominence was based on testing AZT. But Sonnabend and Callen had disputed this view of Fischl's frequently and publicly. They had criticized Fischl for her *lack* of knowledge and expertise, for her incompetence. It was known throughout the AIDS medical community that there was bad blood between them.

In addition, Fischl had identified herself with the PI reactionaries, those principal investigators who were against all the new medical research initiatives proposed by the CRI, ACT UP, and Project Inform. Finally, Fischl herself was hardly a representative of a community-based research organization. She worked out of a big university-backed academic hospital in Miami. The Phase II AZT trials, for which Fischl had a great deal of managerial responsibility, had enrolled almost all white gay males.

The conflict of interest was clear as glass to everyone but those living inside. Margaret Fischl could no more be objective about a proposal for funding coming from Michael Callen and Joe Sonnabend than Larry Kramer could be about Wellcome's David Barry. In this case, the assumption of evenhandedness in a peer review screening was simply ludicrous.

But not to the scientists doing the peer review. Not to the scientific bureaucrats in charge of the money. "I know Margaret and I would be surprised if she let anything influence her," insists Tony Fauci.

Scientists use a double blind in their experiments to prevent any kind of influence on the people in a trial. Neither the subject nor the experimenters know the makeup of the test and control groups during the experiment. The double blind is specifically designed to insulate both the scientists and the patients from their own feelings, prejudices, etc. Scientists desperately want their drugs to succeed. So do patients. They can't help it. The double-blind procedure, as much a canon of science as peer review, was created to deal with exactly the same kind of emotional feelings.

This was not done in the case of Margaret Fischl. In no way should she have been overseeing a peer review panel that judged a proposal by CRI. It was an institutional and personal conflict of interest.

Yet neither Tony Fauci nor Dan Hoth, the head of NIAID's AIDS Program, saw it. They refused to believe that anything could be wrong with their screening system. They denied that NIAID had made any mistake at all.

Fauci called a meeting when the list of winners came out and the CRI wasn't on it. In his office were Dan Hoth, Jack Killen, Bopper Deyton, his assistant adviser for science policy Peggy Hamburg, his deputy director James Hill, and Maureen Myers. Fauci could have overriden the decision and given the CRI funding. He didn't. Why? "They didn't put in a very good application. You can't judge whether you are going to fund somebody in a legal government contract by the fact that they walk around saying, 'Hey, we're the guys who thought about all of this first.' You can't rest on your laurels," says Fauci. "You have to put something on paper that is judged by peers to be of a high enough priority. They didn't do it. They kind of took it for granted that they were going to get it."

Maybe. But what about all the work CRI did on the aerosol pentamidine trial, which was accepted by the FDA? Suddenly, it was all junk. "When you go back and look at what they really did with the aerosolized pentamidine, did they really do clinical research or did they just give some patients . . . [pause] . . . and collect some, whatever it is, and send it down to San Francisco?" asks Fauci. It was a peculiar interpretation of data collected on toxicity that the FDA said was critical to its approval of the drug. Clearly Ellen Cooper didn't think the CRI's work had been junk a year before when the FDA approved the commercial sale of aerosol pentamidine.

In the end, the issue that sank the CRI was control. To both the NIAID bureaucracy, especially Maureen Myers and Dan Hoth, and the PIs who ran their AIDS clinical trials program, the entire community-based research movement, financed by Mathilde Krim's AmFAR and the pharmaceutical industry, was *outside their control.* It threatened their monopoly over patient enrollment and drug trials.

For NIAID, the mere existence of the CRI, with PWAs in key decision-making positions and the FDA accepting its data on aerosol pentamidine, was an implicit criticism of its own failure in its clinical trials network to produce anything after spending hundreds of millions of dollars of taxpayer money.

To the PIs, their whole way of life, their scientific research, was being threatened by the CRI and the community-based research movement. Control over patients, drugs, and, increasingly, drug company money was shifting away from them to the local doctors such as Joe Sonnabend, Barbara Starrett, and Nathaniel Pier and to such activists as Michael Callen.

If there was any doubt about that, it evaporated when NIAID announced the kind of relationship it was going to have with its own new community-based organizations. NIAID funded its own community trials network with a contract system, the very same contract system that the PIs had revolted against back in 1986 because it was so controlling.

This time around, however, the PIs insisted that Dan Hoth use only the contract system. They were opposed to setting up the NIAID community-based trials network from the beginning. They opposed the Watkins commission recommendation for community trials, they hated it when Congress appropriated $9 million for the effort and told NIAID to set it up. The PIs said again and again that they would lose control over their patients to the new community-based organizations. They insisted that they have control over them, and Tony Fauci capitulated to their demands.

The PIs demanded and received guarantees that each of the eighteen new community-based research organizations would consult with them on a continuing basis about everything they were doing, especially about trials and patient accruals. The PIs, in effect, would control patient enrollment in the new community network.

By using contracts, NIAID tightly enforced these rules and regulations on the eighteen groups. They were to have virtually no independence. Instead of empowering local community groups, NIAID and the PIs were actually building a network of dependent organizations, held tightly on a financial leash, that would not challenge the superiority of the traditional university-based, hospital-based clinical system. Blacks, Hispanics and IV users with AIDS were to be enrolled in the satellite NIAID community trials network while the hospital-based PI network continued to dominate the big-time science scene.

A quick check of the medical groups that did receive money from NIAID proves the point. None of the organizations that had true community representation received money. In addition to the CRI, neither Boston's

Community Health Center nor L.A.'s S.W. Community-Based AIDS Trial Group got a penny. The CCC in San Francisco received funding, but it was a more conservative group not controlled by PWAs. By and large, big inner-city public hospitals got most of the NIAID funding. The aim was to use them to increase minority representation within the NIAID trials network. A laudable goal.

But hospitals, including public ones, do not generally give community representatives much power. Many do not even have any such representatives sitting on key committees. They are top-down hierarchies, controlled by the doctors and scientific bureaucrats. Each public hospital was paired with a private, academic hospital, which had all the power, all the control: hardly "community-based" organizations.

That was why CRI was not funded. The CRI was an independent community research group with PWAs in positions of authority throughout the organization. It didn't fit the mold. It was outside the control of the PIs and their NIH allies.

Tony Fauci was walking a very thin line at this point. He was trying to bolster his political position by bringing a few hand-chosen AIDS activists inside the Washington AIDS bureaucracy. Yet each attempt was met by ferocious opposition from the PIs, much of his own staff, and most of the FDA's staff. Fauci depended totally on the PIs for the smooth operation of his clinical trials program. He could kick them around a bit and make threatening noises about contracts, but in the end, he had nowhere else to go.

The PIs had enormous power. They had saved Fauci back in '87 when Dan Hoth brought them in to rebuild NIAID's first trials network that never tested anything. Fauci needed the investigators more than they needed him. After all, the PIs worked in two worlds, the private pharmaceutical company universe of clinical trials and compensation plus the public arena of drug testing. They moved back and forth constantly, without any ethical concerns about conflicts of interest.

To the PIs, Fauci had "gone over to the other side." By the summer of '89, he was backing ACT UP and Project Inform time and again against the biomedical bureaucracy when it came to DHPG, a national drug registry of AIDS trials, placebos, parallel track, and early release of ddI. So when NIAID put its new community-based research group under contract and control, the PIs appreciated Fauci's effort to accommodate them.

Yet by the fall, Fauci and the PIs were fighting again. He was pushing something they considered even worse down their throats. Fauci wanted to get a few AIDS activists into the policy-making apparatus so that PWAs could be seen as having a voice in the scientific and medical decisions. ACT UP's Jim Eigo and New York attorney Jay Lipner already sat on the prestigious Institute of Medicine's Panel on AIDS. Fauci had just nominated Eigo to NIAID's AIDS Research Advisory Committee (ARAC). Martin Delaney also sat on several committees.

None of these groups, however, had line responsibility for the actual operations of the government's AIDS effort. What ACT UP wanted most was a voice in two key organizations: the AIDS Clinical Drug Development Committee, the gateway for all drugs into the AIDS Clinical Trial Group system, and the ACTG itself, which was in overall charge of NIAID's clinical trials. The PIs dominated both the ACDDC and the ACTG. Indeed, the quarterly meetings of the ACTG were composed of the investigators and their staff. The upcoming November meeting was expected to have 820 people.

Mark Harrington had told Tony Fauci in the summer that he wanted to have ACT UP at the next ACTG meeting. Fauci said fine. He committed himself to getting ACT UP into the meeting. But when he went back to Dan Hoth, who ran the AIDS Program two miles down the road, Hoth said no. Hoth said the PIs wouldn't stand for it. *He* didn't like it. Maureen Myers didn't like it either. Fauci told Hoth to work the PIs, gradually get them used to the idea. He told Hoth to tell them that Eigo and Harrington were "good guys," smart enough to understand the science and perhaps even more knowledgeable than some of the researchers when it came to understanding the drug development process.

ACT UP's request remained in limbo for the rest of the summer and early fall. Then, when Fauci went to New York to talk at a weekly ACT UP meeting, Harrington reminded him he'd been told he could attend the next ACTG meeting, three weeks away. Fauci said sure, fine, to Harrington. "It's my personal opinion that you have a lot to bring to these meetings," he said. But privately Fauci was unsure what the response would be from the PI community. Had they changed their mind since the summer?

The answer was swift in coming. It was a simple no. They hadn't changed their opposition to having ACT UP or any other outsiders come to their meeting. They told Hoth who told Fauci that it was their job to do science. They wanted to talk only science at the ACTG meetings, not politics and certainly not the dumb ideas that AIDS activists had: stupid drugs such as AL 721 or ribavirin. As one key member of the ACTG put it: "What are you going to do if you want to have a serious scientific discussion about a promising agent and you've got someone from the Provincetown PWA Coalition who thinks that Peptide T is the greatest thing since sliced bread and says, 'I don't want to talk about anything else'? These people will divert the discussion. They will have other agendas driving them."

Ironically, the ACTG meetings are not formally closed to the press and outsiders. In practice, however, it is impossible to attend unless invited. Fauci tried to explain: "The ACTG meeting is not a closed meeting. . . . [Pause] . . . Well, it is a closed meeting, really technically it isn't, but a lot of people, because no one outside goes, they openly speak about a lot of things that if you had people who were not responsible, they really could distort. You could get somebody who wants to be mischievous, they could call up the newspapers and say this and that."

A high official who attended all the ACTG meetings has a simpler explanation. "It is by invitation only. We have always kept that meeting closed. Anyone who wants to attend has gotta have a very good reason for being there."

Tony Fauci called Mark Harrington and basically disinvited him. It wasn't a good idea to come down just now. The PIs really objected to ACT UP's coming to their party, Hoth told Harrington.

Then Peggy Hamburg, an assistant to Fauci, called Harrington and Rebecca Pringle Smith, an ACT UP member who worked at the Community Research Initiative, and *she* asked them not to show up.

The next day Hamburg and Jack Killen, Fauci's chief assistant, went to New York to attend a scheduled meeting with ACT UP and Bristol-Myers on the early release of ddI. They asked Jim Eigo to use his influence to stop ACT UP from attending the ACTG meeting. Hamburg and Killen said the PIs were paranoid. They would feel inhibited if ACT UP showed up. They reminded Eigo that as a member of the Institute of Medicine's AIDS panel, he could go to the ACTG. They just didn't want people from ACT UP going. "We know *you,* " was the message Fauci recalls being passed on to Eigo. "We know Mark. We know you won't be spouting off to the press about things that may be misrepresented. But the investigators don't know that. It will create a tremendous amount of anxiety there."

Eigo told Hamburg and Killen that the decision to go to the ACTG meeting had been made in committee at ACT UP and he couldn't personally change that. They were going. If they weren't let in, there was going to be a demonstration. ACT UP was going to zap NIAID. Count on it.

Later in the day, Harrington told Fauci that ACT UP believed the only way it would ever get into the ACTG meetings was by precipitating an action. Fauci told him that he respected ACT UP's activist tactics, "but I'm gonna hafta hold the hand of the group [of PIs]."

Fauci then called a meeting with his top staff. He drove the two miles to the AIDS Program center and talked with Dan Hoth, Maureen Myers, and several other people. The major issue was whether they should let ACT UP into the meeting and deal with the PI backlash. Or they could keep ACT UP out of the meeting and risk a big public demonstration. Could the PI backlash be minimized? asked Fauci.

Myers didn't think so. She opposed letting the activists in. She complained that they were being blackmailed. Fauci said it was better than seeing their names in newspaper articles about "closed-door" meetings. That argument carried the day.

Fauci then met with the Executive Committee of the ACTG for several hours before the meeting on Sunday night, trying to cajole them into accepting the AIDS activists into their midst. The Executive Committee was composed of the PI leadership, the very best and the very toughest of the hundred or so researchers working in the ACTG system. They were the true believers in science done the old-fashioned way, their way, without outside political interference in their affairs. It was extremely difficult to persuade them. Dr. Lawrence Corey, from the University of Washington, was the chairman and he was definitely opposed. Marty Hirsch couldn't believe his ears when Fauci suggested inviting ACT UP. Neither could Margaret Fischl.

Fauci had to go back and talk with the Executive Committee at seven the next morning, the morning of the ACTG meeting. "These are good guys," he kept repeating to the PIs. He hammered home his new philosophy toward the AIDS activists. "If you get the right people—and these are the right people—that are intelligent and open-minded and just need to be informed, then it will work ultimately to our benefit to have them inside the tent, not outside," he said.

After several more hours of coaxing, the Executive Committee relented. But they struck a deal. There would be open and closed sessions. ACT UP could attend only the open sessions. There just had to be private meetings where they could talk openly about things. Okay, said Fauci, let me call Harrington and find out if that's agreeable to the ACT UP people. He called. Harrington said yes.

Seven ACT UP members attended. Five were officially from ACT UP.

Two were AmFAR representatives but were quietly members of ACT UP as well.

The meetings went fairly smoothly. No fireworks occurred as PIs and AIDS activists eyed each other across conference rooms. Tony Fauci sighed in relief when it was over. "The meeting went across well," he reports. "The investigators gained the confidence [that] they were dealing with people who would not try to—[pause]. So I think it was a real good step forward. I just got some notes from people who said that, ya know, 'We were skeptical at the beginning but you were right, we should have them there as long as they understand there are things that just should not be discussed openly.'" It was a peculiar concept of science in America: science as a secret society.

The meeting was important for ACT UP. It was clear at the meeting that a serious rift had opened between Tony Fauci and the PIs. After three years and hundreds of millions of dollars, not a single drug had yet come out of NIAID's new clinic trials system. The scientists over at the NCI were snickering at Fauci behind his back, and he knew it. Not one thing out of his ACTG! The pressure was intense on Fauci, and he, in turn, blamed the principal investigators. Where were the drugs he had promised Congress, the AIDS activists, Mathilde Krim?

Fauci lambasted the PIs for not performing. He told them they weren't working fast enough. He complained that they didn't have any interest in running trials of drugs for opportunistic infections. The major achievements of the past year, aerosol pentamidine and DHPG, had not come out of his clinical trials network. Fauci told the PIs they were letting him down.

Both Fauci and Dan Hoth gave this message to the hundreds of PIs and their associates at the meeting. "There was a tone of desperation in their anger and in their pleading," says one PI who attended. "They were saying nothing seemed to be working. There was nothing to show the public that they were succeeding. They had to rescue themselves somehow." The pressure was intense. By the summer of 1990, Fauci would find a way and, of course, it would involve AZT.

At the meeting, Eigo and Harrington also found out that the NIAID clinical trials network was moving all its data gathering and management away from a well-established scientific data management company, down in the Research Triangle next door to Burroughs Wellcome in North Carolina. They were sending it up to Harvard's School of Public Health, home to Marty Hirsch and the Boston "AIDS mafia": Hirsch, Jerome Groopman, William Haseltine, and Max Essex. Together, they received nearly $40 million in AIDS research money, almost all from the NIH. Harvard alone received $32 million in 1989—before data management was moved to its School of Public Health. Ironically, the NIAID clinical trials run in the Boston area had the reputation among AIDS activists as having the worst record on patient enrollment in the country. But NIAID was not about to antagonize the Boston "AIDS mafia."

That move was going to prevent any new trials from opening for a year, at least. And *that* news was met with anger at the meeting of the ACTG's Opportunistic Infections Committee. They were going to be the most affected. Once again, OI was being given short shrift by NIAID.

At the Primary Infection Committee meeting, Eigo and Harrington learned that the four new priority trials were for ddI and ddC. Once again, NIAID was emphasizing AZT-type antivirals over drugs that might work against the infections that actually killed PWAs. It was the same old story. Nothing had changed for years.

The ACT UP people kept hearing in the halls that the PIs were increasingly worried that the new parallel track would drain patients away from their own trials. Bristol-Myers had already signed up twelve hundred people for its two parallel track trials of ddI but only one hundred had enrolled for three of the formal clinical trials. The activists knew that clinical trials had traditionally been slow in enrolling people because they were so terribly designed, but no one had ever told the investigators to change their trial designs, so they simply proceeded, year after year, doing the same things over again. The ddI parallel track was simply throwing the poorly designed clinical trials into stark relief.

In every committee except one, Pediatrics, all the PIs talked about was science. Patient care wasn't on anyone's agenda. It wasn't even in the vocabulary. The unspoken belief was that long-term benefit was best served by getting their science done. Of course, no one had to say that this belief was totally in the interests of the scientists, not necessarily the people with AIDS or other diseases. The Pediatrics Committee was the only one where the kids were the focus of discussion.

This insular arrogance expressed itself best in the attempted sabotage of the parallel track program by the PIs. They used a reporter as their vehicle—Gina Kolata of the *New York Times.*

On November 21, 1989, Kolata wrote a front-page story, "Innovative AIDS Drug Plan May Be Undermining Testing," in which she asserted that the parallel track, designed to increase the availability of experimental drugs, threatened the entire clinical trials system. Kolata, who covered the AIDS beat, said that twenty times as many people were flocking to get ddI in the two new parallel track trials as in the three regular clinical trials of the drug. This was "leaving researchers in despair over whether they will ever be able to complete the formal study." All of Kolata's sources that appeared in print were PIs who had been against the parallel track concept from the very beginning. Kolata became their avenue of attack. The article appeared just three weeks after the parallel track notion was approved in Washington.

Kolata quoted Dr. Douglas Richman of the University of California at San Diego as saying that thirteen hundred patients had already enrolled in the parallel track program and a hundred a day were being added. In contrast, just a fraction of that total had entered the three clinical trials. "As it stands, parallel track will not work," said Richman. "What actually was put into place is an invitation to disaster. It will prevent us from finding drugs that will help people."

Dr. Jerome Groopman of New England Deaconess Hospital said in the article that "People talked about and tried to reassure the academic community that yes, the parallel track will not dismantle our ability to do organized studies. But we have to face this head on. There really are conflicting issues here. If the philosophy is that anyone can decide at any point what drugs he or she wants to take, then you will not be able to do a clinical trial."

Parallel track was clearly threatening the PI monopoly of patients around the country—just as the CRI threatened the PI monopoly over research trials themselves, and as the growing number of buyers clubs threatened medicine's hold over the supply of drugs. This was a fight for power, and the PIs had used the *New York Times* to further their position.

Kolata then went further—this time right off the deep end. The *New York Times* ran a piece by her on the front page called "Odd Surge in Deaths Found in Those Taking AIDS Drug." It purported to show that ten times as many people taking ddI in the parallel track trials were dying as compared with those PWAs taking the same drug in the regular clinical trials. Up to 290 people were dead, and Kolata said that it was the fault of the new, freer testing system.

It was clearly such blatant nonsense that even the PIs who were quoted in the story said that Kolata had got it wrong. As Jim Eigo, Mark Harrington, and Martin Delaney had said time and again to deaf ears, only those PWAs who couldn't get into the clinical trials would go into the parallel track trials. In real life, that meant that only the sickest individuals went into the two parallel track trials. Of course more of them died. They were much sicker to begin with. They didn't die from ddI, they died from AIDS. It was so obvious, it was embarrassing.

The enrollment problems for the ddI clinical trials merely reflected chronic difficulties with accrual problems that had been going on for decades. ACT UP's Iris Long had clearly shown that enrollment was shockingly low for nearly all AIDS drug protocols. In cancer, it usually took two, three, even four years to get enough people to enroll in trials. That was the norm for a life-threatening disease!

In terms of the ddI trials, the three regular clinical trials were far behind in enrollment of PWAs because they literally started after the parallel track trials. A last-minute change in dosage, prompted by fears of higher toxicity for ddI, delayed those three clinical trials by many weeks. The labels had to be changed by Bristol-Myers before anything could take place. The newly rewritten protocols had to be reviewed all over again by the local Institutional Review Boards (IRBs) at the forty-five hospital sites for the ddI trials. In addition, the drug dosages received by many sites wasn't correct and had to be sent back to Bristol-Myers. It all took months.

That was just the beginning. ACT UP and other AIDS activist organizations had put together lists of PWAs eager to join the three clinical trials. They gave these lists to the PIs in charge. But even with the lists of willing participants, the PIs couldn't enroll very many patients. Often it turned out that hospital staffing was inadequate to handle the people. They were able to enroll just a handful of people a week.

As to "cheating," a repeated PI fear, even Bristol-Myers was saying that the PWAs enrolling in the parallel track trials couldn't get into the three clinical trials. They didn't qualify. About 60 percent did not fit the medical criteria; they were too sick or were on other drugs they couldn't stop taking. Another 30 percent simply lived too far away from the nearest clinical trial site. Of the remaining 10 percent, only a fraction might have gone into the formal clinical trials. The goals of parallel track were being met—increased access to treatment for people who couldn't get into clinical trials. Nothing more was happening.

"So what?" was the PI response. The evidence mattered little. They continued to believe blindly that the parallel track was wrong, so wrong that their animosity often suggested they thought there was something evil about the concept and its promoters.

Thomas Merigan, the Stanford PI and chairman of the Primary Infection Committee of Tony Fauci's NIAID clinical trials network, complained at the time to an audience of PIs in Washington that his own trial for ddC (yet another cousin to AZT) was suffering because of the parallel track. He said that the parallel track "for ddI is drawing patients away from our trials. There is a temptation for our patients to leave the program—an unfortunate loss. . . . There are early signs of a downturn in accrual. Most of our Phase I or II studies are pausing in accrual. The ddC studies are not accumulating many patients. We need to define a window of opportunity for ddC. In the study of ddC for long-term AZT users, six sites are willing to participate, but only two may accumulate patients—it hasn't opened yet."

Merigan also told a high NIAID official that he "wants to put into place an oversight system to see to what extent the initiative of these protocols [parallel track] affects other therapeutic studies, not just ddI." Merigan hinted at what he had in mind when he told the PIs at the ACTG meeting that "We're going to monitor on a monthly basis the comparative accruals in the ddI studies and expanded access. We're going to look at enrollment by zip code catchment areas. We may need to use this information to argue against the use of Treatment INDs at the start of Phase II—after all, *we're* the people most affected by it."

It was a fascinating insight into the way researchers viewed their work. Merigan was saying that the PIs were most affected by the new parallel track idea. Not a word about patients was said, not a word about treatment was said. People with AIDS and others with diseases were perceived as fodder to be experimented *on.* Control of this human fodder by these investigators was absolutely necessary to continue their research. They were part of the scientific method. They certainly were not perceived as ill people who needed greater access to treatment. Merigan stripped them of their humanity and made them part of *his* laboratory work, the work of *his* cohorts, the researchers. It was a damning exercise in selfishness. It was also an exercise in ignorance.

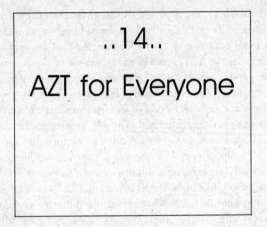

# ..14..
# AZT for Everyone

They couldn't remember a precedent. It had never happened to them before. Tony Fauci, director of NIAID, *personally* calling at ten o'clock in the morning to announce the results of a drug trial. No director of an NIH institute had ever contacted the press like that.

These thoughts passed through the minds of about a dozen journalists on the "AIDS beat" in early August 1989. Fauci got on the phone with Marilyn Chase of the *Wall Street Journal,* perhaps the best AIDS reporter in the country. He also talked to Marlene Cimons in the Washington bureau of the *L.A. Times.* He made phone calls to the *New York Times,* the *Boston Globe,* and the big three TV networks.

Fauci wasn't the only high official at NIAID working that morning. Dan Hoth, head of the AIDS Clinical Trials Program, was punching away at his telephone as well. He called ACT UP's Jim Eigo and about a dozen or so other AIDS activists with the news.

"It's really significant," Fauci told one and all. NIAID's clinical trial number 016 was pretty important. That was the AZT trial of 713 persons who had only mild symptoms to see whether the drug slowed down the progression to the more serious infections associated with full-blown AIDS. "It did," said Fauci, sometimes whispering to the reporter, sometimes practically shouting. Fauci offered to fax the press release immediately. He had most of the numbers already at hand but he did still need a few. A number of reporters wanted him to read the press release there on the phone. He did.

After three years, Tony Fauci finally had some good news to spread from his woebegone clinical trials program. True, it was still about that same drug, AZT, that NIAID was always talking about. But this time the data was significant. And it was *his* data, from *his* trials network, not Burroughs Wellcome's or the NCI's.

Protocol 016 enrolled people with T-4 cell counts between 200 and 800 and a few mild symptoms of early AIDS. It was a placebo trial, with half getting the full dose of 1,200 milligrams of AZT and half getting a sugar pill. The trial indicated that the people helped most were those with T-4 cell counts below 500. These people also showed significantly less toxicity than did PWAs with full-blown AIDS and severe infections. To Fauci, that meant that people should get tested immediately and start using AZT once they started showing the first signs of the disease, a status then called ARC, for AIDS-Related Complex. But there was something in Fauci's voice that implied this was not all. There was even more to come. His voice suggested "stay tuned" as he talked to reporters around the country.

Tony Fauci didn't see anything wrong with the head of an NIH institute personally publicizing the results of a drug trial. Should he be touting what, after all, the taxpayers had been paying him to do for years? To Fauci, the answer was an unambiguous yes. After four long years of nothing, after the public humiliation he had suffered at the hands of Congressmen Weiss and Waxman, Fauci felt cocky. Sam Broder wasn't the only guy around the NIH who could produce. Fauci could now point to a definite "product" of his institute's work—an improved treatment.

For Margaret Fischl, the PI on trial 016, it was great news. She, of course, had been the chief PI for the Phase II study of AZT. This was a second "win": one for Burroughs Wellcome, the private sector, and now one for NIAID, the public sphere. Her star was really rising in the field. For David Barry at Wellcome, it was wonderful news too. When NIAID broke the code on 016, the potential market for AZT immediately increased many times over. There were far more people with mild symptoms of AIDS than with the full-blown disease. Yet Barry was restrained, as if he were holding back, as if he were waiting for another shoe to drop.

It did two weeks later. On August 17, the biggest, most important NIAID clinical trial, of protocol 019, was ended. Nothing approached 019 in terms of the priority Tony Fauci and the clinical trials group gave it. It had 3,200 people in it, practically half of all the subjects enrolled in all of NIAID's system. It was a classic double-blind, placebo-controlled trial that started back in July 1987 and was known inside the NIH and within gay communities from coast to coast simply as "the asymptomatics." Protocol 019 tested AZT to see if it delayed the onset of AIDS symptoms in people who were infected with the virus but who were not showing any clinical evidence of the disease. They hadn't got sick in any way.

The good news was that AZT did just that. According to Fauci, the two-year-old trial showed that AZT really delayed the progression of asymptomatic people with the AIDS virus to symptomatic illness. Specifically, AZT delayed progression of the disease for persons whose T-4 cell count had fallen below 500 per cubic millimeter. Only half as many progressed to early AIDS symptoms as those taking a placebo.

There was even better news. The people participating in 019 were divided into three groups. One received 1,500 milligrams of AZT a day, another 500 milligrams and a third placebo. To the surprise of the researchers, the progression to AIDS symptoms was the same for both groups taking the actual drug. The lower dose worked just as well as the full dose. Even better, the lower dose also sharply cut toxic side effects. Much less bone marrow was eaten away, reducing the anemia associated with AZT. The NIAID press release announcing the end to trial 019 recommended very early testing and treatment with AZT. Now anyone who was seropositive should get on the drug, advised NIAID.

That meant a bonanza for Burroughs Wellcome. Tony Fauci's clinical trials system had just increased the potential market for AZT by over 2000 percent! Before, only about half of all PWAs could stand taking AZT, especially at full dose. At the time, about 50,000 had full-blown AIDS. Some 20,000 paid for it privately, while another 5,000 were supported by the government, for a total of 25,000 people taking AZT in the summer of 1989. Now, a much larger percentage would be able to take the drug. And those were just the people who actually had AIDS.

There were approximately 1.5 million people in the United States alone infected with the AIDS virus. At any one time about 600,000 either had mild symptoms of the disease or were immune-suppressed so that their T-4 cell counts had dropped below 500 even though they weren't yet showing any signs of disease. Now all 650,000 might be considered the market for AZT. That was just for the United States. There was Europe, Latin America, Asia, and Africa too. The market might be as big as 4 or 5 million. Maybe even 10 million. Who knew?

Wellcome, of course, was cautiously ecstatic. The company didn't know just how many additional people would use AZT, but there was a good chance now that AZT might become one of the world's biggest profit-making drugs.

During the week after Fauci made the announcement, the shares of Wellcome stock on the London exchange jumped 45 percent, from $8.32 to $12.10. Estimates of Wellcome's potential profit from AZT ranged up to $2 billion annually by 1995. The more conservative analysts settled on $1 billion by 1992. The financial pages were full of stories comparing Burroughs Wellcome with another big British drug company, Glaxo, which saw its stock price jump twelvefold, adjusted for inflation, in the 1980s from just one drug. Its antiulcer drug Zantac was a global pharmaceutical best-seller, with sales of $1.6 billion in 1989. Even at $12.10, Burroughs Wellcome became one of the top dozen British companies in terms of stock market value. Amazing for a drug company that was still 75 percent held by a private charitable foundation.

In all the excitement, the newspapers didn't pick up reports of a similar trial of AZT in Europe. Ironically, only *Science,* the trade magazine of the science profession, did. A full-page article in November stated simply that European scientists didn't believe the results of trial 019. They thought Tony Fauci's clinical trials group had drawn erroneous conclusions.

The *Science* piece described how the Americans and Europeans, looking at the exact same data, came to very different conclusions about AZT. It took French and British scientists working on Concorde 1, a trial closely patterned after protocol 019, three months to gain access to the NIAID data. But once they got it, the European scientists were puzzled.

Jean-Pierre Aboulker, the PI for the French side, said that "the results we have seen do not allow us to give a strict recommendation to give AZT [to asymptomatics]." Ian Weller, the British PI, believed the reason for stopping trial 019 and for the recommendation to give AZT very early in the United States stemmed from political pressure, not scientific proof.

Weller said that because the average amount of time spent by an enrolled person in the trial was only a year, there was no data available on long-term effects of the drug. There might even be long-term harm done to patients. In addition, the data showed that 9 percent of the asymptomatic people progressed to mild AIDS symptoms within a year if they did not take AZT. For those taking AZT, half as many, or 4.5 percent, developed these mild AIDS symptoms.

To Weller, this showed that over 90 percent of the people not taking AZT were still healthy a year later. For the others, the 4.5 percent, there were many drugs far better able to control early infections than AZT. Bactrim and aerosol pentamidine were superior in preventing *Pneumocystis carinii* pneumonia, for example, than was AZT. Zovirax was certainly better than AZT at curbing the various herpes infections that befall PWAs early in the disease.

So to the British and French it made no sense to give AZT to asymptomatics as Fauci and Dan Hoth had recommended in August. It was far too early in the course of the infection, especially because the AIDS virus had proved to be resistant to AZT over time. "The worry is that when [the patient] really needs the drug, it is not going to be of benefit," said Weller.

Criticism of both trials 016 and 019 grew over the winter months. Margaret Fischl and Paul Volberding, respective PIs for the two trials, found themselves increasingly on the defensive. In March, the *Journal of the American Medical Association* came out with a full-page story on the controversy. It said that yet another large-scale study of AZT on asymptomatics, this one at the Veterans Administration, didn't show any real effect on symptom-free people with the AIDS virus. Dr. John Hamilton, cochair of VA study 298, was quoted as saying that after *two years*, there was "no statistically significant difference in progression to AIDS" for patients with T-4 cell counts between 200 and 500. He said that deaths were virtually identical for those taking AZT and those getting the placebo.

The *JAMA* article hit hard at the real-life implications of the figures given in NIAID trial 019. Skeptics, it said, pointed out that according to the NIAID data, one hundred patients would have to take AZT for a year to prevent only four infections that could be better treated with other drugs. In addition, the article pointed out that even Paul Volberding had concluded in his written report on trial 019 that questions of long-term benefit, toxicity, survival, and resistance to AZT remained unanswered.

The bottom line was that great uncertainty surrounded the NIAID trials. The value of early treatment was very much open to doubt. Even Douglas Richman, one of the original PIs for the AZT Phase II study and an AZT career man, said at the time that "thoughtful, intelligent, and ethical" physicians might want to let PWAs who were stable at T-4 cell counts close to 500 "choose not to" take AZT. It was a convoluted way of saying that Burroughs Wellcome's huge new market for AZT, the AIDS asymptomatics, might not benefit much from the drug and that it might actually do them more harm than good in the long run.

Some physicians, including Donna Mildvan, questioned whether they should give AZT to their patients who were stable, even if their T-4 cell counts were down to 400 or even 300. AZT's therapeutic powers were transient anyway. Why waste it earlier in the disease when the patient was not getting worse?

But infected people for the most part didn't want to hear about any limitations on AZT. They *wanted* to believe that it was a magic bullet. They besieged their doctors and demanded AZT, even if they were still healthy and not suffering any symptoms. About 13,000 PWAs started taking AZT for the first time in the fall of 1989, pushing Wellcome's total market up to 40,000.

The American public didn't get to hear much about the controversy, either. For the most part, the doubts expressed about the results of trial 019 by French, British, and American scientists were ignored by the press and other media. The general impression left in the collective consciousness was that AZT was a great treatment, if not a cure, for everyone infected with the AIDS virus. The notion went undisputed.

The only fight was over price. The acceptance of NIAID's conclusion about AZT, that it helped asymptomatics, had enormous public policy implications. Who was going to pay for all that AZT? The cost would average $5 to $10 billion a year, according to the *Journal of the American Medical Association.* Already, the government was Wellcome's largest single customer, paying $320 million in 1988 in subsidies to patients through Medicaid and in federal grants to the states for the purchase of the drug. That didn't count what NIAID paid Wellcome for the AZT used in trials 016 and 019. Nearly 4,000 people were enrolled.

With the market for AZT exploding exponentially, demand for Wellcome to lower its price soared. At that point, Wellcome was pricing AZT very high as an orphan drug, when the truth was that the drug now had a mass market. Drugs sold under the orphan drug status were supposed to be for rare diseases afflicting 200,000 people or less. The AIDS market was now 600,000 to 1 million.

Congressman Henry Waxman threatened to hold hearings on the price of AZT. He met with Wellcome officials several times, each time requesting information on the cost of manufacturing the product. Each time he was refused. Wellcome has never broken out its costs to make AZT. Consequently, it has never revealed the profit margin on the drug. Waxman was furious.

He wasn't the only one. ACT UP was born in March of '87 in a demonstration against the price of AZT. Several months after that Wall Street demonstration, Wellcome cut the price by 20 percent, from about $10,000 annually to about $8,000 for the retail buyer. In early September of '89, ACT UP went into action on Wall Street again. Peter Staley, a former bond trader on the street, and six other men, all dressed in suits, entered the New York Stock Exchange wearing false name tags supposedly from the investment house of Bear Stearns. At 9:29, a minute before trading was supposed to begin, they chained themselves to a banister on the balcony overlooking the trading floor. Staley and the others then unfurled a banner that read SELL WELLCOME, and used emergency marine foghorns to prevent any communication on the floor. Outside, some one thousand protesters marched. The exchange traders went wild with fury until Staley was taken away by the police. Wellcome didn't budge.

Then Henry Waxman wrote a letter to T. E. Haigler, the president of Burroughs Wellcome USA. He complained about the high price of AZT. He said that trials 016 and 019 had opened an enormous market for Wellcome. If the company didn't lower its extremely high price for AZT, it would cost the government and the American taxpayers billions of dollars. Waxman then said he wanted a response by the upcoming Friday or he would schedule hearings.

To Waxman's surprise, T. E. Haigler walked into his office in Washington, D.C., that Friday, along with David Barry and a few other Wellcome people. Haigler was wearing a big smile. Before Waxman could even extend his hand for the perfunctory shake, Haigler announced that Wellcome was going to cut the price of AZT by 20 percent. He paused and waited for a good pat on the back from Waxman. The price of AZT was now down to $6,200 a year for the full dose, $3,100 for a half dose.

Without skipping a beat, Waxman said, "That's a good first step. But you can do better than that." They were still talking billions and billions of dollars of public money for one drug. It wasn't nearly good enough. The whole health care system of the country was falling apart because of the burdens imposed by the spread of AIDS. This was going to put a tremendous financial burden on everyone.

Haigler's smile vanished and he left the congressional office crestfallen.

What Waxman missed in that encounter was that while Wellcome was cutting the price of AZT under heavy public pressure, it was raising the price of another key AIDS drug, acyclovir, sold as Zovirax, used to fight herpes infections such as CMV and shingles. Zovirax is much more than an AIDS drug. Herpes infections affect millions of Americans. Wellcome cut the price of AZT by 20 percent twice, in 1987 and 1989, lowering the price per capsule from $1.80 to $1.50 to $1.20. As the price of AZT was being cut, the price of Zovirax was quietly raised over the years. In 1985, when it was introduced, Zovirax cost 43 cents per capsule. By 1989, it was up to 56 cents, a hike of 30 percent.

Zovirax is Burroughs Wellcome's largest-selling product. In the fiscal year ending August 1989, worldwide sales for Zovirax totaled $491 million while AZT came to $225 million. The United States accounted for over 80 percent of the totals. For 1990, it is estimated that Zovirax sales will approach $600 million and AZT will rise to nearly $300 million. If the public funding can be found to pay for the 600,000 asymptomatics with the AIDS virus who are now eligible for AZT, the drug's likely sales will jump to several billion dollars a year.

But even with AZT not yet a mass market drug, AIDS has already become a lucrative disease for Burroughs Wellcome. If the projected sales of Zovirax, AZT, Septra, and several other key anti-AIDS drugs are totaled, they will come to approximately $1 billion in 1990. That total could easily rise to $5 billion by middecade.

In a strange way, the financial fate of Burroughs Wellcome has become intricately intertwined with that of AIDS. The private British charity that was established to promote biomedical research went public and sold 25 percent of its stock in February 1986, right after the first person took AZT in the Phase II trial. The stock price has moved with the winds of fortune for AZT ever since. For a whole constellation of political, medical, and business reasons, those winds of fortune are blowing very strong.

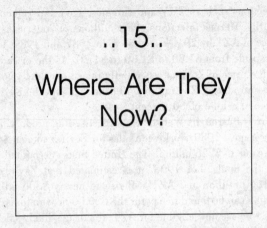

# ..15..

# Where Are They Now?

The state of the AIDS epidemic as it enters its second decade is limbo. There is a pause for both scientists and AIDS activists as they decide on direction and tactics for the nineties. Much was won and done in the eighties. Much more was not.

Some of the greatest success came in the personal careers of a handful of researchers who rode AIDS and AZT to the top. Sam Broder was appointed director of the National Cancer Institute when his mentor, Vincent DeVita, left. He's still enthusiastic about AZT, the drug that made his reputation at the NIH. He even remains loyal to Suramin, for which the NCI requested funds to try to show that the drug is good for something, this time fighting cancer. Some drugs never get on the list of compounds to be tested for efficacy at the NIH, such as AL 721, because as the acronym says, they were "Not Invented Here." Others, those that were, never seem to leave.

What Broder is not enthusiastic about is Burroughs Wellcome. He's furious with the company. While his fight with Wellcome revolves around credit for the development of AZT, his revenge has been focused on potential private profits. Through his efforts, the Federal Technology Transfer Act has been passed by Congress. It encourages NIH scientists to quickly patent their discoveries for the government. Then the FTTA requires the NIH to adopt a resonable-price clause in all its licensing agreements with private companies. No more $10,000 price tags on drugs if the NIH can beat the pharmaceutical companies to the patent office.

Broder's agenda at the NCI includes FDA bashing, to break the regulatory agency's stranglehold on drug development and to speed up access to treatment for people with AIDS and other diseases. He is also in favor of using surrogate markers instead of clinical death to measure a drug's effectiveness. Finally, Broder is addressing the serious problem of slow enrollment in cancer trials, a phenomenon highlighted by ACT UP's criticism of the glacial pace of enrollment in AIDS trials. New trial designs with the patient in mind, not just the principal investigator, will be encouraged. All three efforts are to be lauded.

As an officer in the Public Health Service, Broder was promoted to rear admiral.

Tony Fauci was perceived as so successful in certain Republican political circles that he was, at one point, seen as a potential candidate for director of the entire NIH. He told everyone that his first love is AIDS research and turned the offer down. The story was a bit more complex, and included a political litmus test on abortion by the Bush administration that practically all scientists considered a political invasion of their turf. A number of powerful PIs around the country, angry with Fauci for supporting changes in their closed, insular medical world, also lobbied against him.

Fauci's NIAID clinical trials system continues to rely on AZT for most of its protocols. It has stopped testing any new drugs for opportunistic infections for at least a year because it decided to transfer its data management to Harvard. No provision was made for any temporary data collection and analysis while the switch was being made—yet another typical NIAID management maneuver. In the course of that one year, the number of people with AIDS will double to 200,000.

ACT UP demonstrated against the NIH and against Fauci in particular on May 21, 1990, charging that $1 billion had been spent on testing drugs and only AZT has been approved, again and again. On the defensive, Fauci then said that NIAID had done many things, including proving that ribavirin, dextran sulfate, and AL 721 were not effective. Of course, no Phase II efficacy trial of AL 721 has ever been done, and there are dozens of anecdotes suggesting just the opposite. It was a "misstatement" from the man who talked about "debunking" AL 721.

David Barry has done very well. His career has skyrocketed as fast as the profits made by Burroughs Wellcome on AZT. He was promoted to president of research, basically the head of all research and development by the company in the United States. It was no accident that Barry replaced Howard Schaeffer, the man who developed Zovirax, the antiherpes drug, who retired. Barry also replaced Schaeffer on the parent foundation's board of directors in London. Burroughs Wellcome clearly rewards people who create products that make profits for the company. David Barry knew the rules of the drug development game and played the shrewdest hand of anyone.

Now Barry's greatest challenge may be before him. New data indicate that a rare cancer, non-Hodgkin's lymphoma, is increasing rapidly in long-term survivors of AIDS. The aggressive cancer appears to increase with the length of diagnosis and the time PWAs are on AZT. It is not known whether the cancer is caused simply by the passage of time and the decline in the body's immune system or by AZT.

According to Jerome Groopman, a key PI for AZT at New England Deaconess Hospital in Boston, the question is whether AZT acts to enhance the cancer or whether the cancer is the outcome of prolonged immune deficiency due to AIDS. His gut feeling is that it isn't AZT.

Barry will need more than gut feelings, however. The huge market for AZT opened up by NIAID trials 016 and 019 may come to nothing if the drug is shown to be a factor in this rapidly growing lymphoma. Putting infected people with few signs of AIDS on AZT may not be such a good idea after all. Barry will have to sort this out.

Joe Sonnabend has been redeemed. Forever the outsider because of his belief that the AIDS virus alone does not cause AIDS, that a cofactor has to be present, Sonnabend has seen his hypothesis adopted by none other than Robert Gallo and Luc Montagnier, plus a growing number of NIH researchers. At the Sixth International AIDS Conference in San Francisco in June 1990, Montagnier said he now believes the AIDS virus needs the help of a microbe called a mycoplasma to transform itself into a killer of human cells. In essence, Montagnier said that AIDS is caused not by a single virus acting alone but by a microbe and virus working together.

Keeping to the traditional way American scientists have treated the French when it came to AIDS, Montagnier was given a relatively minor speaking slot at the San Francisco conference. The American Medical Association stepped in and cosponsored a late-night news conference for Montagnier, where he presented his views.

Gallo was another convert. He was the biggest proponent of the single AIDS virus idea, made famous with his quote "HIV [AIDS virus] kills like a truck." In the popular magazine *Discover*, Gallo said that the AIDS retrovirus "goes into hiding" once it invades the human body. "It remains in the T cell until the cell is kicked into action by another infection. Then the virus comes out of hiding, reproduces and spreads."

Keeping to his arrogant style, Gallo went on to say that "Only a few months ago, it was shown that if a person infected with HIV is also infected with human leukemia virus, the development of AIDS is strikingly enhanced. To my knowledge, this is the first clear evidence of a cofactor in AIDS." Gallo also said that a new kind of herpes virus, Human Herpes Virus #6, or HHV-6, acts as a cofactor to the AIDS virus. The leukemia and herpes viruses have one thing in common. They were discovered in Gallo's own lab.

Joe Sonnabend, of course, had been discussing cofactors as part of the pathogenesis of AIDS as far back as 1981. He published articles on cofactors in 1982. That Gallo is now discovering cofactors and proclaiming the discovery his own is just one more example of the incredible hubris of the man.

Joe Sonnabend never could get any government funding for his research. The NCI, at Gallo's urging, requested millions of dollars to investigate viruses that might act as cofactors in AIDS. Each dollar was a redemptive nod to Sonnabend for his original work on the cause of AIDS.

The entire foundation of the scientific explanation of AIDS is actually under attack. Examples have been found of men with Kaposi's sarcoma and no AIDS virus. KS was one of the earliest opportunistic infections to be associated with AIDS, back in the early eighties. No one seems to know what to make of the anomaly. Then there is the mysterious "viruslike agent" Dr. Shih-Ching Lo of the Armed Forces Institute of Pathology says is found in many PWAs. It may be a cofactor. It may play a more fundamental role, as Lo suggests.

Sonnabend continues to work as a community doctor and to do drug testing at the Community Research Initiative. Bernie Bihari is now executive director of the CRI. Tom Hannan, one of the founders, is out. Hannan's departure was not friendly. In fact, it almost marked the demise of the CRI. It did mark a definitive split between East and West Coast factions in the AIDS activist movement.

In the late spring of 1989, Project Inform's Martin Delaney launched a secret clinical trial of Compound Q, a drug derived from the Chinese cucumber. Earlier, it had been shown that in the test tube, Q selectively killed macrophage cells infected with the AIDS virus. If that proved true in humans, a drug had been found that could kill up to three-quarters of the virus in the body.

NIAID launched a Phase I safety study under Paul Volberding of AZT fame. But that would take a year. Meanwhile, the AIDS underground was being flooded with smuggled Q and bootleg Q. Delaney decided to do a quick combination safety/treatment trial without telling the FDA. Hundreds of PWAs were taking it anyway, and there were reports of severe toxicity and even deaths.

Joe Sonnabend and Mike Callen were asked by Delaney to have the CRI join in the underground experiment. They refused. All CRI drug tests had to be FDA approved. Moreover, Sonnabend and Callen believed that Delaney's Q clinical trial could be dangerous. It wasn't being tested for safety first before being administered as treatment. The two were being done at the same time. It also hadn't been cleared by the FDA. Hannan, however, disagreed and proceeded to help Delaney on his own.

When Robert Bazell, the science reporter for NBC, broke the news of Delaney's Compound Q tests, all hell broke loose. The FDA investigated, reports of people dying flashed through the news, and Joe Sonnabend and Michael Callen publicly lambasted Delaney. Then it turned out that nearly the entire staff of the CRI had participated in the New York arm of the Delaney experiment. They were furious at Sonnabend and Callen. Several left. The CRI survived, but barely, then recouped and returned to testing promising drugs with pharmaceutical company support. It has a dozen drug trials either under way or about to be launched.

But the bad blood between the CRI's Callen and Sonnabend and Project Inform's Delaney remains. The public feud was very bad politics for the AIDS activist movement, regardless of the value of the Compound Q trial. So far, Q has not turned out to be a magic bullet, but it has shown some efficacy. It is, however, toxic and must be supervised properly, which is what Delaney has done from the beginning.

Callen is burned out for the moment. He has resigned from the CRI and all other AIDS organizations and plans to move out to Los Angeles. Why Los Angeles? "Because no one knows me out there," he says.

Arnold Lippa moved to Malibu in 1988 after he was forced out of Praxis. He became president of a small biotech company called Vega Biotechnologies. Now he heads another start-up that is developing a hearing aid that works through bone vibrations rather than moving through nerves. If it works, tens of thousands of deaf people may be able to hear again.

AL 721 continues to be tested in Israel, Germany, and France. The Weizmann Institute has regained control of the license for the compound and plans to give it to a large German pharmaceutical company. Sales of bootleg AL 721 in Germany have continued to be high. Ironically, scientific investigation at the NIH has shifted to the cell membrane. Sam Broder has finished a Phase I safety trial for CD4, which might prevent the AIDS virus from attaching to human T-4 cells. The concept is similar to the process by which AL 721 is said to work as an antiviral.

Mathilde Krim continues to do the pragmatic thing. AmFAR has given nearly $25 million to support small AIDS research projects around the country. It gave another $1 million to the community-based research organizations it originally funded along with the CRI. The money was a godsend because very few of these groups received any money from the new NIAID community-based program. NIAID financed mostly hospitals and established organizations run out of hospitals. The funding was specifically placed under the control of the usual batch of powerful PIs and their elite academic institutions. This, of course, was in contradiction to the original intent of the president's AIDS commission, which had pointed to the CRI, organized with PWAs on all decision-making committees, as the model for community-based research organizations. Of course, that concept was too much of a threat to the PIs and their allies within NIAID.

Jim Eigo, Mark Harrington, and Iris Long of ACT UP and Martin Delaney have made revolutionary changes in the biomedical research world. The latest and perhaps the most important was announced in late May 1990. The Department of Health and Human Services said it was making the parallel track concept official. Not only will people with AIDS be able to get early access to experimental drugs if they cannot get into regular clinical trials, but people with cancer and other illnesses will also. It puts choice back into the hands of the patient and the community doctor. It takes control away from a small band of PIs. If implemented, the HHS decision can be a monumental change for the better in medical science.

Eigo, Harrington, and Delaney continue to be slowly incorporated into the biomedical establishment. They sit on dozens of NIAID, FDA, and other government AIDS advisory committees. ACT UP continues to hold demos outside the NIH buildings, but several members are already on the inside. It is not clear how much influence they will ever have. Right now, they are seen as "Fauci's boys" by the PIs who dominate these committees and who hate the very idea of outsiders sitting in on their discussions. The PIs retain enormous power.

Larry Kramer has just finished a screenplay and is working on a novel. He has had serious disagreements with several ACT UP leaders over the direction of the organization and has moved inward toward his art for the time being.

There is a new angst, a sorrow, that sneaks into Larry Kramer, unheralded. He is still a volcano of anger. But now his body sags a little from time to time and his voice, naturally strong and loud, weakens. Kramer has tended, over the years, to reflect the movement he has helped create and nurture.

Kramer is still the same man who shouted "murderer" at Ellen Cooper in front of a thousand people at the Fifth International Conference on AIDS in Montreal. His *Normal Heart* continues to be staged around the country, and generates controversy wherever it is played.

Yet there is a stepping back and viewing of himself by himself that is uncharacteristic. So much has happened over the past decade. So much has not.

Kramer has been the chief chronicler of the AIDS epidemic through its long years. He is the oracle who speaks the truth. He can't help it. His furies are always there. Through *Faggots, The Normal Heart,* and countless articles, Kramer has set down the unvarnished truth—and paid the penalty that anyone pays when he sets himself that task.

Today, in his living room, where the GMHC and ACT UP were born, where Molly still messes around in his writing, Kramer is growing weary. He talks of personal limitations, what *can't* be done. "I like Joe [Sonnabend]. He's a very nice man, Joe. Joe is almost like a tragic hero. There is a group of people who, from the very beginning, have had a sense of what was going on.

"We had flaws in our character and I include myself in that group. Because of that, we weren't listened to. I'm basically impatient and combative and not a very good negotiator. Joe cares so passionately about it that he gets angry too.

"Anybody who has been passionately involved in this for a long time is going crazy in their own way.

"The gay community doesn't have any leaders. We don't have a Jesse Jackson, we don't have a Gloria Steinem, we don't have a Cardinal O'Connor. We don't have a NOW, we don't have a B'nai B'rith, we don't have a National Rifle Association. We have very few lobbyists in Washington. It costs a hundred thousand dollars a year to have a lobbyist in Washington. That's all. Every gay community in every city could raise that money.

"What we're great at is things like the [NAMES Project Memorial] Quilt and making people cry. We're not very good politically. We are the *most disorganized of any minority.* The blacks are better organized. The Hispanics are better organized.

"There's a big Republican contingent within the gay community. They all voted for Ronald Reagan. If I were a conservative gay person and very rich, there has never been a gay organization that I would feel was trustworthy enough to give my money to.

"Columbus, Ohio, has a huge gay population that is very rich. Money is raised there, but quietly. L.A. has a huge gay population with lots of money. Heads of film studios are gay. Yet there hasn't been a single [Hollywood] movie about AIDS.

"Most people are in the closet. I mean, they may be open but not really open. They don't want to make waves. They feel powerless. When you've been discriminated against all your life, its real hard to change that mindset."

Kramer's face changes for just a moment. He smiles and opens his arms that have wrapped themselves around his chest. "Thank God for the young people of ACT UP. Every week I walk into ACT UP on Monday night thinking there is not going to be anybody there. But every week there are even more people."

But then it is over and Kramer returns to his monologue of what it's been like in the AIDSies. "The frontline doctors are all burned out. In New York, doctors are so busy they don't have enough time for their patients. They don't have time to read up on the latest stuff so they're afraid to give it to you. Their patients often know more about new drugs than they do. There are so many AIDS cases in the city that there are waiting lists to get into a *hospital.*

"In the middle of all this, we destroy our own. It's Michael Callen bad-mouthing Martin Delaney. For what? To what end? It only hurts us.

"You see, we don't have the *time.* We don't have time." Larry Kramer becomes very quiet, exhausted. He looks down at Molly, who has jumped into his lap. There is silence. A long pause as he cradles his Molly. "We don't have the time. Last November, I tested positive."

# Epilogue

It is a polite fiction that the NIH does public health. It will receive about $9 billion from Congress in 1991 to do medical research that is supposed to benefit the public. Three-quarters of it will be sent to principal investigators in their elite academic institutions around the country. In true trickle-down fashion, a portion of that money will actually go to meet the medical needs of people. But by and large, PIs do their own kind of science and, more often than not, their experiments have little to do with either health or the public. They test drugs by private pharmaceutical companies for personal gain, for money that goes to their universities, and for power.

They use taxpayer dollars to design experiments in fields that are in fashion, that are primarily basic and not applied science, that will enhance their professional careers through publications and prizes. This is the real PI game. This is what principal investigators actually do day in and day out. There is nothing wrong with their goals. It is just deceitful. The leading borders of certain kinds of science get pushed out but public health does not generally benefit.

Scientists do what they do totally without oversight because Congress and the public have accepted their argument that only they are knowledgeable enough to police themselves. The United States has never accepted this kind of argument from its military; it should not accept it from its biomedical establishment.

In the case of the disease AIDS, and probably in cancer, heart disease, Alzheimer's, and others, a very small number of PIs, a dozen or two, have enormous power that they misuse. Their intentions are good, but the road to hell is paved with good intentions. Again and again, conflicts of interest have arisen in AIDS. Scientists who have made their entire careers in AZT have sat on committees voting on potential commercial competitors. Scientists who have had financial dealings with Burroughs Wellcome or other pharmaceutical companies have come to dominate the government's entire clinical trials network. Hundreds of millions of dollars have been spent on their AIDS drug trials only to see them chronically underenrolled because of poor design. Many are never properly enrolled. Yet they go on and on. What happens to that money? Where does it go? Who is responsible? No one.

Nowhere is there accountability. The NIH extramural programs, especially NIAID's AIDS Program, may well become known as the HUD of the nineties, in which billions of taxpayer dollars have disappeared into the private projects of a handful of scientists who insist they know what is best for the health of the country. It is simply not true; they don't.

There are dozens and dozens and dozens of drugs that may be far better than AZT against AIDS that are not being tested because of the structure of the nation's biomedical system. There are probably hundreds of drugs for opportunistic diseases that are similarly being ignored because PIs have their own scientific agenda, which is not necessarily the same as the country's.

The FDA condones and contributes to this secret scientific world within a world. It is prepared to make behind-the-scenes deals on the levels of proof it will accept for new drugs. It is willing to have its own officials who have been colleagues of, even coauthors with, private corporate executives intervene for the acceptance of that drug company's product by FDA advisory committees. This was clearly the case with AZT. How many other drugs were passed in that fashion? How many, such as AL 721 or Peptide T, were denied a fair chance because their company sponsors didn't have the right connections?

Burroughs Wellcome and a small number of other top drug companies understand the system. It is clear that they know how to make it work. Small start-up companies don't have much of a chance. Even if they are more creative, they can't cut through the invisible web of relationships and arrangements that regulate drug development.

It is true that Wellcome is making enormous profits off AZT. Perhaps it is profiteering, perhaps not. But Wellcome at least delivers for the cash, something the NIH cannot claim to do. AZT is probably an overpriced mediocre drug that offers some short, transitory benefit to PWAs. But, Sam Broder's claims notwithstanding, it was Wellcome that developed the antiviral, whatever its effectiveness. Wellcome also developed acyclovir, or Zovirax, and Septra. Of the important drugs now in use to combat AIDS, Wellcome has developed most of them all except for aerosol pentamidine. That drug came out of community-based effort paid for by LyphoMed, a private pharmaceutical house. The CRI, the CCC, and other community-based groups, supported solely by private pharmaceutical companies and private fund-raising, are busy testing all kinds of drugs and combinations of drugs. Where are the government drugs?

The NIH and the science community in general are usually portrayed as under siege by political ideologues or by government tightwads who don't provide enough financing for worthy projects. In the case of AIDS, both were certainly true in the early years of the Reagan administration. It hasn't been the case since 1985.

The real problem with biomedical research today is lack of accountability. The generals are in charge of the war against AIDS and they are losing it. ACT UP, the CRI, Project Inform, AmFAR have consistently shown over recent years that people with the disease, their doctors, and their advocates know more about treatment than do ivory-tower PIs hidden away from the realities of life and driven by careers that don't reward them for furthering the public health. The changes in trial design, the beginning of parallel track, the curbing of placebos, the use of surrogate markers instead of death in tests, the quick testing of drugs at the community level, are all revolutionary research initiatives that should have been taken years ago. If they are widely implemented they will speed up the development of drugs for every disease and will open access to treatment for millions of people. None of them came from within the scientific community, from among the PIs. They came from a handful of people, most of whom are racing with death for control of their own lives.

# Sources

In addition to the interviews that form that core of the reporting for *Good Intentions*, a wealth of printed material, some of it public, much of it not, provided critical information. This material was found in Congressional testimony and internal NIH documents.

For an inside look at the NIH, there is nothing better than Stephen Strickland's *Politics, Science and Dread Disease: A Short History of U.S. Medical Research Policy* and *The Story of the NIH Grants Program.* Richard Sorian's *The Bitter Pill: Tough Choices in America's Health Policy* is perhaps the best analysis of what happened to the nation's health care under the Reagan Administration.

Of course, no book dealing with AIDS can be written without owing a huge debt of gratitude to Randy Shilts's *And the Band Played On.*

The following is a brief list of printed sources ordered by category.

## CONGRESS

Kaposi's Sarcoma and Related Opportunistic Infections: Hearing Before the Subcommittee on Health and the Environment of the Committee on Energy and Commerce, House of Representatives, April 13, 1982.

Acquired Immune Deficiency Syndrome—AIDS: Hearing Before the Subcommittee on Health and the Environment of the Committee of Energy and Commerce, House of Representatives, September 17, 1984.

The Public Health Service's Response to AIDS, Office of Technology Assessments, Joint Hearing Before the Subcommittee of the Committee on Government Operations and

# SOURCES

the Committee on Energy and Commerce, House of Representatives, February 21, 1985.

AIDS Issues: Hearings Before the Subcommittee on Health and the Environment of the Committee of Energy and Commerce, House of Representatives, July 22, 1985.

Research and Treatment for Acquired Immune Deficiency Syndrome, July 29, 1985.

Protection of Confidentiality of Research Subjects and Blood Donors, November 1, 1985.

Testimony of Dr. David Barry, Vice President of Research, Burroughs Wellcome, July 1, 1986, Before the House Committee on Government Operations on the Status of AIDS Drug Development.

Letter to Senator Lowell Weicker from Congressman Henry A. Waxman, August 13, 1986, expressing his concern over the number of requests from constituents, their friends, and total strangers for admission in NIH clinical trials.

Testimony of T. E. Haigler, Jr., President and CEO of Burroughs Wellcome Co., March 10, 1987, Before the House Committee on Energy and Commerce, Subcommittee on Health and the Environment.

Hearings Before the Subcommittee on Health and the Environment of the Committee on Energy and Commerce, House of Representatives, Cost and Availability of AZT— March 10, 1987; AIDS and Minorities—April 27, 1987; AIDS Research and Education—Sept. 22, 1987. U.S. Government Printing Office.

Therapeutic Drugs for AIDS: Development, Testing and Availability: Hearings Before a Subcommittee of the Committee on Government Operations, House of Representatives, April 28, 29, 1988.

Letter by Congressman Henry A. Waxman, Chairman, Subcommittee on Health and the Environment, to Dr. Anthony Fauci, NIAID, May 11, 1988, expressing his dismay at the delays in the AIDS drug-development program.

Reply by Dr. Anthony Fauci, NIAID, to Congressman Waxman, June 27, 1988.

Hearings Before the Subcommittee on Health and the Environment of the Committee on Energy and Commerce, House of Representatives, Pending AIDS Legislation—September 29, 1987; Public Health Service Update on the AIDS Epidemic—October 19, 1988; The Needs for AIDS Research Activities—March 15, 1988.

AIDS Drugs: Where Are They? Seventy-third Report by the Committee on Government Operations, October 19, 1988.

Children and HIV Infection: Hearings Before the Human Resources and Intergovernmental Relations Subcommittee of the Committee on Government Operations, House of Representatives, February 22, 23, 1989.

Opening Statement by Henry A. Waxman: Hearings on the Parallel Track Proposal for Drug Development, Committee on Energy and Commerce, Subcommittee on Health and the Environment, U.S. House of Representatives, July 19, 1989.

# SOURCES

## BOOKS

Kramer, Larry. *Reports from the Holocaust.* New York: St. Martin's Press, 1988.

Sorian, Richard. *The Bitter Pill: Tough Choices in America's Health Policy.* New York: McGraw-Hill Book Co., 1988.

Shilts, Randy. *And the Band Played On: Politics, People and the AIDS Epidemic.* New York: St. Martin's Press, 1987.

Shinitzky, Meir, ed. *Physiology of Membrane Fluidity.* Vols. 1 and 2. Boca Raton: CRC Press, 1984.

Strickland, Stephen P. *Politics, Science and Dread Disease: A Short History of U.S. Medical Research Policy.* Cambridge, Mass.: Harvard University Press, 1972.

Strickland, Stephen P. *The Story of the NIH Grants Program.* Washington, D.C.: National Library of Medicine, 1989.

## COMMUNITY PUBLICATIONS

ACT UP/NY. *AIDS Drugs Now.* May 2, 1989. Testimony in Front of the Interim Report to the National Committee to Review Current Procedures for Approval of New Drugs for Cancer and AIDS [the Lasagna Committee].

ACT UP/NY. *A National AIDS Treatment Research Agenda.* Issued at the Fifth International Conference on AIDS, Montreal, June 1989.

*AIDS Treatment News.* Published biweekly by John S. James in San Francisco.

*AIDS Treatment Registry.* Directory of AIDS/HIV Clinical Trials Open in New York and New Jersey. August 1989. Dr. Iris Long, David Kirschenbaum, Julie Fishman, Mark Malano, Gary Kleinman, Michael Cowan.

*AIDS Treatment Registry.* Directory of AIDS/HIV Clinical Trials Open in New York and New Jersey. Vol.1. Oct. 5, 1989. Dr. Iris Long, David Kirschenbaum, Julie Fishman, Mark Malano, Gary Kleinman, Michael Cowan.

American Foundation for AIDS Research. *AIDS/HIV Experimental Treatment Directory.* May 1989.

Callen, Michael, ed. *AIDS Forum: Diverse Views About Acquired Immune Deficiency Syndrome.* Vol. 1, No. 1. January 1989.

Callen, Michael, ed. *AIDS Forum: Diverse Views About Acquired Immune Deficiency Syndrome.* Vol. 1, No. 2. March 1989.

GMHC. *Treatment Issues.* Newsletter on experimental AIDS therapies.

People With AIDS Coalition, Michael Callen, ed. *Surviving and Thriving with AIDS: Hints for the Newly Diagnosed.*

# SOURCES

People With AIDS Coalition, Michael Callen, ed. *Surviving and Thriving with AIDS. Volume 2: Collected Wisdom*, especially "The Lipid Story," by Suzanne Phillips.

The National Committee to Review Current Procedures for Approval of New Drugs for Cancer and AIDS [the Lasagna Committee]. January 4, 1989. Testimony by Dr. Broder, Dr. Chapner, Dr. Fauci, Dr. Young.

# NIH PUBLICATIONS

*AIDS Clinical Trials Program.* Report of the AIDS Clinical Trials Advisory Group of the National Institute of Allergy and Infectious Diseases. December 1987.

*ACDDC Meeting Minutes 2/26/87.* Minutes of the AIDS Clinical Drug Developm~ Committee meeting, giving priority ratings to AL 721, isoprinisine, and ribavirin.

NIAID. *AIDS Clinical Trial Units (ACTU'S).* A list of NIAID's clinical trial sites and principal investigators.

NIAID. *AIDS Clinical Drug Development Committee.* A list of members.

A list of all committee members of all NIAID ACTG committees, including the Executive, Biological Response Modifier, Immunology, Neurology, Oncology, Opportunistic Infection, Pediatrics, Pharmacology/Pharmacokonetics, Primary Infection, and Virology Committees.

AIDS Research Exchange. *Update on Aerosolized Pentamidine: Treatment IND Approved.* NIAID. April 1989.

# FDA

Minutes of the FDA Anti-Infective Drugs Advisory Committee of the Department of Health and Human Services, Public Health Service, Food and Drug Administration meeting on recommending that the FDA grant Burroughs Wellcome permission to sell AZT. 8:30 A.M., January 16, 1987.

Minutes of the second FDA Anti-Infective Drugs Advisory Committee of the Department of Health and Human Services, Public Health Service, Food and Drug Administration meeting on recommending that the FDA grant Burroughs Wellcome permission to sell AZT. 8:30 A.M., May 13, 1988.

# SOURCES

## AL 721

*Absorption and Dissemination of Phosphatidyl Chlorine and Phosphatidyl Ethanolamine in AL 721.* Meir Shinitzky. January 1987. Interim report carried out under a grant from Praxis Ltd. from January 1986 to January 1987 at the Weizmann Institute of Science.

"HIV Envelope Membrane as a Potential Site for Antiviral Drugs." C. A. Klempner, F. T. Crews, J. Laurence, D. I. Scheer, M. E. Weksler, A. S. Lippa. Paper presented at the American Society for Microbiology, Atlanta, Georgia, March 1–6, 1987.

"Lipids Are Major Components of Human Immunodeficiency Virus . . . Modifications of HIV Lipid Composition, Protein Structure and Infectivity by AL 721, a Unique Lipid Mixture." The original letter (before it was toned down) sent into the *NEJM*. F. T. Crews, J. Laurence, D. I. Scheer, P. Sarin, B. McElhaney, A. S. Lippa.

*A Study of AL 721 and HIV Infected Subjects with Generalized Lymphadenopathy Syndrome.* Michael H. Grieco, M.D.; Michael Lange, M.D.; Elena Buymovici-Klien, M.D.; Arthur England, M.D.; George F. McKinley, M.D.; Kenneth Ong, M.D.; Craig Metroka, M.D., Division of Allergy, Clinical Immunology and Infectious Diseases, Medical Service, St. Luke's–Roosevelt Hospital.

## CURRICULUM VITAE

Dr. David Barry, Burroughs Wellcome.

Dr. Samuel Broder, National Cancer Institute.

Dr. Anthony Fauci, National Institute of Allergies and Infectious Diseases.

## THE NEW ENGLAND JOURNAL OF MEDICINE

"Effects of a Novel Compound (AL 721) on HTLV-111 Infectivity in Vitro." 313, No. 20.: 1289–90. P. S. Sarin, R. C. Gallo, D. I. Scheer, F. Crews, A. S. Lippa.

"The Efficacy of Azidothymidine (AZT) in the Treatment of Patients with AIDS and AIDS-Related Complex." 317: 185–91. July 23, 1987. Margaret A. Fischl, M.D.; Douglas D. Richman, M.D.; Oscar L. Laskin, M.D.; Robert T. Schooley, M.D.; George G. Jackson, M.D.; David Durack, M.B., D. Phil.; Dannie King, Ph.D.; and the AZT Collaborative Working Group.

"Federal Spending for Illnesses Caused by the Human Immunodeficiency Virus." William Winkenworder, M.D.; Austin R. Kessler, M.B.A.; Ronda M. Stolick, B.S.E. Special article. June 15, 1989.

# SOURCES

"The Toxicity of Azidothymidine (AZT) in the Treatment of Patients with AIDS and AIDS-Related Complex." 317: 192–217. July 23, 1987. Douglas D. Richman, M.D.; Margaret A. Fischl, M.D.; Micheal H. Grieco M.D., J.D.; Michael S. Gottlieb, M.D.; Paul A. Volberding, M.D.; Oscar L. Laskin, M.D.; John M. Leedom, M.D.; Jerome E. Groopman, M.D.; Donna Mildvan, M.D.; Martin S. Hirsch, M.D.; George G. Jackson, M.D.; David T. Durack, M.B., D. Phil.; Sandra Nusinoff-Lehrman, M.D.; and the AZT Collaborative Working Group.

"Zidovudine in Asymptomatic Human Immunodeficiency Virus Infection: A Controlled Trial in Persons with Fewer Than 500 CD-4 Positive Cells per Cubic Millimeter." Paul A. Volberding, M.D.; Stephen W. Lagakos, Ph.D.; Matthew A. Koch, M.D.; M. S. Carla Pettinelli, M.D., Ph.D.; Maureen Myers, Ph.D.; David K. Booth, P.A.; Henry H. Balfour Jr., M.D.; Richard C. Reichman, M.D.; John A. Bartlett, M.D.; Martin S. Hirsch, M.D.; Robert L. Murphy, M.D.; W. David Hardy, M.D.; Ruy Soeiro, M.D.; Margaret A. Fischl, M.D.; John G. Bartlett, M.D.; Thomas C. Merigan, M.D.; Newton E. Hyslop, M.D.; Douglas D. Richman, M.D.; Fred T. Valentine, M.D.; Lawrence Corey, M.D.; and the AIDS Clinical Trials Group of the National Institute of Allergy and Infectious Diseases.

## SECURITIES AND EXCHANGE COMMISSION

10-K for the Praxis Corporation for the fiscal year ending June 30, 1986.

10-K for the Ethigen Corporation for the fiscal year ending June 30, 1987.

10-K for the Ethigen Corporation for the fiscal year ending June 30, 1988.

## PAPERS

"Correlations Between Membrane Viscosity, Serum Cholesterol, Lymphocyte Activation and Aging in Man. B. Rivnay, S. Bergman, M. Shinitzky, and A. Globerson. *Mechanisms of Aging and Development* 12 (1980): 119–26. Lausann: Essevier Sequota S.A.

"Possible Reversal of Tissue Aging by a Lipid Diet." M. Lyte and M. Shinitzky. Presented by M. Shinitzky, January 1984, Zurich. Meeting on Alzheimer Disease: Advances in Basic Research and Therapies.

## OTHER

Bihari, Dr. Bernard. Letter dated November 6, 1989, faxed to Dr. Anthony Fauci, M.D., National Institute of Allergy and Infectious Diseases, NIH Building #31, Room 7A03,

# SOURCES

Bethesda, Md. 20892. Explains why the Community Research Initiative was refused NIAID community-based research funding.

Bihari, Dr. Bernard, and Ronald English, President of the Board of Directors of the Community Research Initiative. Letter dated November 30, 1989, faxed to Dr. Anthony Fauci, M.D., National Institute of Allergy and Infectious Diseases, NIH Building #31, Room 7A03, Bethesda, Md. 20892.

Michael Callen. Testimony at FDA Hearings, Rockville, Md., May 1, 1989. Callen describes his discussion with Dr. Anthony Fauci two years earlier concerning aerosol pentamidine and asking for FDA approval of the drug.

Crewdson, John. "The Father of Human Retrovirology." *Chicago Tribune.* November 19, 1989. Article on Robert Gallo.

Shinitzky, Dr. Meir, and Dr. David Samuel, Departments of Isotope Research and Membrane Research, The Weizmann Institute of Science, Rehovot, Israel. "AL721: A Novel Membrane Fluidizer." Paper sent to Lida Antonian and Arnold S. Lippa, Matrix Research Laboratories, Inc.

Wellcome plc. Annual Report. 1989.

# Index

# INDEX

# INDEX

# INDEX

# INDEX

# INDEX

# INDEX

# FOR THE BEST IN PAPERBACKS, LOOK FOR THE

In every corner of the world, on every subject under the sun, Penguin represents quality and variety—the very best in publishing today.

For complete information about books available from Penguin—including Pelicans, Puffins, Peregrines, and Penguin Classics—and how to order them, write to us at the appropriate address below. Please note that for copyright reasons the selection of books varies from country to country.

---

**In the United Kingdom:** For a complete list of books available from Penguin in the U.K., please write to *Dept E.P., Penguin Books Ltd, Harmondsworth, Middlesex, UB7 0DA.*

**In the United States:** For a complete list of books available from Penguin in the U.S., please write to *Dept BA, Penguin,* Box 120, Bergenfield, New Jersey 07621-0120.

**In Canada:** For a complete list of books available from Penguin in Canada, please write to *Penguin Books Ltd, 2801 John Street, Markham, Ontario L3R 1B4.*

**In Australia:** For a complete list of books available from Penguin in Australia, please write to the *Marketing Department, Penguin Books Ltd, P.O. Box 257, Ringwood, Victoria 3134.*

**In New Zealand:** For a complete list of books available from Penguin in New Zealand, please write to the *Marketing Department, Penguin Books (NZ) Ltd, Private Bag, Takapuna, Auckland 9.*

**In India:** For a complete list of books available from Penguin, please write to *Penguin Overseas Ltd, 706 Eros Apartments, 56 Nehru Place, New Delhi, 110019.*

**In Holland:** For a complete list of books available from Penguin in Holland, please write to *Penguin Books Nederland B.V., Postbus 195, NL-1380AD Weesp, Netherlands.*

**In Germany:** For a complete list of books available from Penguin, please write to *Penguin Books Ltd, Friedrichstrasse 10-12, D-6000 Frankfurt Main I, Federal Republic of Germany.*

**In Spain:** For a complete list of books available from Penguin in Spain, please write to *Longman, Penguin España, Calle San Nicolas 15, E-28013 Madrid, Spain.*

**In Japan:** For a complete list of books available from Penguin in Japan, please write to *Longman Penguin Japan Co Ltd, Yamaguchi Building, 2-12-9 Kanda Jimbocho, Chiyoda-Ku, Tokyo 101, Japan.*